Traditional Chinese Acupuncture

Traditional Chinese Acupuncture

Volume I Meridians and Points

J. R. Worsley

Founder and President, College of Traditional Chinese Acupuncture U.K.
Professor of the College of Chinese Medicine (China);
Hon. Professor of the Department of Oriental Medicine, Won Kwang University, Korea;
Vice-President of The World Academic Society For Acupuncture;
Hon. President, Compagnonnage d'Acupuncture Traditionnelle;
Founder President, Traditional Acupuncture Society;
Founder President, Traditional Acupuncture Institute, U.S.A.

ELEMENT
Shaftesbury, Dorset • Rockport, Massachusetts
Brisbane, Queensland

First published in Great Britain in 1982 by
Element Books Limited

This edition first published in 1993 by
Element Books Limited
Shaftesbury, Dorset SP7 8BP

First published in the USA in 1993 by
Element Books, Inc.
PO Box 830, Rockport, MA 01966

First published in Australia in 1993 by
Element Books Limited for
Jacaranda Wiley Limited
33 Park Road, Milton, Brisbane 4064

Reprinted 1995

Anatomical illustrations by Denys Baker
Design by Humphrey Stone
Printed in Singapore

British Library Cataloguing in Publication
Data available

Library of Congress Cataloging
Data available

ISBN 0–906540–03–8

Contents

Preface

As with any book, the author is charged with the responsibility of what to include and what to omit. Therefore, keeping in mind the fact that this book is intended as a guide to the acupuncture points and the meridians of Ch'i energy, I have chosen not to embark in this volume on the task of explaining the natural laws or conveying specific information about patrons, pulses, treatment techniques, traditional diagnosis, officials or spirits of the points. Although these are not subjects which can be properly understood and felt merely from the written word, I shall in due course write further volumes to aid those actively involved in studying them. Using any of this material without adequate training can be dangerous.

I have therefore in this volume selected information concerning meridians and points which will aid students in their studies and also serve as reference for qualified practitioners. With that in mind, it will be noted that I have endeavoured to keep the format of the book simple and practical. The information relating to each of the meridians is accompanied by appropriate illustration. In the main text, each illustration is therefore relevant only to the text on the opposite page.

I have included comment about each point in order that it may be understood and chosen not simply by formula but with greater sensitivity to its proper function. Each point has its own character, its own quality of expression, and, when called upon at the appropriate time and in an effective manner, it will contribute precisely that function, that character and that expression to the healing process.

JRW
The College of Traditional Acupuncture U.K.
Royal Leamington Spa, Warwickshire, England
1981

Acknowledgements

I wish to extend my gratitude to two members of the Faculty of The College of Traditional Acupuncture U.K., namely Judy Becker Worsley and my son, John Worsley, who have spent countless hours proofing, typing, re-writing, indexing, etc., and without whose untiring efforts this volume would not have been possible.

I also wish to express my thanks to two other members of the Faculty, namely Alan Hext for proofing the drawings and indexing and Allegra Wint for proofing the meridian pathway descriptions and point locations.

Finally, I would like to express my heartfelt thanks to Denys Baker for all the effort he has put into the wonderful illustrations and to John Moore for all his help and guidance in making this publication possible.

Traditional Chinese acupuncture, when practised correctly according to natural laws, is one of the most beautiful systems of medicine known to man. It is both an art and a science. The fundamental principle of its practice is the giving of constant attention to diagnosis and treatment of the causes rather than the symptoms of disease.

When acupuncture is used to treat only labelled diseases or immediate symptoms, it is called 'local doctor', symptomatic or formula acupuncture. There are certain circumstances when this use is appropriate but it should be borne in mind that, when practised in the East, it is employed in the great majority of cases at the very onset of illness because people there consult their local doctors at the first sign of trouble. Even then, it is usually only administered to give temporary comfort and relief until such time as any serious underlying cause can be diagnosed and treated by a fully trained and experienced doctor.

Nevertheless, it should be added that, in certain cases where the patient visits the local doctor at the immediate onset of the symptoms, the preliminary treatment which gives relief and comfort sometimes enables the body to overcome the cause of the illness itself. Symptomatic acupuncture is therefore not to be totally dismissed as ineffective in certain circumstances.

In the West however, at present, people tend to visit the acupuncture practitioner only when Western medicine has failed and their illnesses, more often than not, have existed for some considerable time and may well have reached chronic stages. For this reason, acupuncture treatment in Western society is more appropriate and effective when given by practitioners well trained and experienced in the ancient and comprehensive science of traditional acupuncture.

To apply local doctor or symptomatic acupuncture techniques in cases of long-standing or serious illness can at best only give temporary relief through the removal or suppression of the obviously troublesome symptoms. At worst, it can be dangerous because such practices will very likely fail to rectify the underlying cause which may then continue to persist unidentified and unchecked. Temporary elimination of symptoms does not constitute effective cure.

A local doctor can be trained in first aid techniques in a matter of a few months. The full training of a traditional acupuncturist can take many, many years. This is because he or she is required to comprehend thoroughly a complete system of medicine which takes into account the functioning of the whole person—body, mind and spirit. (Also, in the training, each practitioner must become versed in basic Western medical science.) In order to achieve this, it is not only necessary to understand the practice of traditional acupuncture but also the system of philosophy which underlies it.

The Taoist concept of health, illness and cure

Tao is the Chinese character which, approximately translated, means 'The Way'. It is the expression of a subtle concept which Lao Tzu, the

Taoist sage of the sixth century B.C., said could not be spoken of, only lived. Following The Way means treading a path through nature's eternal changes, acknowledging in all living things their essence or true spirit. To interpret the Tao is almost impossible but it indicates the path which we travel from birth to death, that path which, if followed, allows us to acknowledge who we are and allows us to appreciate all creatures as living in harmony.

Traditional Chinese acupuncture is a form of health care and healing which seeks to harmonise the human being with the Tao. The practitioner is ever mindful and trusting that nature, allowed to work and flow unimpeded, leads the patient to health in body, mind and spirit, just as the rivers flow naturally and effortlessly towards the ocean. 'Easy is right' said another Chinese sage, Chuang Tzu. Disease is the result of violating natural laws, of falling out of harmony with the Tao. Losing The Way means losing the inherent ability of the body, mind and spirit to adjust readily to the changing environmental and social circumstances. Failure to adjust causes constrictions and blockages within, interventions which then disrupt the flow of vital and healing energy, a situation which increases vulnerability. The body becomes diseased, the mind uneasy, and the spirit withdraws. If it withdraws completely, death prevails.

The traditional acupuncturist is therefore carefully trained to understand the laws of nature, to diagnose in acknowledgement of them and to work therapeutically to restore their effectiveness. In doing so, the life force, the Ch'i energy as it is called, is able to cure the causative factor of the disease. The continuing flow of this energy is the essential prerequisite of good health. One must be mindful of the fact that in all systems of healing, from the ancient traditional Chinese methods to the modern technical, scientific methods of the Western trained practitioner, neither man nor woman has the power to cure disease. At best, all she or he can do is assist nature in the cure. Therein lies one of the main foundations of Chinese traditional medicine. It is only possible to reinforce the body's own defence mechanism to overcome the disease in the most natural of natural ways.

Ch'i energy gives all life the strength to follow the Tao. Traditional acupuncture treatments should always encourage the recipient to realise this inherent principle so that he or she may gain a genuine appreciation of the remedial and worthwhile benefits of being in harmony with nature.

The Yin and Yang aspects of Ch'i energy

Ch'i energy is the life force which creates and maintains all living forms. Yin and Yang are the two aspects of that energy. Both are always present and together they represent the dual nature of all events and situations. They function in relation to each other so that one cannot be separated or isolated from the other. Everything that lives demonstrates the presence of Yin and Yang, and never is anything comprised solely of one or the other. They complement each other as night and day, as winter and summer, as female and male, as moon and sun.

Balance is, however, crucial to a good state of health. If Yin and Yang are in harmony, there can be no disease. But if serious imbalance occurs, then the body, mind and spirit systems become disturbed and disrupted, and disease ensues.

Yin energy rises from the earth and creates Yang energy, Yang energy descends from the heaven and penetrates the earth, recreating in turn Yin energy. Together they keep the cycles of all living processes in motion.

In both men and women, the direction of flow of the Yin aspect is up the inside of the legs and thorax, and thence centrifugally out on the anterior surface of the (upraised) arms towards the sky. The Yang energy flows centripetally down the posterior surface of the (upraised) arms to the chest or back, and then down the outside of the legs to the earth.

When the energies of Yin and Yang are in balance, the organism is in a state of free and stable flow, a situation which promotes the health and integrity of the body and mind. When the balance is upset, and the pathways of energy are constricted or blocked, then disease assails the weakened areas of the organism. Ultimately the energy system breaks down and death supervenes.

It is worth noting that in all aspects of Chinese medicine the practitioner contemplates the individuality of the patient. It is not possible within this system to treat all people the same. It must be borne in mind that each person is a unique individual, the like of which God the Creator has never made before and will never make again. We are each of us as different as chalk from cheese and therefore this system demands that the practitioner investigates the cause of disease as being unique in each individual in his or her care. Thus one can appreciate the importance of the personal relationship and rapport that needs to be established between practitioner and patient.

The Meridians and Points

The Ch'i energy follows specific pathways, called 'meridians', throughout the body. These meridians are sometimes near the skin surface – 'superficial pathway' – and sometimes deep inside the body – 'deep pathway'.

There are twelve principal meridians, each of which is assigned a name and number. The order of the meridians – indicated by consecutively ascending Roman numerals – is dictated by the sequence in which the Ch'i energy follows a complete cycle throughout the body. Six of them carry predominantly the Yang qualities of energy and six the Yin qualities.

I	Heart Meridian	Lesser Yin
II	Small Intestine Meridian	Greater Yang
III	Bladder Meridian	Greater Yang

IV	Kidney Meridian	Lesser Yin
V	Circulation-Sex Meridian	Absolute Yin
VI	Three Heater Meridian	Lesser Yang
VII	Gall Bladder Meridian	Lesser Yang
VIII	Liver Meridian	Absolute Yin
IX	Lung Meridian	Greater Yin
X	Colon Meridian	Sunlight Yang
XI	Stomach Meridian	Sunlight Yang
XII	Spleen Meridian	Greater Yin

There are in addition two special meridians, numbered XIII and XIV, called Conception Vessel and Governor Vessel respectively.

At certain specific locations along the meridian pathways the energy may be effectively regulated. These locations are called 'points'.

The points are again named and numbered. The ascending sequence of numbers indicates the direction of energy flow, the first point being at the beginning of the meridian.

In the text which follows therefore, III 7, for example, indicates the seventh point on the Bladder Meridian; or XII 14 means the fourteenth point on the Spleen Meridian.

Elements

Each meridian is not only associated with either Yin or Yang but also with one of the five 'elements' – traditionally named fire, earth, metal, water and wood – which indicates the particular properties of the energy being transmitted by the meridian. The elements are also assigned associated colours (which are used where appropriate throughout the following text).

I	Heart	Fire (Red)	VII	Gall Bladder	Wood (Green)
II	Small Intestine	Fire (Red)	VIII	Liver	Wood (Green)
III	Bladder	Water (Blue)	IX	Lung	Metal (White)
IV	Kidney	Water (Blue)	X	Colon	Metal (White)
V	Circulation-Sex	Fire (Red)	XI	Stomach	Earth (Yellow)
VI	Three Heater	Fire (Red)	XII	Spleen	Earth (Yellow)

In addition to the characteristic elemental nature of the complete meridian, each of the meridians has one point—'command point'—associated with each of the elements. For example, the elemental nature of the Heart Meridian is fire; its third point is water, its fourth metal, its seventh earth, and so on.

Terminology used to describe location of points

Although the anatomical description given in the text is as accurate as possible, final location of the points in practice must depend on palpation since the exact position of some of them varies slightly from one individual to another.

The descriptions used refer to the human body in the erect posture, with the arms down by the sides and with the palms of the hands facing forwards.

In traditional Chinese medicine, the stance adopted for descriptive purposes is the erect posture with the arms raised above the head, palms of the hands facing forwards. This is indicative of the centrifugal and centripetal flows of energy, mentioned earlier, where the Yin and Yang qualities of energy flow 'from earth to heaven' and 'from heaven to earth' respectively. Modern convention, however, makes it more convenient to use the arms-lowered stance.

The terms 'anterior' and 'posterior' are used to describe the front and back respectively of the body or limbs.

When describing the hand, 'palmar' and 'dorsal' are used in place of anterior and posterior respectively. For the foot, 'plantar' and 'dorsal' are similarly employed.

The 'median' plane is a sagittal (vertical) plane which passes through the centre of the trunk and divides the body into superficially symmetrical right and left halves. It therefore cuts a line both along the anterior and posterior surface of the body, a line called 'the median line'. The terms 'medial' (nearer to the median line) and 'lateral' (further from the median line) are also used.

The terms 'superior' and 'inferior' indicate levels relatively above and below a given point; 'proximal' and 'distal' indicate nearness to and distance from a given point.

'Abduction' means movement of a limb away from the median line (in a coronal plane) whilst 'adduction' means movement towards the median line. 'Supination' and 'pronation' are respectively medial and lateral rotation of the forearm; 'flexion' and 'extension' are limb movements in a sagittal plane, superiorly and inferiorly respectively.

Anatomical Chinese Inch

In traditional Chinese medicine, the basic unit of measurement is known as the Anatomical Chinese Inch—the ACI. This is used to assist in the location of acupuncture points on all parts of the body. It is a relative unit of measurement because it varies according to the size of the individual and according to the part of the body concerned.

The various lengths of different parts of the body are divided into a certain number of equal portions, each portion being 1 ACI. Anatomical illustration in the following text includes ACI 'grids' where appropriate. A composite of all the ACI grids is illustrated on page 315.

The anatomical divisions, and the number of ACI measures in each one, are as follows:

Forearm The distance from the crease at the flexure of the wrist to the crease at the flexure of the elbow is 12 ACI.

Upper Arm The distance from the anterior crease at the flexure of the elbow to the anterior crease of the axilla is 9 ACI.

Lower Leg The distance from the prominence of the medial malleolus to the medial extremity of the knee crease is 15 ACI. The

distance from the prominence of the lateral malleolus to the lateral extremity of the knee crease is 16 ACI.
Thigh The distance from the medial extremity of the knee crease to the medial extremity of the groin is 13 ACI.
Abdomen The distance from the superior edge of the pubic symphysis to the centre of the umbilicus is 5 ACI. The distance from the centre of the umbilicus to the xiphisternal joint is 8 ACI.
Chest The distance from the xiphisternal joint to the suprasternal notch is 8 ACI. The distance from the anterior median line to the paramedian nipple line is 4 ACI.
Back The distance from the posterior median line to the medial border of the scapula is 4 ACI.
Head The distance from the intervertebral depression between the first and second cervical vertebrae and the point between the medial extremities of the eyebrows on the anterior median line is 15 ACI. The points III 3 to 8 and VII 16 to 18 are located in relation to these ACI as illustrated. The distance from the intervertebral depression between the first and second cervical vertebrae and the intervertebral depression between the seventh cervical and the first thoracic vertebrae is 3 ACI. The distance from the posterior median line to the prominence of the mastoid process is 4½ ACI.

Acupuncture techniques: needle and moxibustion

Two basic techniques are used in acupuncture practice to regulate the flow of energy at meridian points. The first involves the insertion of very fine acupuncture needles. The second, moxibustion, entails the application of a fine impulse of heat at the point. In the following text, use of the needle is represented by the symbol ⊥ and the use of moxibustion by the symbol △.

According to the meridian point being treated, there are recommended depths to which the needle may be safely inserted. The measure of needle depth is called a 'fen'. One fen is the equivalent of one tenth of an ACI. This indicates that the needle depth to be used is calculated in relation to the build of the person being treated. In the following text, each point has a designated, recommended needle depth. For example, I 7 is assigned ⊥3, meaning that three fen is the recommended depth for the seventh point on the Heart Meridian. In some cases, a double figure is given; for example, ⊥ 2–3 at point I 8. This indicates a minimum and a maximum depth. The former should be sufficient to obtain the appropriate effect with the average person; the latter is the limit of penetration beyond which the needle would pass through the point.

Needle treatment is contra-indicated for certain points. This prohibition is represented in the text by the capital letter X. Further, the letters XP means that the use of the needle is forbidden at that point during pregnancy. XP used with a number—for example, XP4—indicates that that point should not be used for needle treatment as of the fourth month of pregnancy.

Moxibustion is effected by the slow burning of a small cone of a herb (*Artemesia vulgaris latiflora*) on the skin surface over the acupuncture point. The combination of heat and herbal properties stimulates or supplies energy at the point. The number of moxa applications at a particular point is indicated in the text by the moxa symbol △, followed by the appropriate number. Again, a double number—for example, △ 3–7—recommends the minimum and maximum number of moxa applications according to the degree of effect required.

Moxa is also contra-indicated for certain points. △X means moxa is forbidden; △XP that moxa is forbidden during pregnancy; △XP with a number that moxa is forbidden as of that month of pregnancy.

Content of the book

The fourteen meridians are treated in conventional sequence. Each meridian section is divided into three parts.

The first part illustrates and describes the complete **Pathway**—both deep and superficial—of the particular meridian in relation to other points and the internal organs.

The second part illustrates and describes each **Point Location** on that meridian in relation to underlying skeletal and muscular structure, and in relation to arteries, veins and nerves. Please note that in all cases, the written location is the definitive source of information in finding each point.

The third part, **Point Description**, gives basic information about the character and particular properties of each point, including its number, its name in English and Chinese, its location and specific elemental association (if any), and the recommended needle and moxa indications appropriate for that point.

Although the illustrations show the meridians on only one side of the body, these pathways do, in fact, travel bilaterally.

The main section of the book is followed by thirty appendices. These are compiled to permit ready access to additional point information; also to enable quick reference to point relationships and properties either not evident or not easily retrievable from the main text. Following the appendices, there are three full-page composite illustrations of the fourteen superficial pathways, showing all the meridians and points.

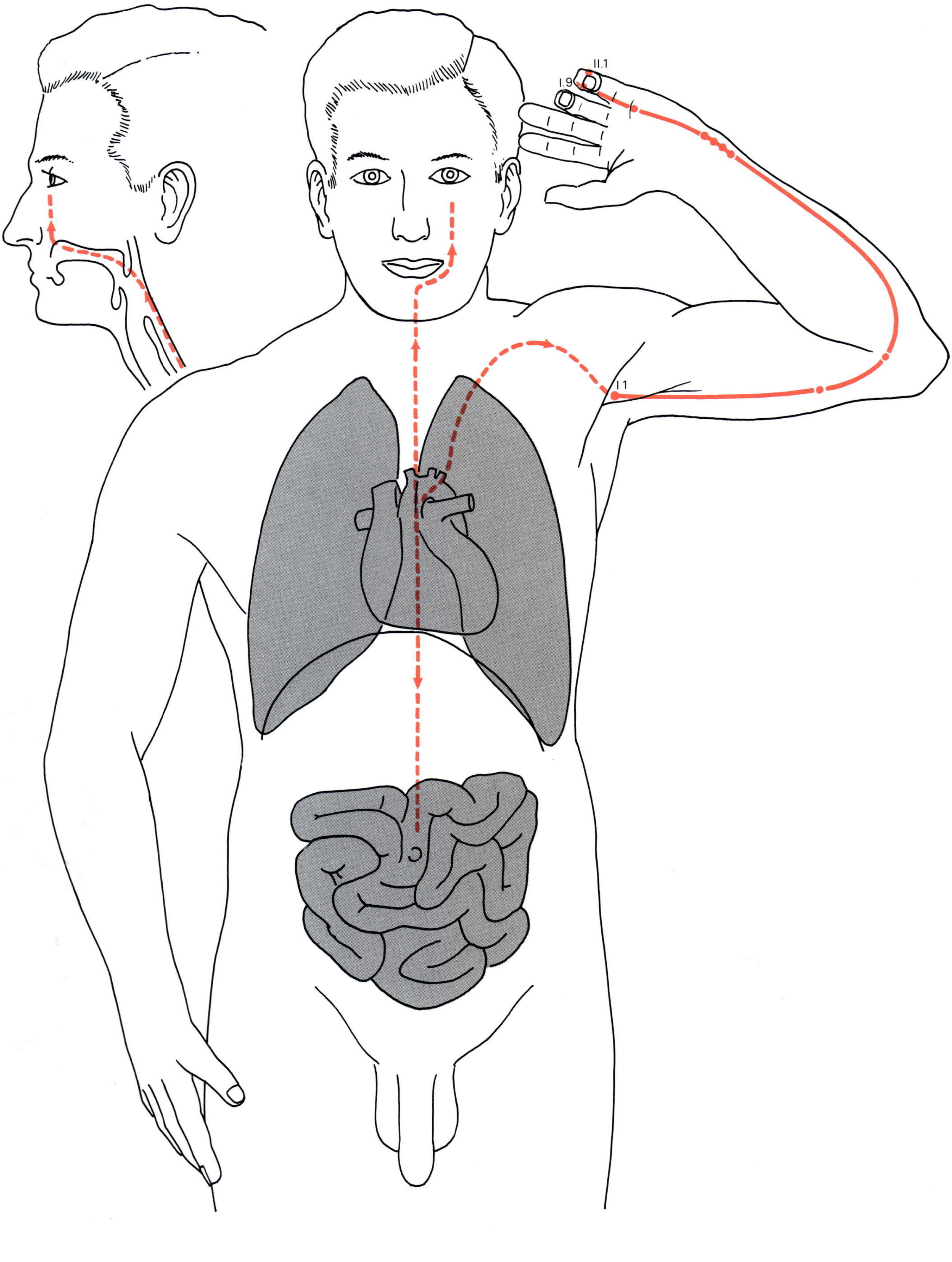
II.1
I.9
I.1

The heart meridian begins at a deep level in the tissue of the heart itself. A deep pathway travels down the median line, through the diaphragm into the abdomen and connects with the small intestines.

Another deep branch travels superiorly alongside the oesophagus, over the pharynx, round the angle of the mouth and up to the optic foramen.

A third pathway ascends along the aorta, passes into the lungs and runs laterally along the subclavian artery to the axilla, where the meridian becomes superficial at the entry point, I 1.

The meridian continues down the medial border of the biceps to the flexure of the elbow, anterior to the medial epicondyle of the humerus. It travels along the medial border of the ulna to the lateral side of the pisiform bone. Crossing the wrist, it runs over the palm of the hand between the fourth and fifth metacarpal bones and along the radial side of the little finger, ending at the radial nail point, the exit point, I 9. From here it connects to the first point of the small intestines, II 1, the ulnar nail point of the little finger.

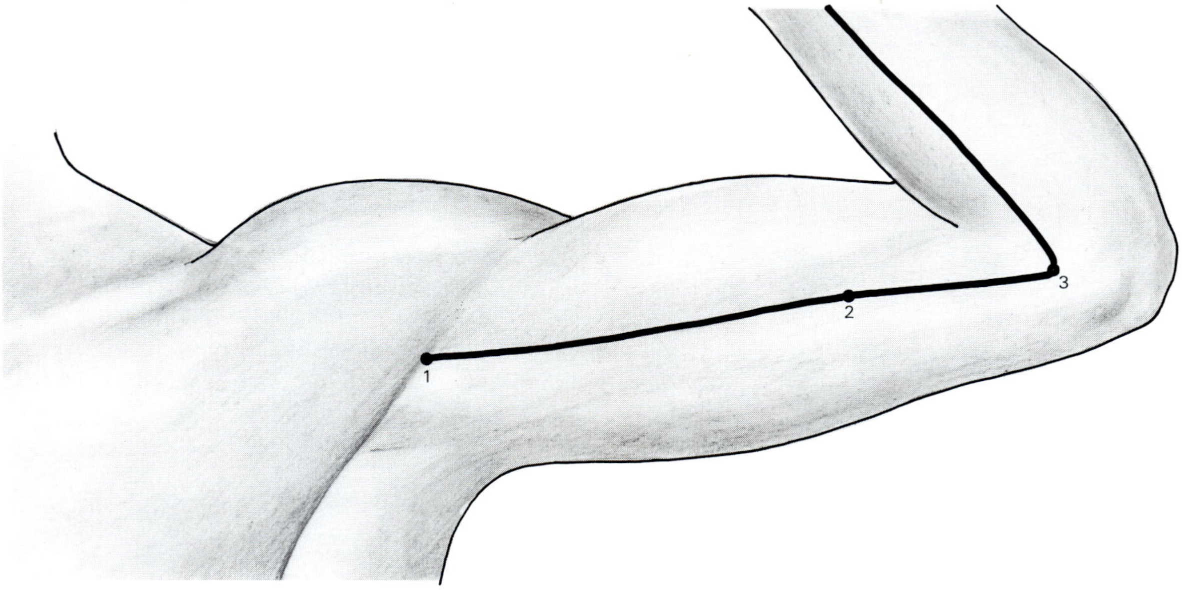
1
2
3

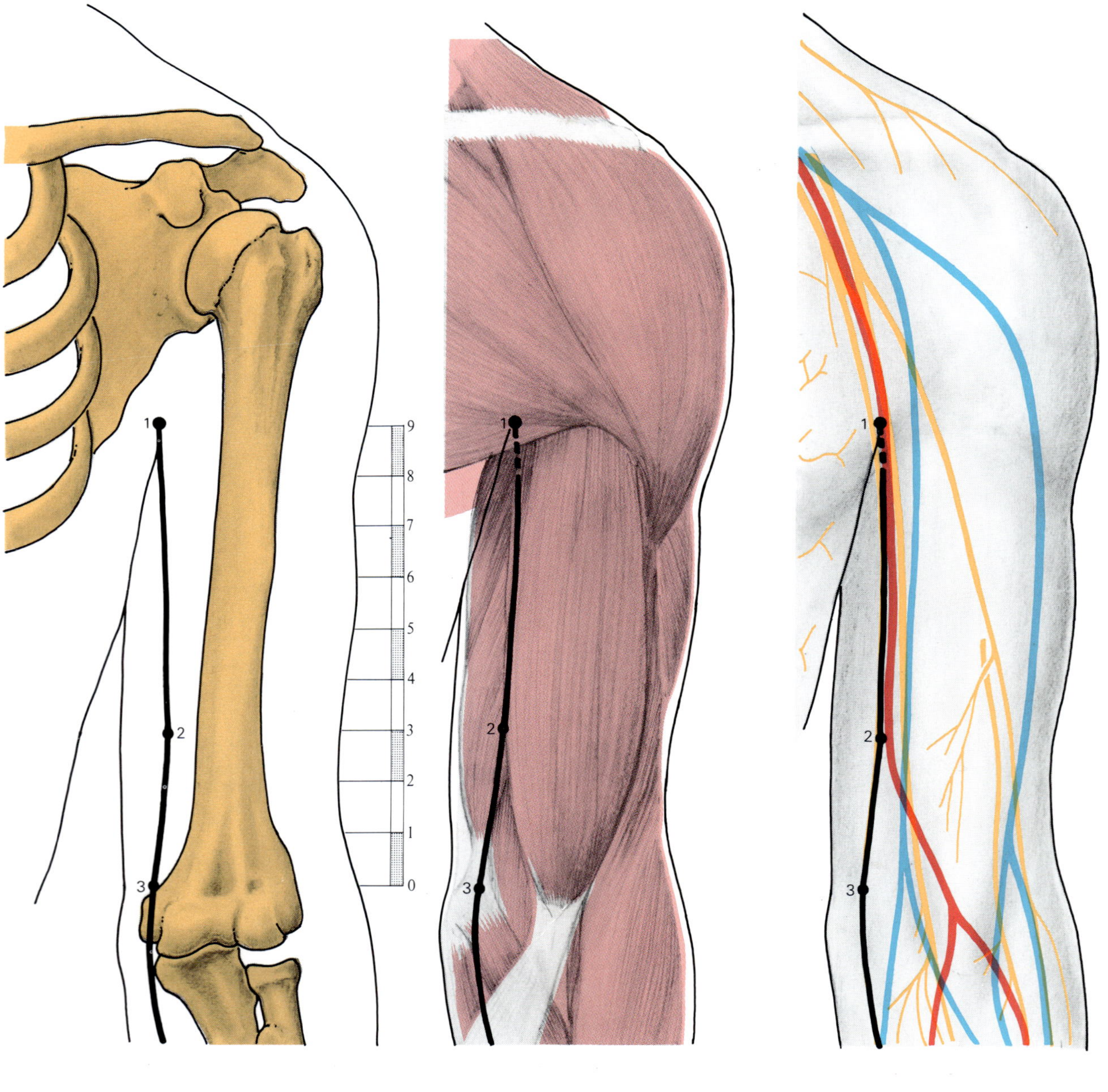
1
2
3
9
8
7
6
5
4
3
2
1
0
1
2
3
1
2
3

I 1 In the axilla, upon the axillary artery. To expose the point, semiabduct the arm and palpate the artery.

I 2 On the medial surface of the arm, 3 ACI proximal to the flexure of the elbow, upon the brachial artery.

I 3 Close to the medial end of the elbow crease when the arm is slightly flexed, approximately half-way between the medial epicondyle of the humerus and the tendon of the biceps.

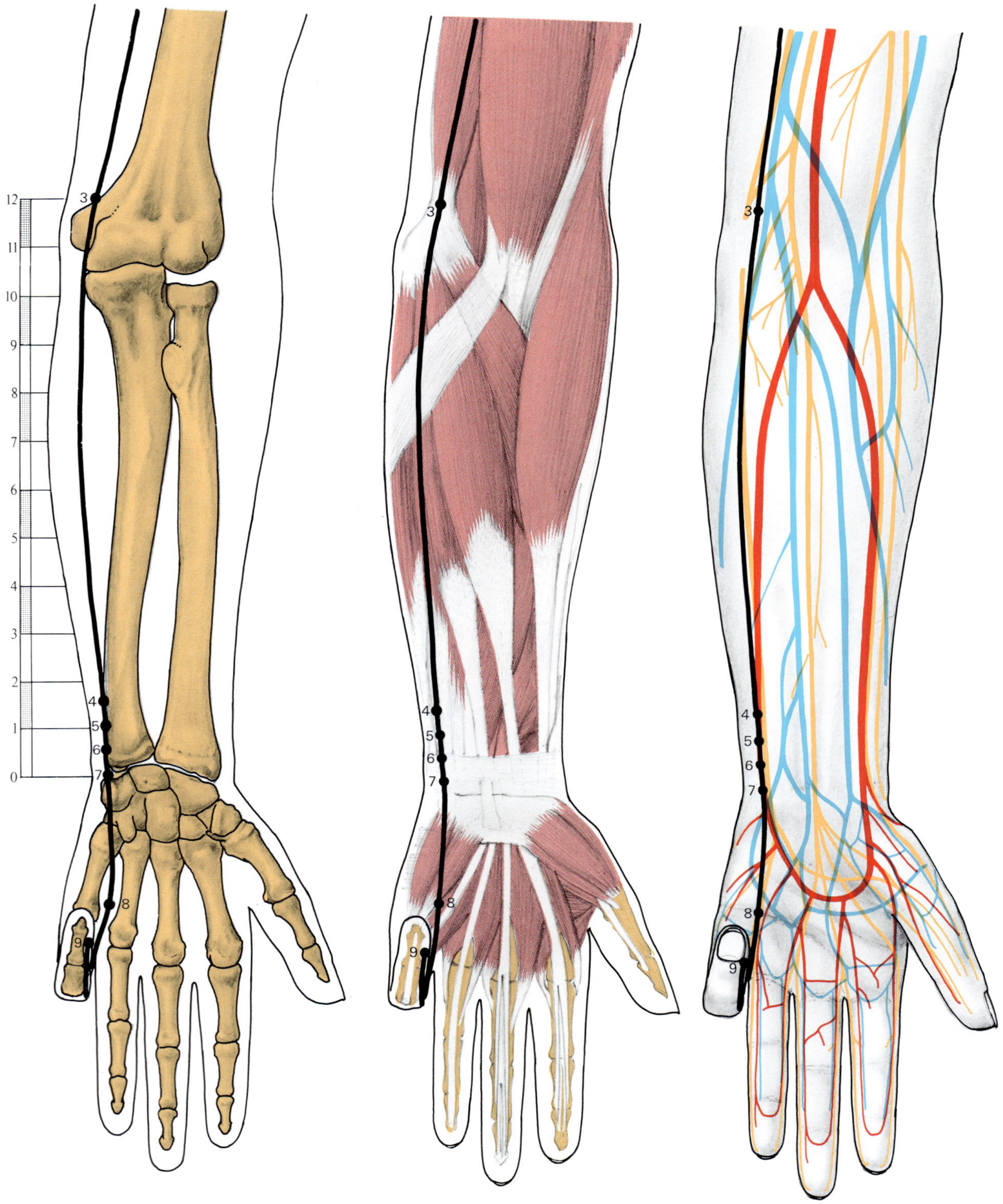
3
4
5
6
7
8
9
12
11
10
9
8
7
6
5
4
3
2
1
0

I	3	Close to the medial end of the elbow crease when the arm is slightly flexed, approximately half-way between the medial epicondyle of the humerus and the tendon of the biceps.
I	4	On the anterior surface of the forearm, $1\frac{1}{2}$ ACI proximal to I 7, upon the ulnar artery.
I	5	On the anterior surface of the forearm, 1 ACI proximal to I 7, upon the ulnar artery.
I	6	On the anterior surface of the forearm, $\frac{1}{2}$ ACI proximal to I 7, upon the ulnar artery.
I	7	On the crease of the flexure of the wrist, on the proximal radial side of the pisiform bone, upon the ulnar artery.
I	8	On the palmar surface of the hand, between the fourth and fifth metacarpal bones, on the distal transverse crease, or the 'heart line' of the hand.
I	9	Radial nail point of the little finger.

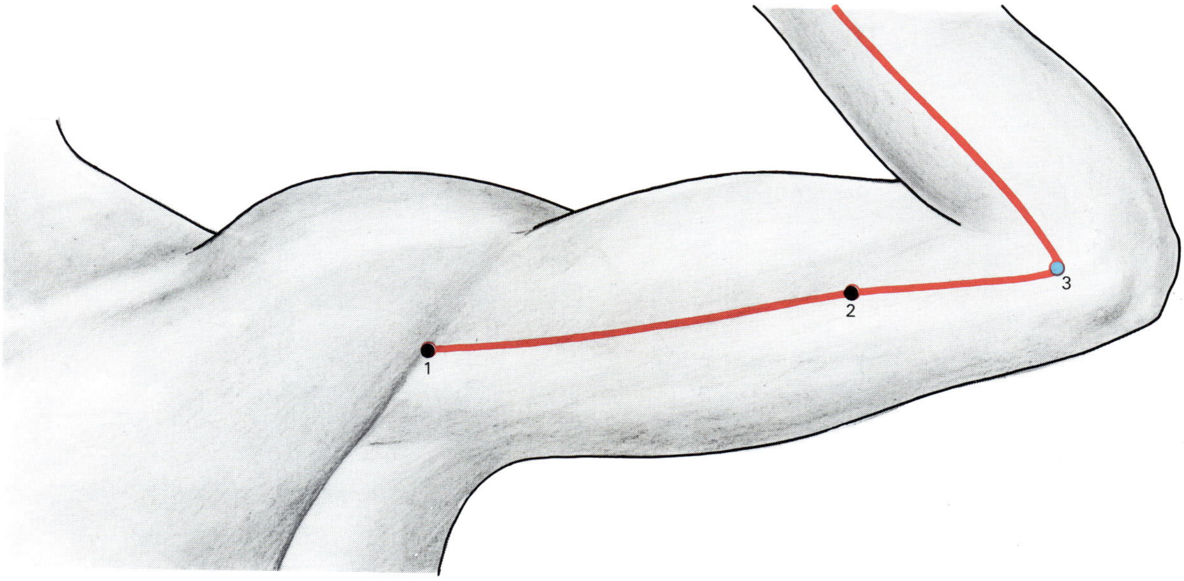
1
2
3

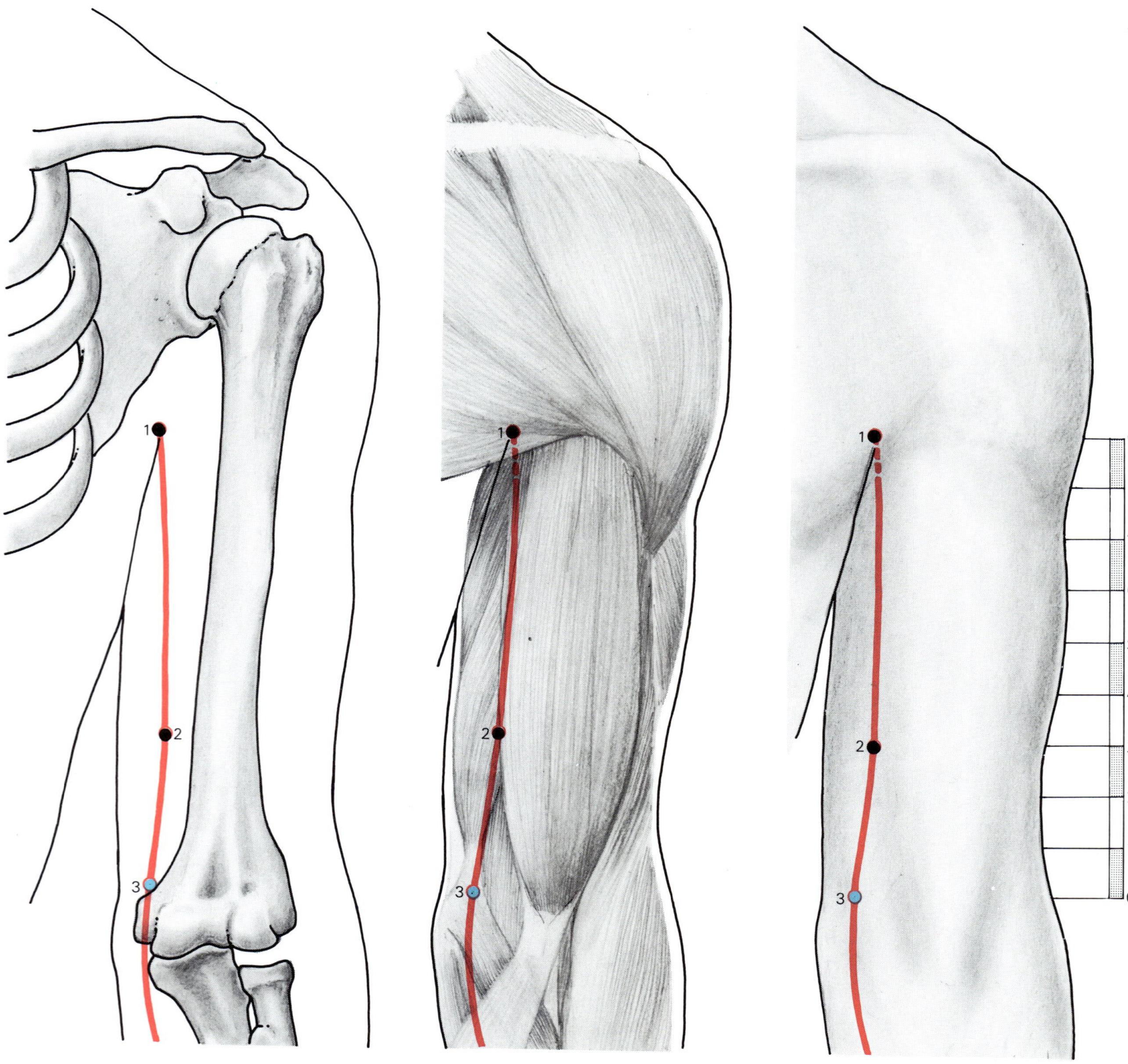
1
2
3
1
2
3
1
2
3
9
8
7
6
5
4
3
2
1
0

I **1** **Utmost Source** (Chichuan)

⊥ 5 Entry
△ 5

In the axilla, upon the axillary artery. To expose the point, semiabduct the arm and palpate the artery.

First Aid: drowning, fainting, heart failure

I **2** **Blue-Green Spirit** (Chingling)

⊥ X
△ 5

On the medial surface of the arm, 3 ACI proximal to the flexure of the elbow, upon the brachial artery.

I **3** **Little Sea** (Shaohai)

⊥ 3–5 Water
△ 3–7

Close to the medial end of the elbow crease when the arm is slightly flexed, approximately half-way between the medial epicondyle of the humerus and the tendon of the biceps.

Point of Ho (Autumn)

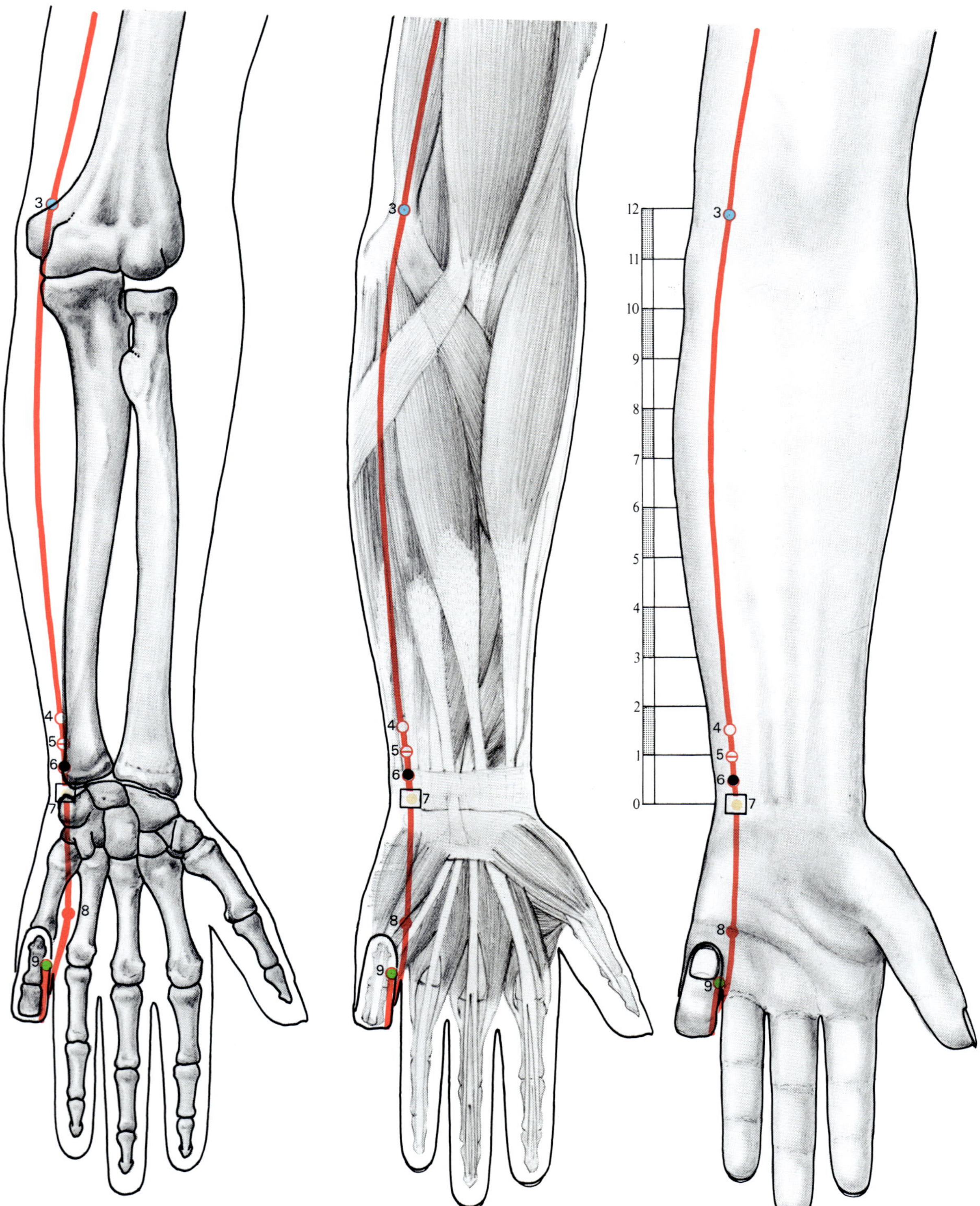
3
4
5
6
7
8
9
3
4
5
6
7
8
9
12
11
10
9
8
7
6
5
4
3
2
1
0
3
4
5
6
7
8
9

I **4** **Spirit Path** (Lingtao)

○ ⊥ 3 Metal
△ 3–5

On the anterior surface of the forearm, 1½ ACI proximal to I 7, upon the ulnar artery.

Point of Ching (late Summer)

I **5** **Penetrating Inside** (Tungli)

⊖ ⊥ 3 Junction
△ 3–5

On the anterior surface of the forearm, 1 ACI proximal to I 7, upon the ulnar artery.

I **6** **Yin Mound** (Yinhsi)

⊥ 3
△ 3–7

On the anterior surface of the forearm, ½ ACI proximal to I 7, upon the ulnar artery.

I **7** **Spirit Gate** (Shenmen)

● ⊥ 3 Earth
△ 5–7 Sedation
□ Source

On the crease of the flexure of the wrist, on the proximal radial side of the pisiform bone, upon the ulnar artery.

Point of Yu (Summer)
First Aid: anxiety, electric shock, fainting, heart failure, hysteria, shock, tooth extraction

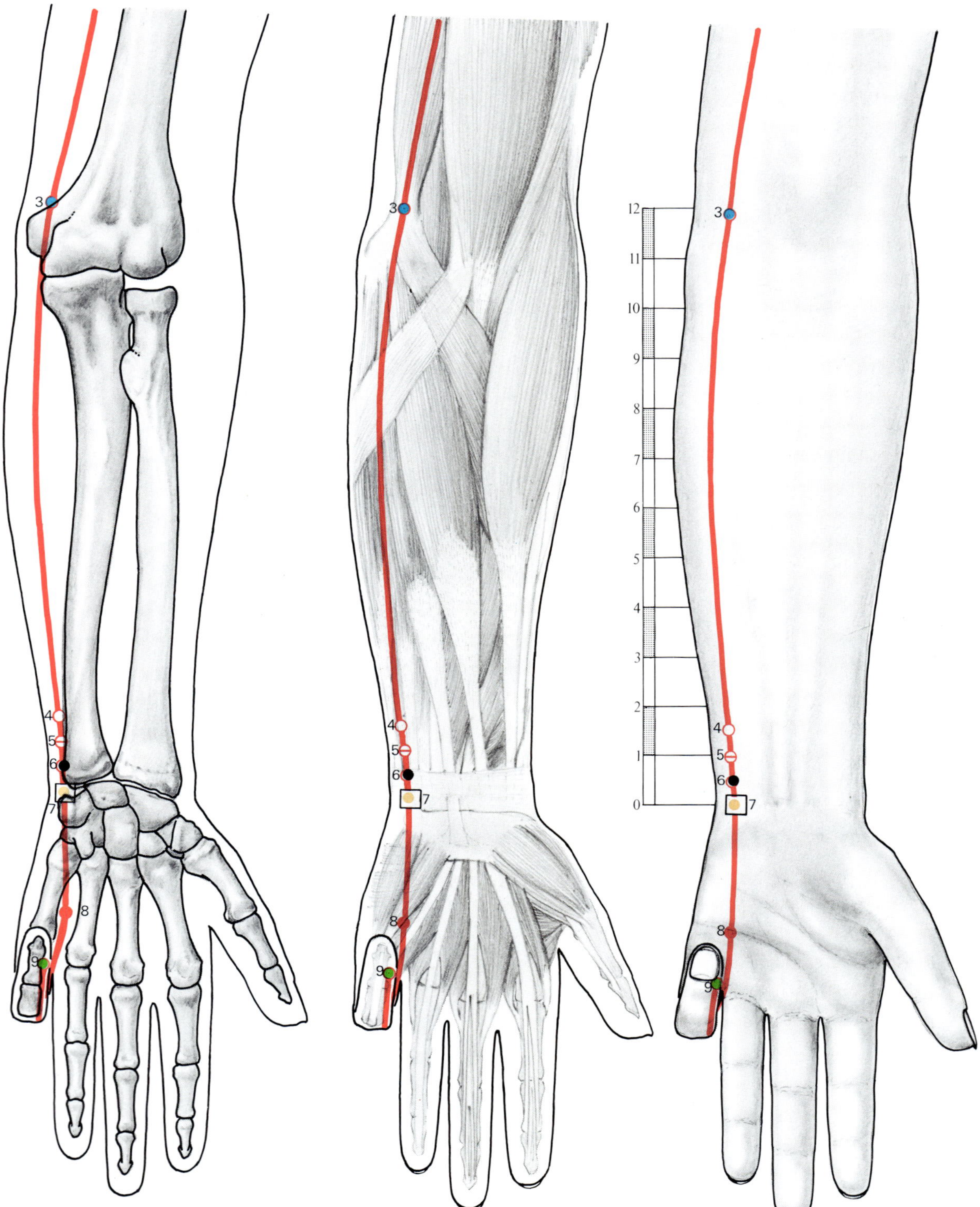
3
4
5
6
7
8
9
3
4
5
6
7
8
9
12
11
10
9
8
7
6
5
4
3
2
1
0
3
4
5
6
7
8
9

I **8** **Lesser Palace** (Shaofu)

⊥ 2–3 Fire
△ 3–5 Horary 11 a.m.–1 p.m.

On the palmar surface of the hand, between the fourth and fifth metacarpal bones, on the distal transverse crease, or the 'heart line' of the hand.

Point of Yung (Spring)

I **9** **Little Rushing In** (Shaochung)

⊥ 1 Wood
△ 3–5 Tonification
Exit

Radial nail point of the little finger.

Point of Cheng (Winter)

■ II Small Intestine Meridian

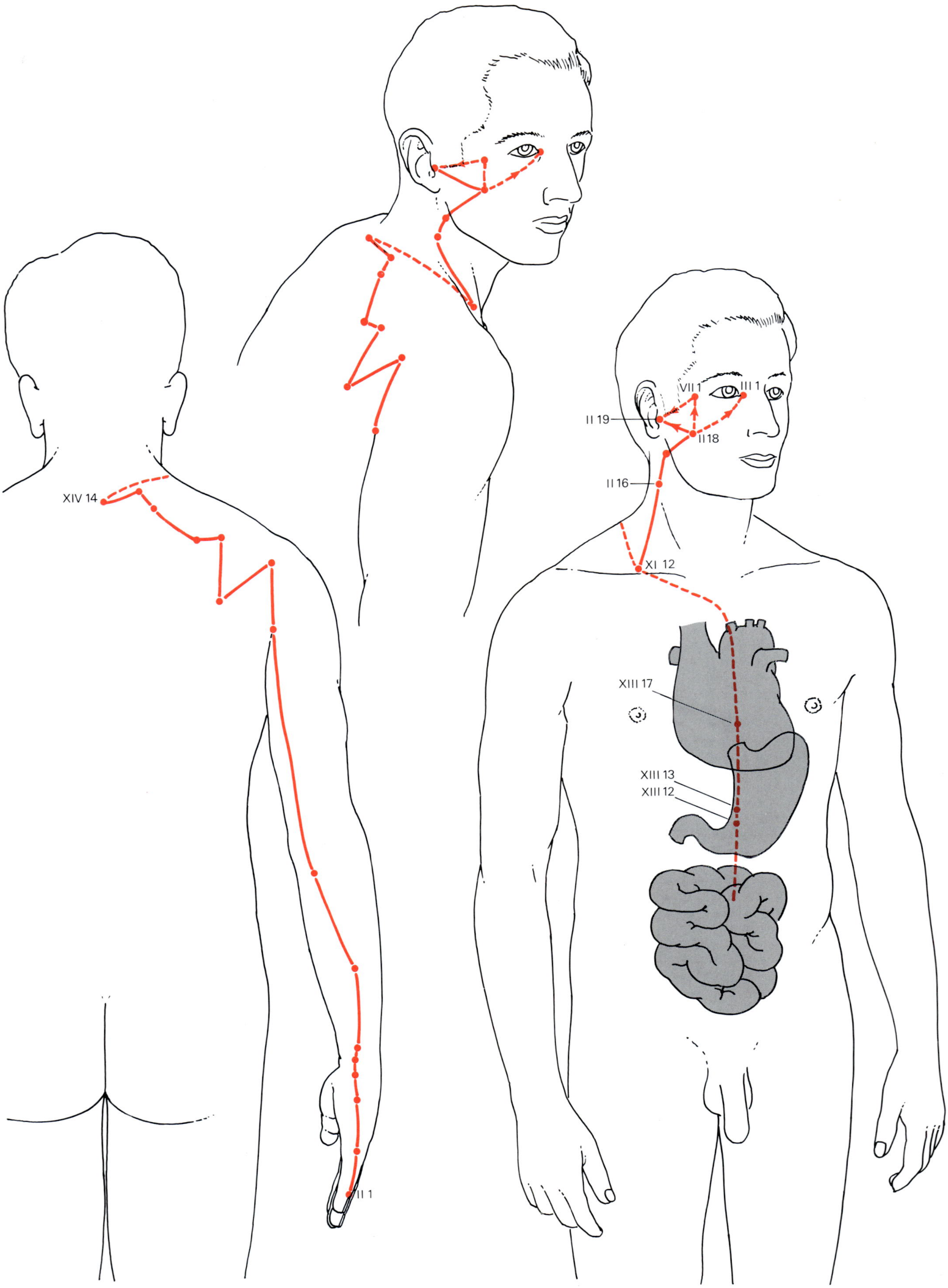

The small intestine meridian begins as the superficial pathway at the ulnar nail point of the little finger, the entry point, II 1. It travels along the medial border of the little finger and the fifth metacarpal bone, runs slightly posterior over the styloid process of the ulna, and up the ulnar side of the extensor carpi ulnaris to the elbow, where it passes between the olecranon and the medial epicondyle of the humerus. It continues up the medial posterior surface of the arm to the inferior edge of the acromion. It then drops down on to the scapula, ascends again and travels medially, superior to the spine of the scapula, and arrives at the median line below the seventh cervical vertebra, at XIV 14. From XIV 14 the pathway becomes deep and runs anteriorly over the shoulder to the supraclavicular fossa, at XI 12. Here the pathway divides.

One branch continues as the deep pathway, first to the heart at XIII 17, then it descends along the oesophagus, penetrates the diaphragm in the median line, passes through the stomach, at XIII 13 and XIII 12, and connects with the small intestines.

The other branch continues as the superficial pathway, ascending the neck along the sternocleidomastoid through II 16, and crossing over the mandible as it ascends the cheek to II 18 and turns laterally to end in front of the tragus of the ear at the exit point, II 19. A deep branch ascends from II 18 to the lateral canthus of the eye at VII 1, to end at II 19. Another deep branch leaves the superficial pathway at II 18, to ascend close to the nose and on to the medial canthus of the eye at III 1, where it connects with the bladder meridian.

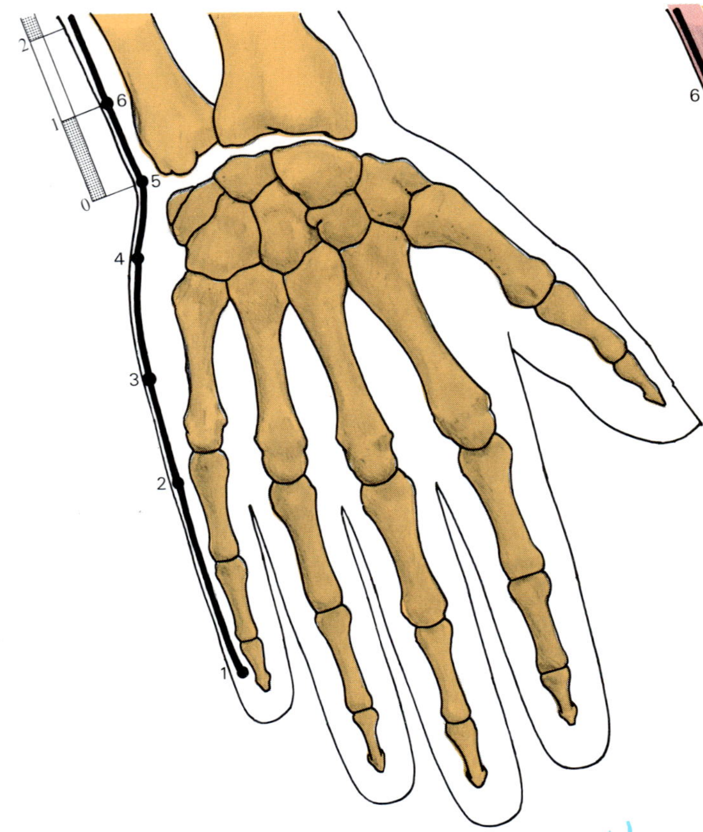
2
1
0
6
5
4
3
2
1

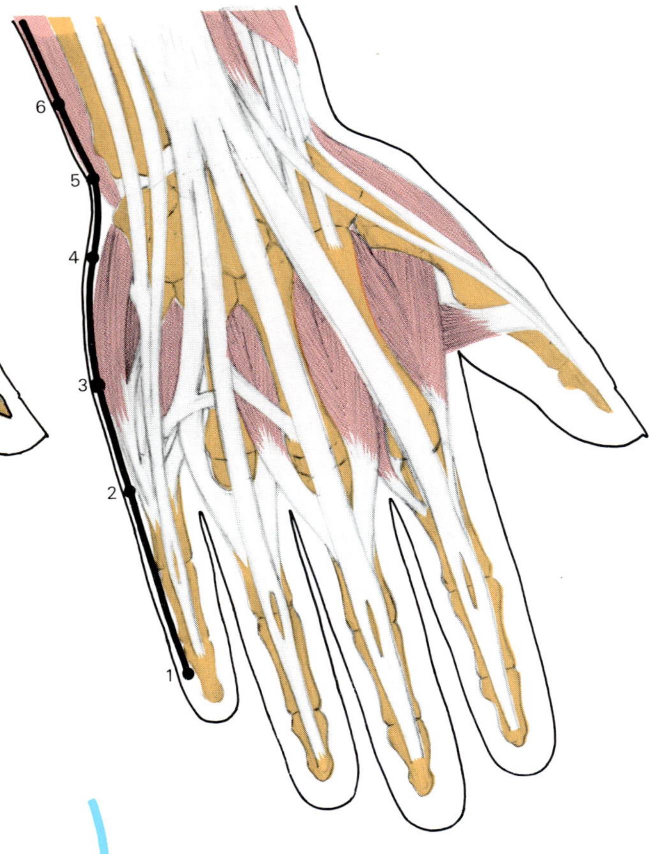
6
5
4
3
2
1

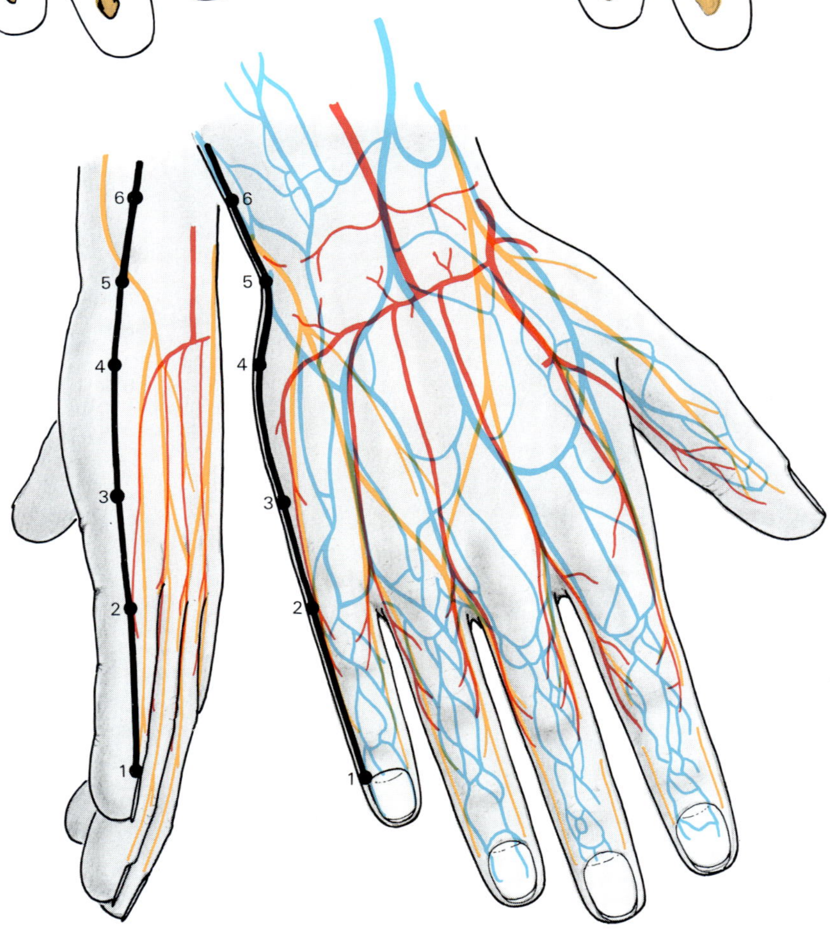
6
5
4
3
2
1
6
5
4
3
2
1

II 1 Ulnar nail point of the little finger.

II 2 On the ulnar edge of the hand, just distal to the base of the proximal phalanx of the little finger.

II 3 On the ulnar edge of the hand, approximately half-way along the fifth metacarpal bone. (Feel along the bone for the notch).

II 4 On the ulnar edge of the hand, in the hollow between the proximal end of the fifth metacarpal bone and the triquetral bone.

II 5 On the ulnar edge of the hand, in the hollow between the triquetral bone and the head of the ulna.

II 6 On the ulnar surface of the forearm, 1 ACI proximal to II 5, just proximal to the head of the ulna.

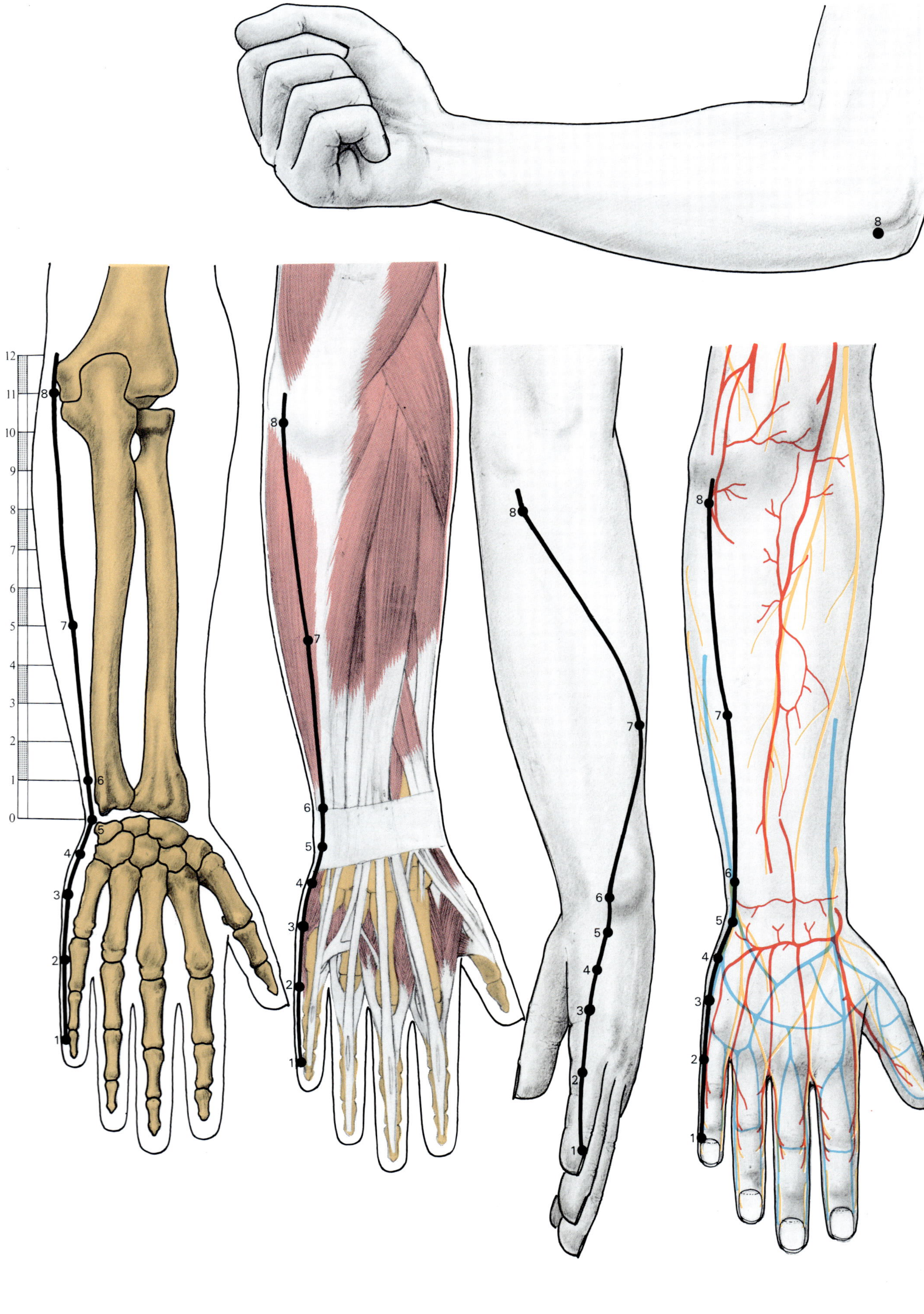

II 6 On the ulnar surface of the forearm, 1 ACI proximal to II 5, just proximal to the head of the ulna.

II 7 On the posterior surface of the forearm, 5 ACI proximal to the flexure of the wrist. With the arm extended and the forearm pronated, it lies in the seam between the ulna and the extensor carpi ulnaris.

II 8 On the posteromedial surface of the forearm, 1 ACI distal to the hollow between the medial epicondyle of the humerus and the olecranon when the forearm is semiflexed.

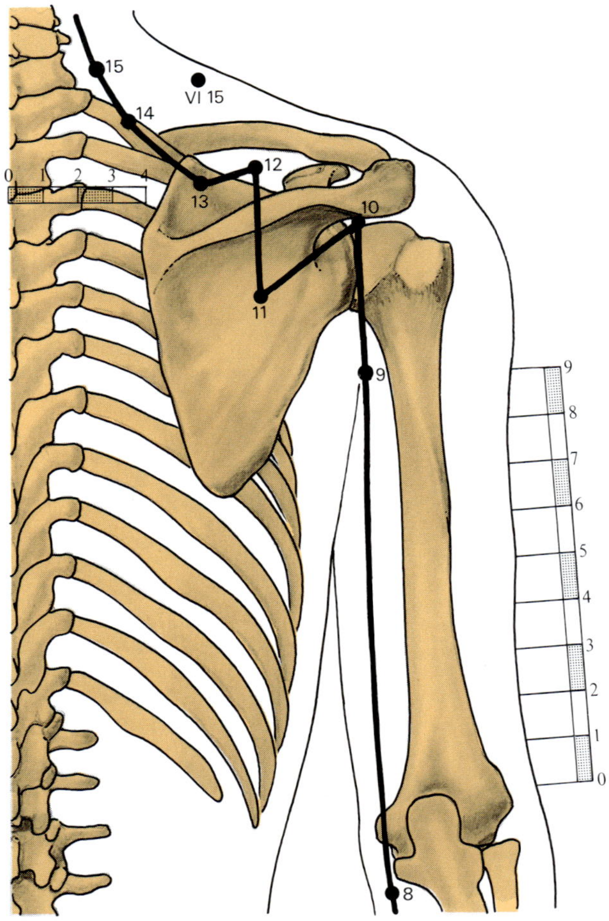
15
VI 15
14
12
13
0 1 2 3 4
10
11
9
9 8 7 6 5 4 3 2 1 0
8

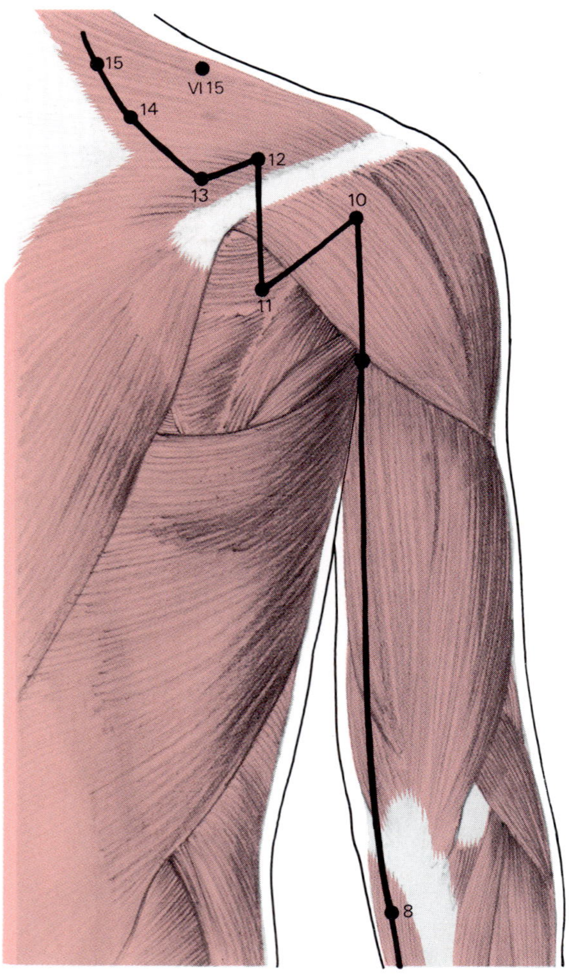
15
VI 15
14
12
13
10
11
8

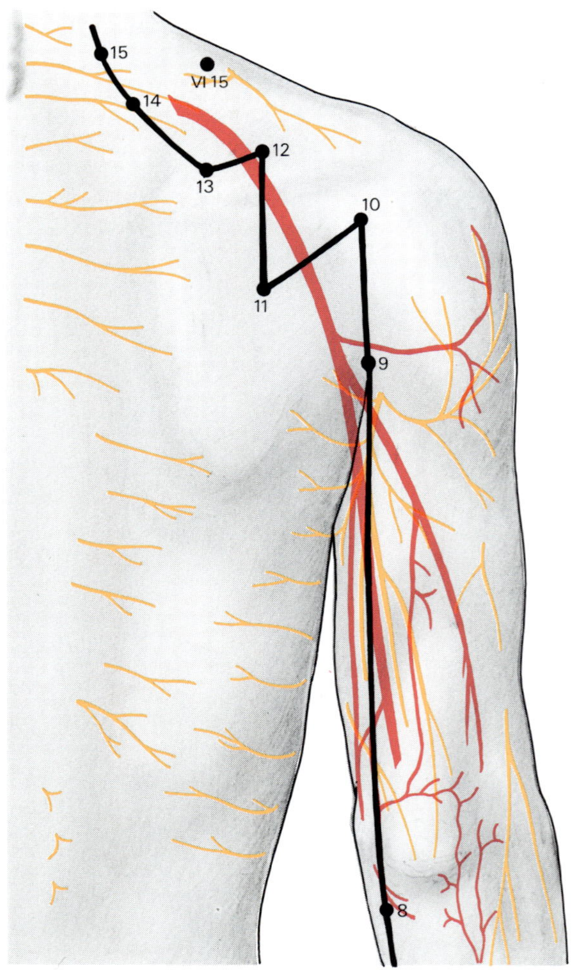
15
VI 15
14
12
13
10
11
9
8

II	8	On the posteromedial surface of the forearm, 1 ACI distal to the hollow between the medial epicondyle of the humerus and the olecranon when the forearm is semiflexed.
II	9	On the posterior surface of the shoulder, at the superior end of the axillary fold.
II	10	On the posterior surface of the shoulder, in the depression inferior to the acromion, directly superior to II 9.
II	11	On the back, in the middle of the scapula, approximately 1½ ACI inferior to the inferior edge of the middle of the scapular spine.
II	12	On the back, approximately 1 ACI superior to the superior edge of the middle of the scapular spine.
II	13	On the back, mid-way between II 12 and the medial border of the scapula, about 1 ACI superior to the superior edge of the scapular spine, in line with VI 15 and VII 21.
II	14	On the back, 3½ ACI lateral to the tip of the spinous process of the first thoracic vertebra.
II	15	On the back, 2½ ACI lateral to the tip of the spinous process of the seventh cervical vertebra.

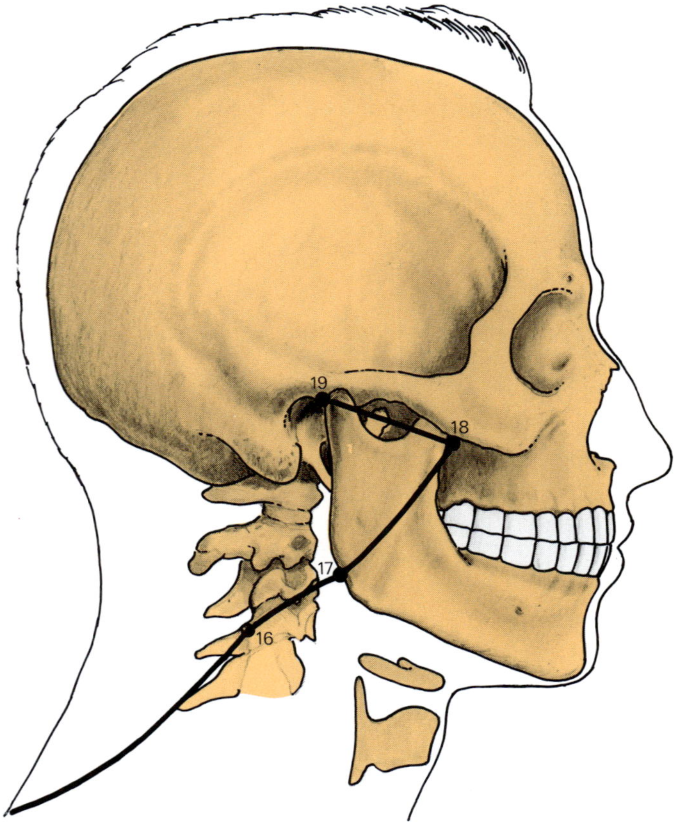
19
18
17
16

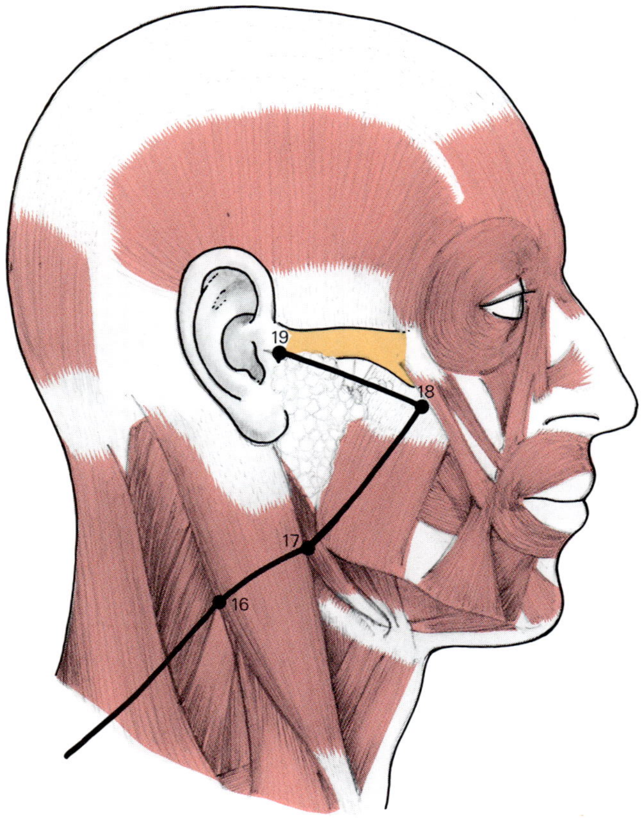
19
18
17
16

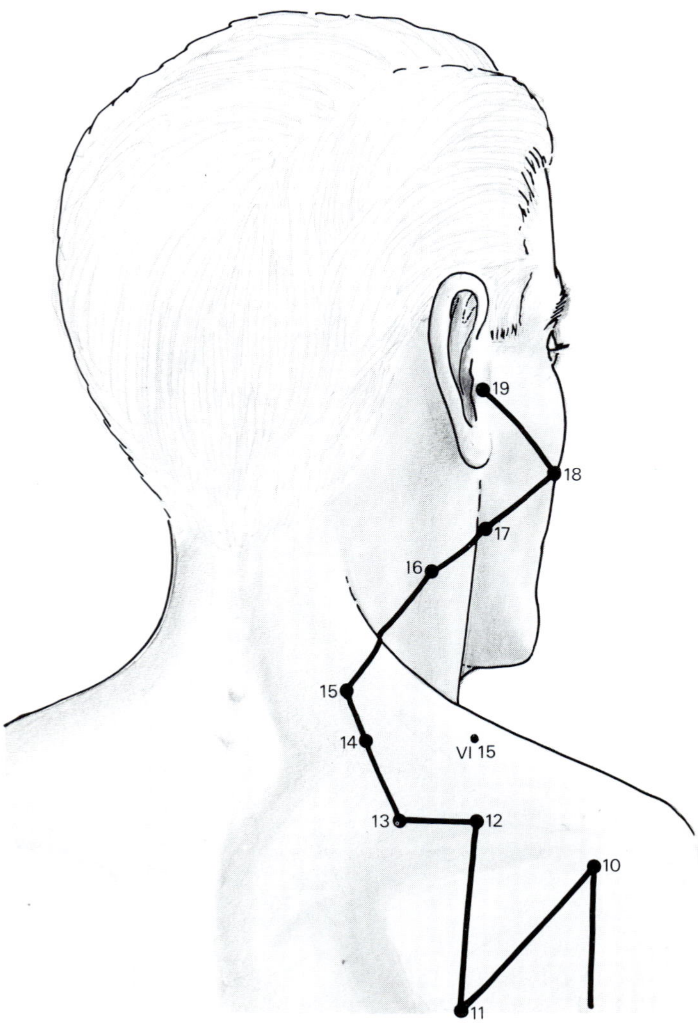
19
18
17
16
15
14
VI 15
13
12
10
11

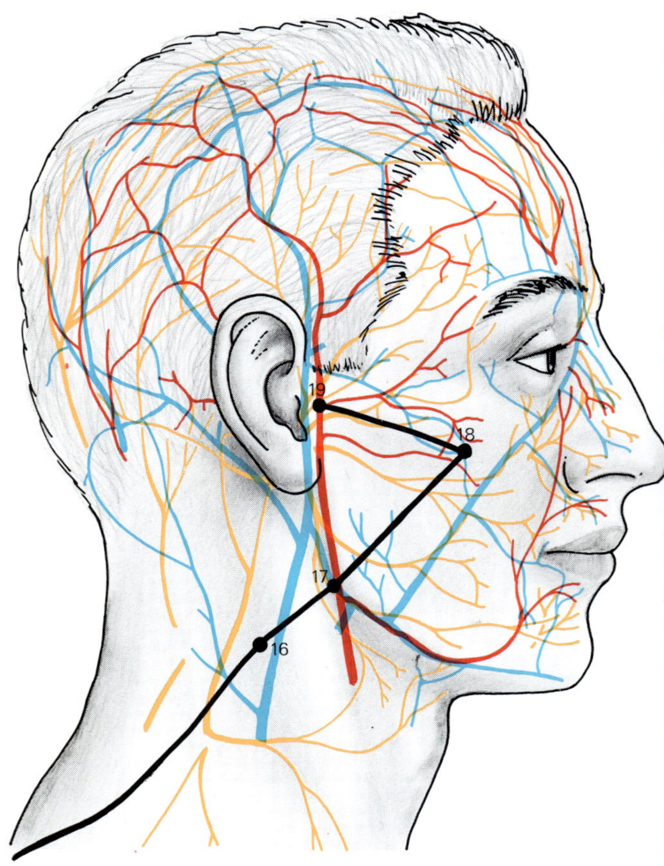
19
18
17
16

II 16 On the lateral surface of the neck, at the posterior border of the sternocleidomastoid, at the level of the laryngeal prominence.

II 17 On the posterior edge of the mandible, in the notch of the bone, slightly superior to the angle of the mandible.

II 18 On the cheek, inferior to the lateral canthus of the eye, in the angle of the zygomatic bone and the mandible.

II 19 Anterior to the tragus of the ear, on the superficial temporal artery, in the depression formed when the mouth is open.

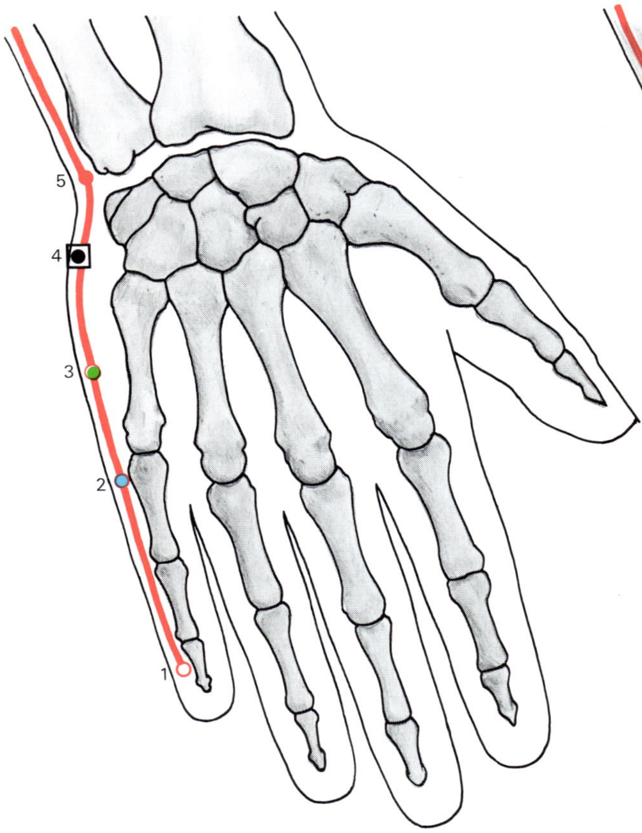
5
4
3
2
1

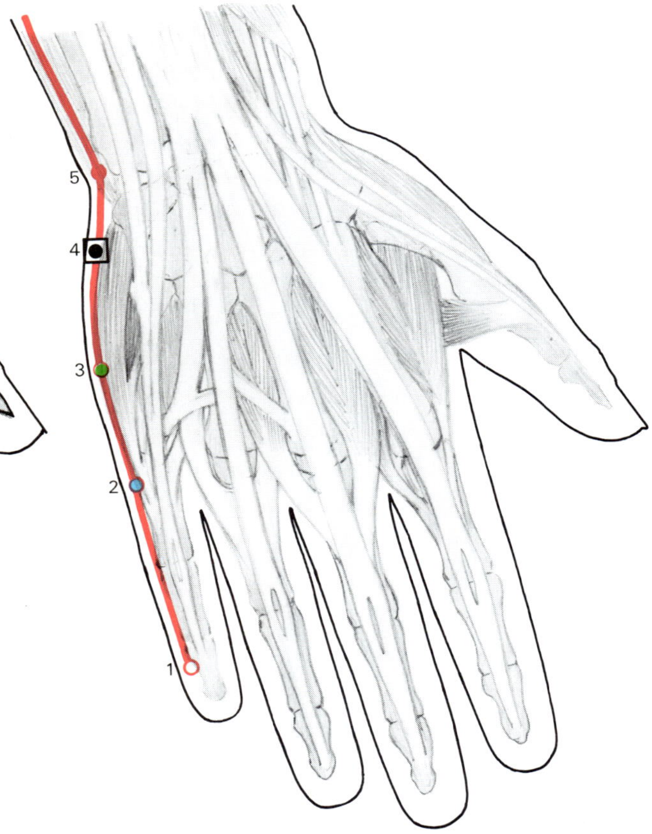
5
4
3
2
1

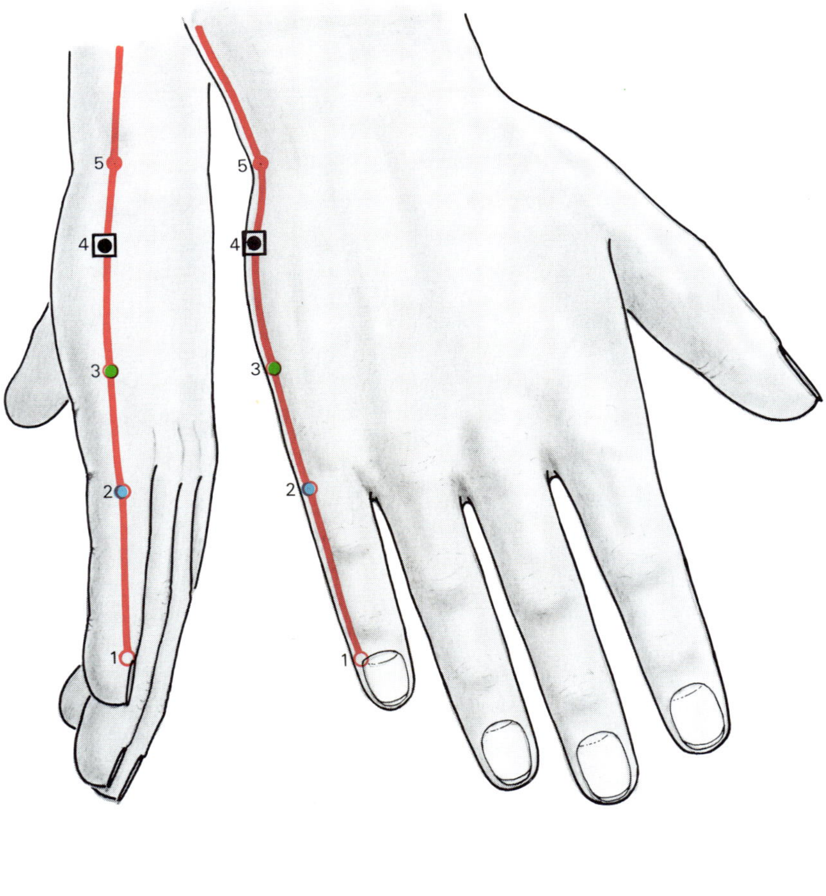
5
4
3
2
1
5
4
3
2
1

	II	**1**	**Little Marsh** (Shaotse)
○	⊥	1	Metal
	△	3–5	Entry

Ulnar nail point of the little finger.

Point of Cheng (Winter)

	II	**2**	**Forward Valley** (Chienku)
●	⊥	1	Water
	△	3–7	

On the ulnar edge of the hand, just distal to the base of the proximal phalanx of the little finger.

Point of Yung (Spring)

	II	**3**	**Back Ravine** (Houhsi)
●	⊥	3	Wood
	△	3–7	Tonification

On the ulnar edge of the hand, approximately half-way along the fifth metacarpal bone. (Feel along the bone for the notch).

Point of Yu (Summer)
Master Point of Du Mo
Coupled Point of Yang Qiao Mo
First Aid: convulsions, earache, exhaustion, insensibility

	II	**4**	**Wrist Bone** (Wanku)
□	⊥	3	Source
	△	3–7	

On the ulnar edge of the hand, in the hollow between the proximal end of the fifth metacarpal bone and the triquetral bone.

	II	**5**	**Yang Valley** (Yangku)
●	⊥	2	Fire
	△	3–7	Horary 1 p.m.–3 p.m.

On the ulnar edge of the hand, in the hollow between the triquetral bone and the head of the ulna.

Point of Ching (late Summer)

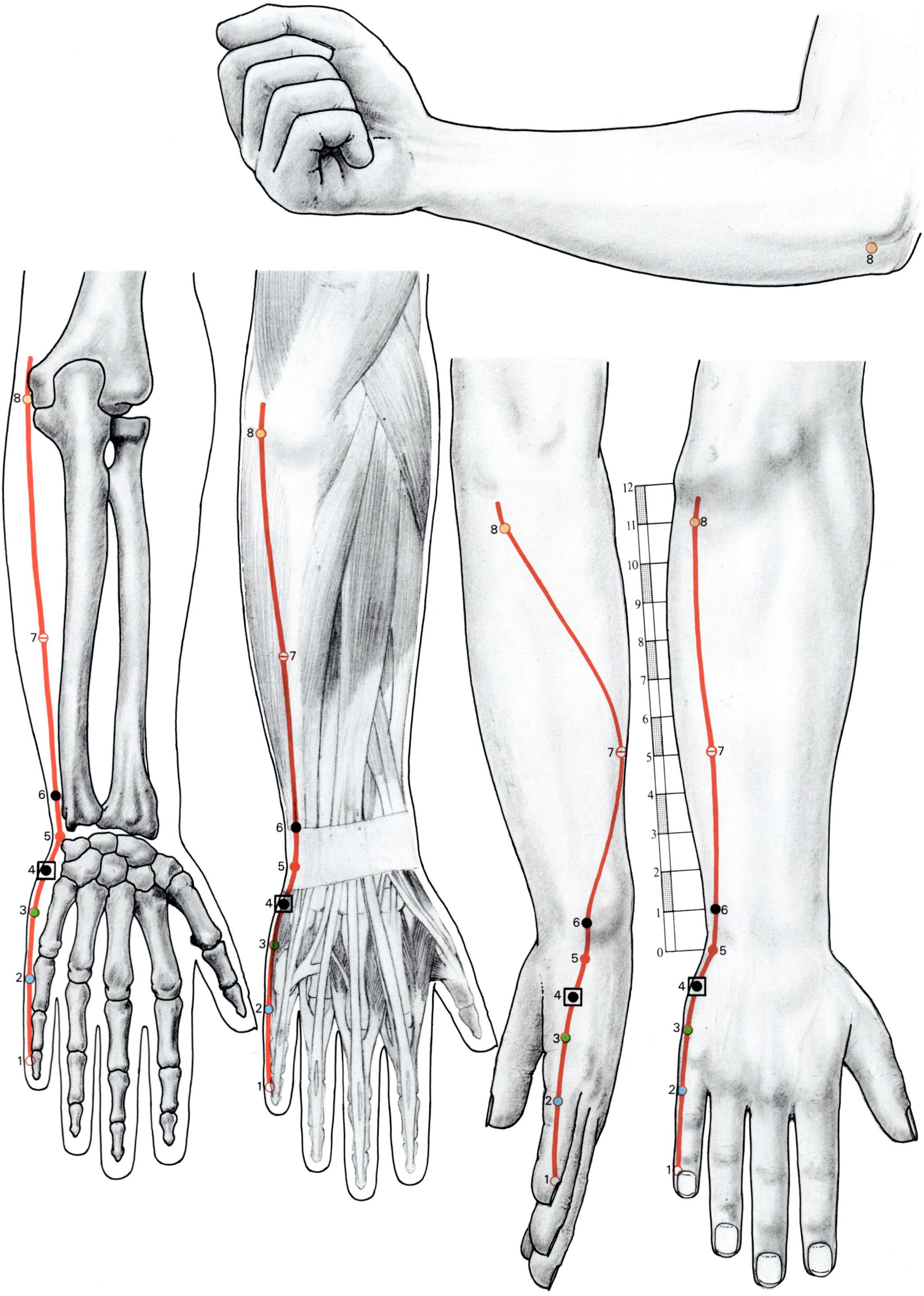

8
8
7
6
5
4
3
2
1
8
7
6
5
4
3
2
1
8
7
6
5
4
3
2
1
12
11
10
9
8
7
6
5
4
3
2
1
0
8
7
6
5
4
3
2
1

II **6** **Nourishing The Old** (Yanglao)

⊥ 3
△ 3–5

On the ulnar surface of the forearm, 1 ACI proximal to II 5, just proximal to the head of the ulna.

II **7** **Upright Branch** (Chihcheng)

⊖ ⊥ 3 Junction
△ 3–7
XP6

On the posterior surface of the forearm, 5 ACI proximal to the flexure of the wrist. With the arm extended and the forearm pronated, it lies in the seam between the ulna and the extensor carpi ulnaris.

Greater Assembling Point of the head and neck

II **8** **Small Sea** (Hsiaohai)

● ⊥ 2 Earth
△ 3–5 Sedation

On the posteromedial surface of the forearm, 1 ACI distal to the hollow between the medial epicondyle of the humerus and the olecranon when the forearm is semiflexed.

Point of Ho (Autumn)
First Aid: haemorrhage

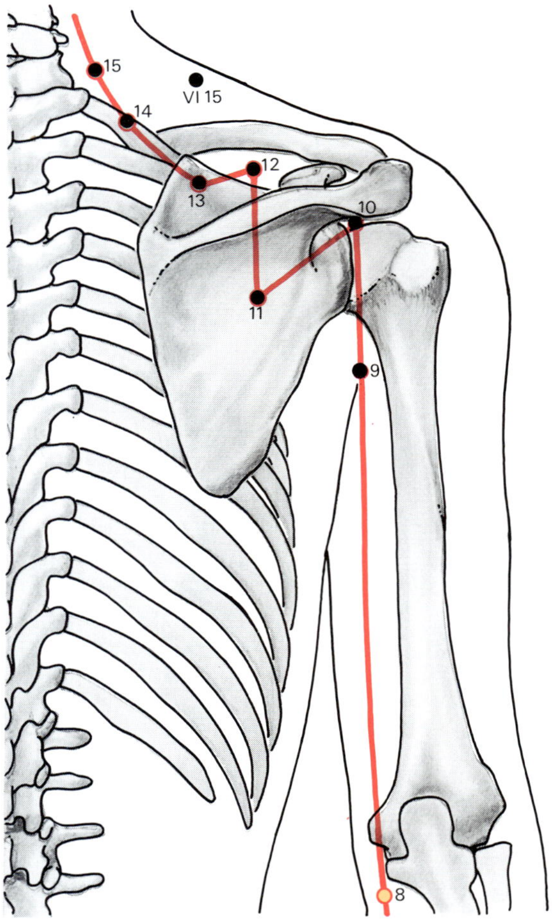
15
14
VI 15
13
12
10
11
9
8

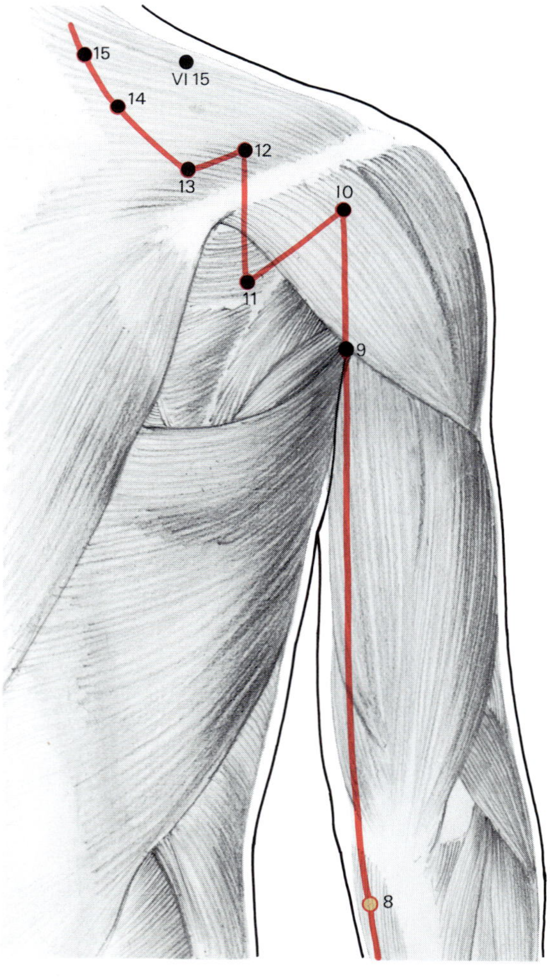
15
VI 15
14
13
12
10
11
9
8

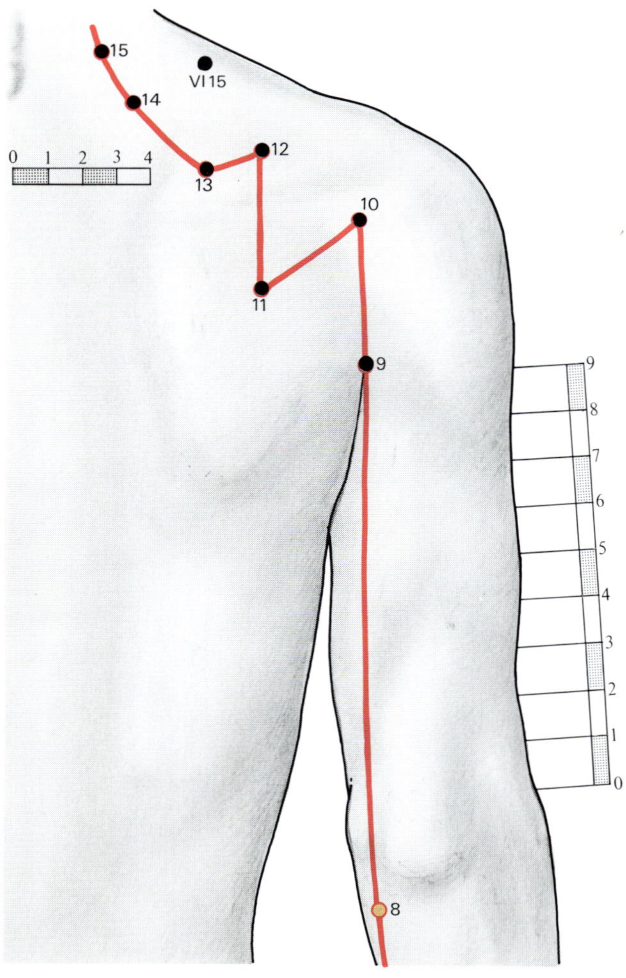
15
VI 15
14
13
12
0 1 2 3 4
10
11
9
8
9
8
7
6
5
4
3
2
1
0

II **9** **Upright Shoulder** (Chienchen)

⊥ 5–7
△ X

On the posterior surface of the shoulder, at the superior end of the axillary fold.

II **10** **Shoulder Blade** (Naoshu)

⊥ 5–7
△ 3–7
XP6

On the posterior surface of the shoulder, in the depression inferior to the acromion, directly superior to II 9.

Point of Yang Wei Mo
Point of Yang Qiao Mo

II **11** **Heavenly Ancestor** (Tientsung)

⊥ 5
△ 5–7

On the back, in the middle of the scapula, approximately $1\frac{1}{2}$ ACI inferior to the inferior edge of the middle of the scapular spine.

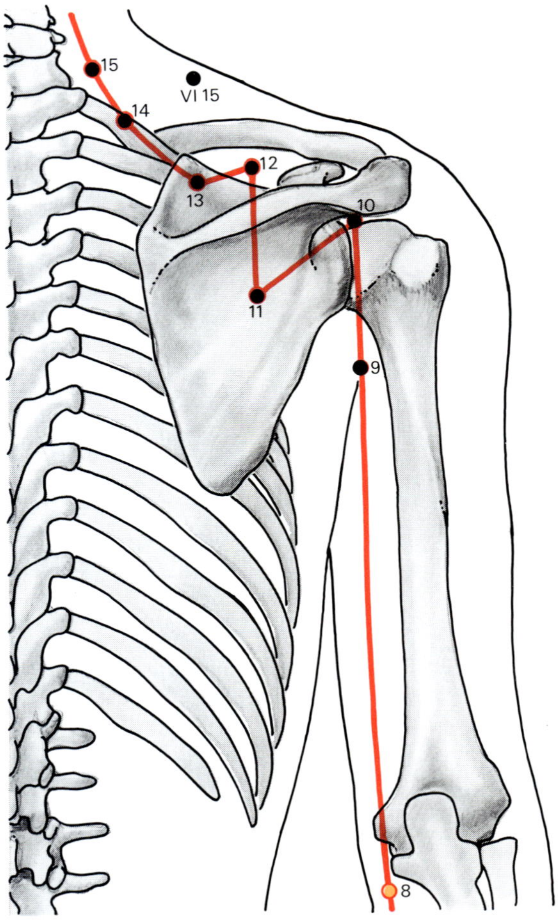
15
VI 15
14
12
13
10
11
9
8

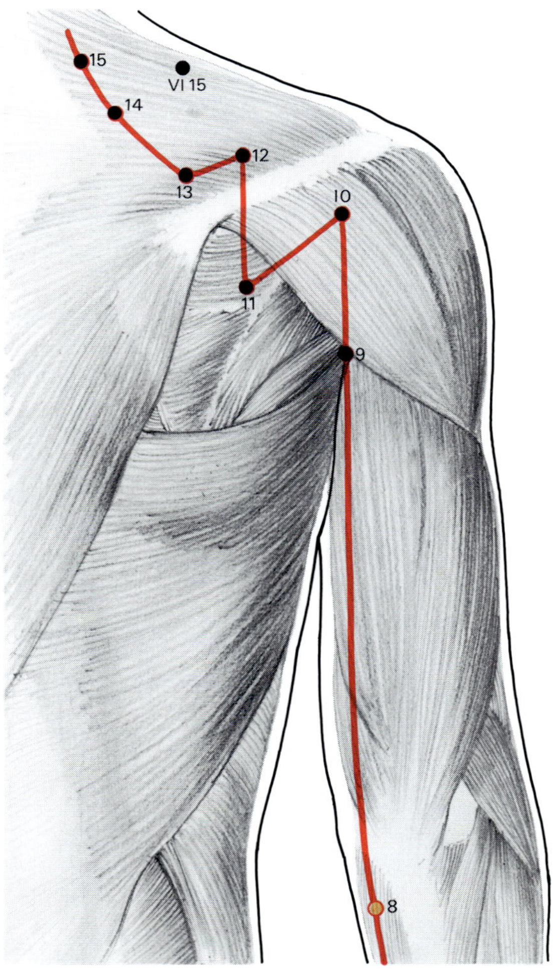
15
VI 15
14
12
13
10
11
9
8

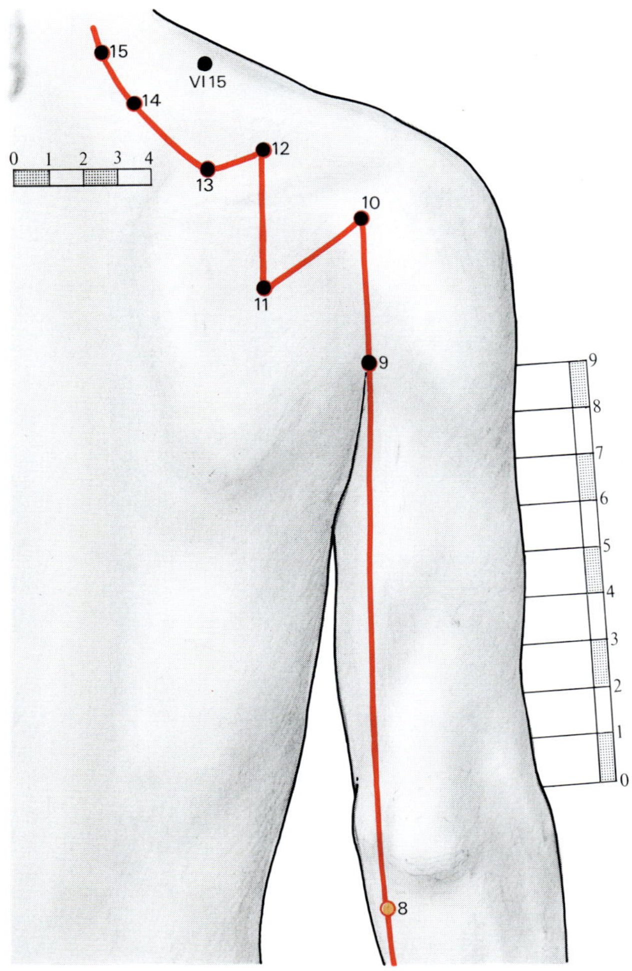
15
VI 15
14
0 1 2 3 4
12
13
10
11
9
9
8
7
6
5
4
3
2
1
0
8

II **12** **Grasping The Wind** (Pingfeng)

⊥ 5
△ 7

On the back, approximately 1 ACI superior to the superior edge of the middle of the scapular spine.

II **13** **Crooked Wall** (Chuyuan)

⊥ 5
△ 3–7

On the back, mid-way between II 12 and the medial border of the scapula, approximately 1 ACI superior to the superior edge of the scapular spine, in line with VI 15 and VII 21.

II **14** **Outside The Shoulder Correspondence** (Chienwaishu)

⊥ 6
△ 3–10

On the back, $3\frac{1}{2}$ ACI lateral to the tip of the spinous process of the first thoracic vertebra.

II **15** **Middle Of The Shoulder Correspondence** (Chienchungshu)

⊥ 3–6
△ 5–10

On the back, $2\frac{1}{2}$ ACI lateral to the tip of the spinous process of the seventh cervical vertebra.

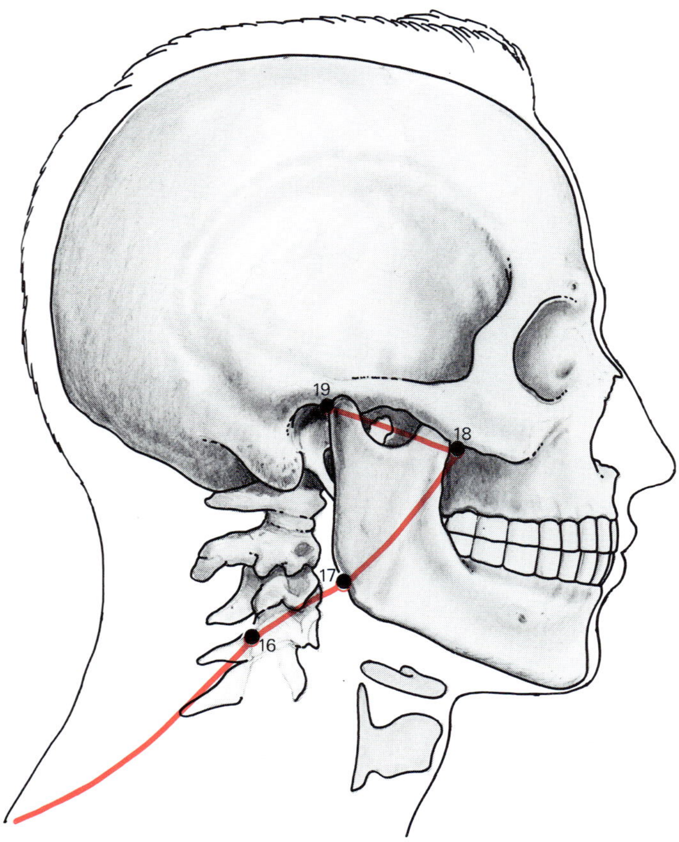
19
18
17
16

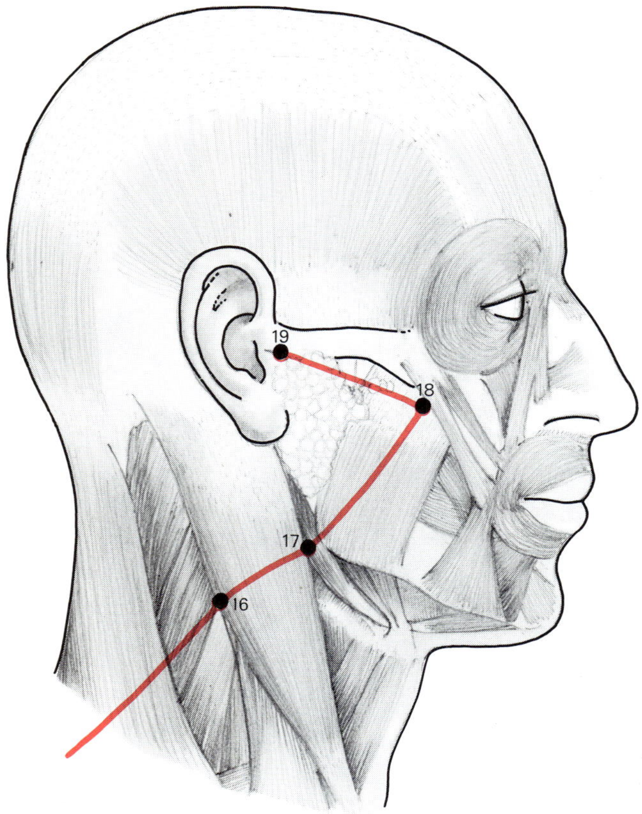
19
18
17
16

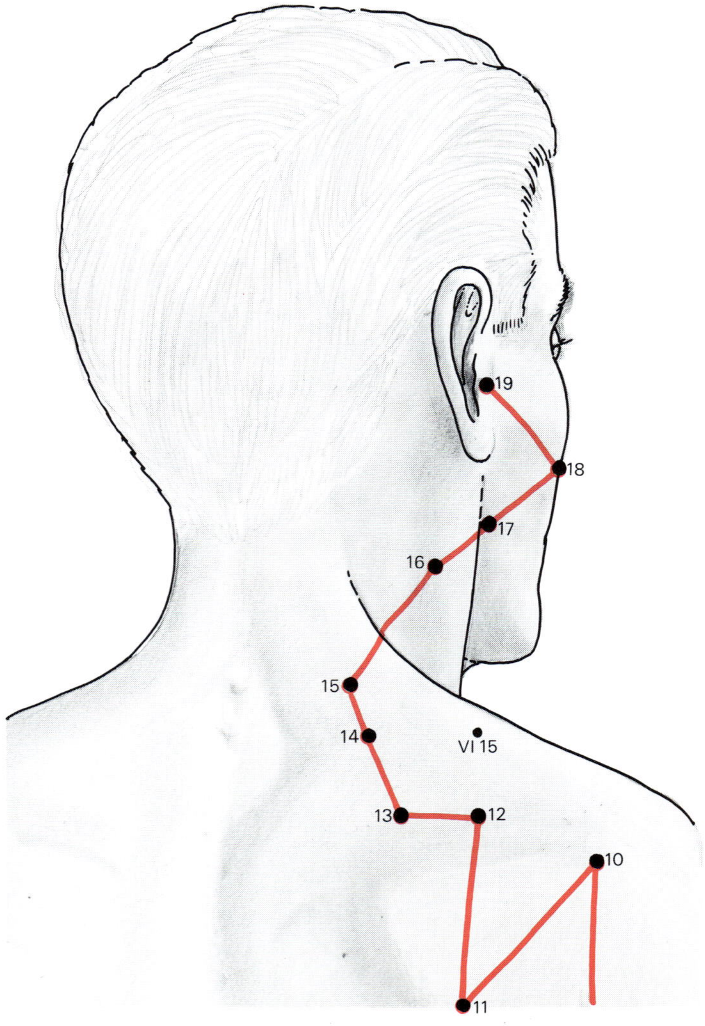
19
18
17
16
15
14
VI 15
13
12
10
11

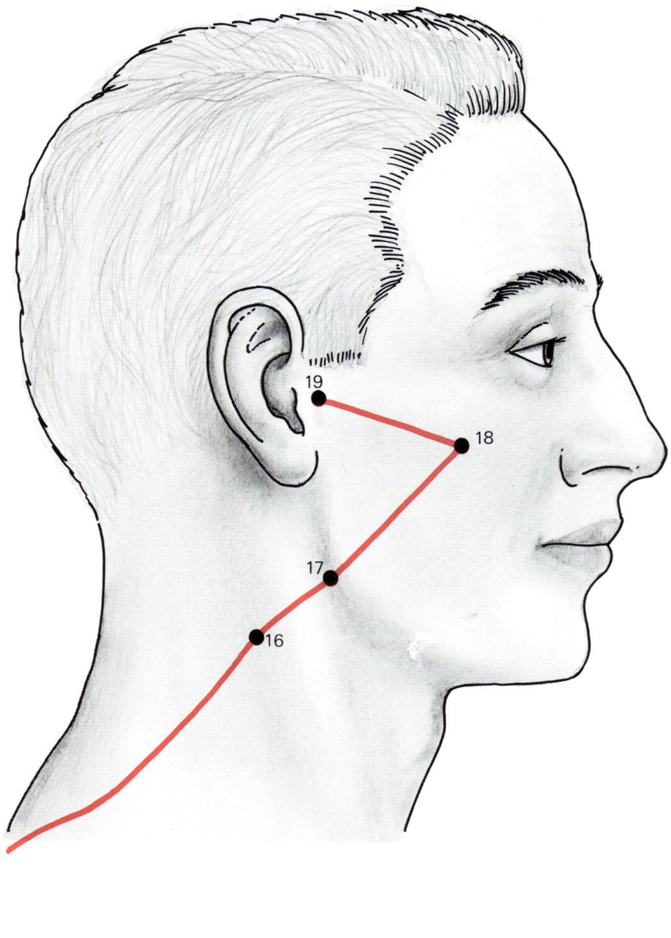
19
18
17
16

II **16** **Heavenly Window** (Tienchuang)

⊥ 3
△ 3

On the lateral surface of the neck, at the posterior border of the sternocleidomastoid, at the level of the laryngeal prominence.

Window of the Sky

II **17** **Heavenly Appearance** (Tienjung)

⊥ 3
△ 3–5

On the posterior edge of the mandible, in the notch of the bone, slightly superior to the angle of the mandible.

Window of the Sky

II **18** **Cheek Bone** (Chuanliao)

⊥ 3
△ X

On the cheek, inferior to the lateral canthus of the eye, in the angle of the zygomatic bone and the mandible.

II **19** **Listening Palace** (Tingkung)

⊥ 2–3 Exit
△ 3–5

Anterior to the tragus of the ear, on the superficial temporal artery, in the depression formed when the mouth is open.

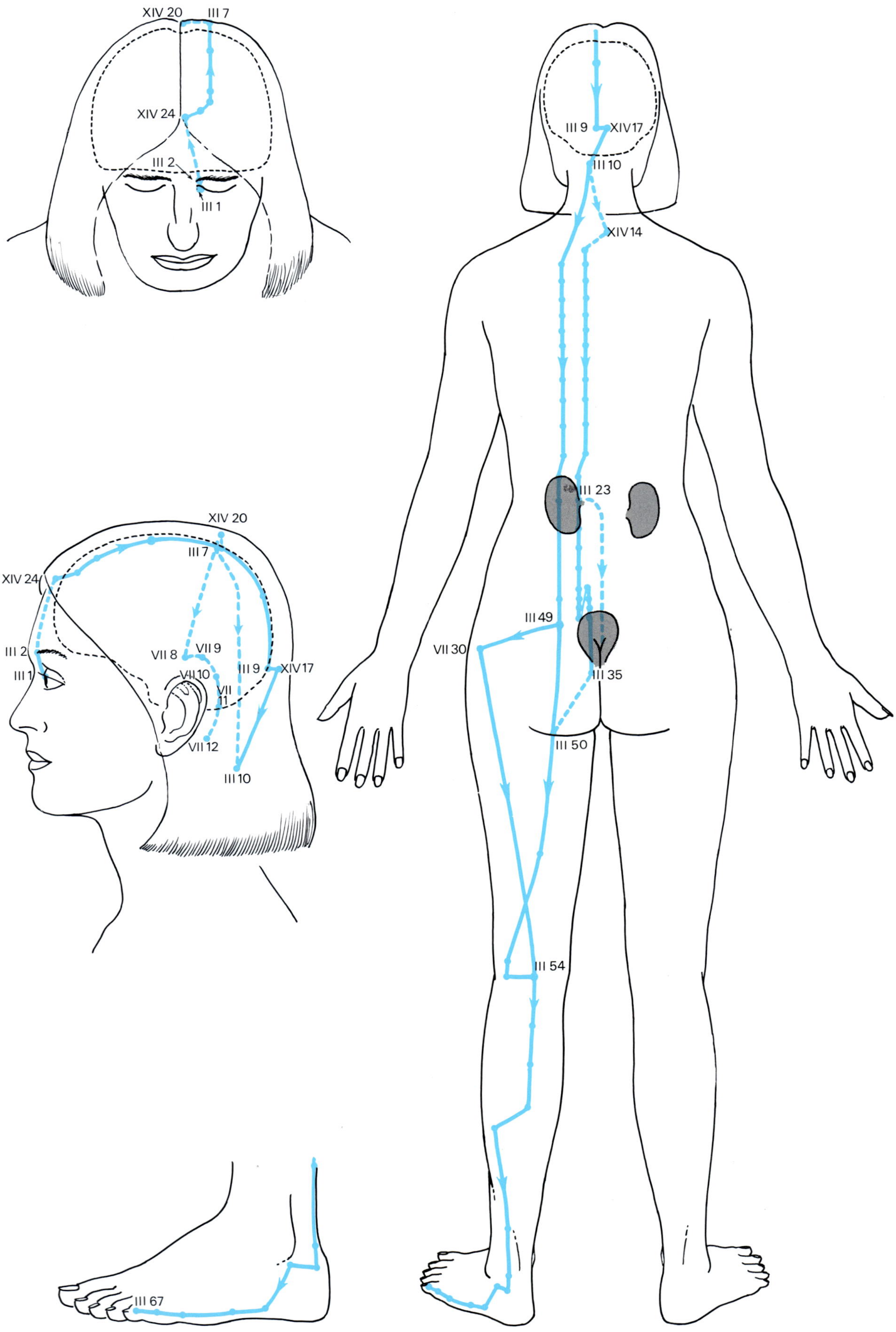
XIV 20
III 7
XIV 24
III 2
III 1
III 9
XIV17
III 10
XIV 14
III 23
XIV 20
III 7
XIV 24
III 2
III 1
VII 8
VII 9
VII 10
VII 11
III 9
XIV17
VII 12
III 10
III 49
VII 30
III 35
III 50
III 54
III 67

The bladder meridian begins as the superficial pathway at the medial canthus of the eye, at the entry point, III 1. It ascends by the medial extremity of the eyebrow, at III 2, to the mid point at XIV 24; then travels over the frontal bone, lateral to the median line, to the vertex of the skull, at III 7.

Here a deep branch emerges which goes to the median line, at XIV 20, and then laterally and inferiorly posterior to the ear, connecting with points VII 8, 9, 10, 11 and 12.

A second branch of the superficial meridian enters the brain from III 7 and emerges to meet the superficial pathway at the nape of the neck. The superficial pathway continues over the head, lateral to the median line. It connects from III 9 to XIV 17, at the median line at the occipital bone, then travels obliquely laterally to the base of the occipital protruberance, at III 10. The meridian now divides and descends the back in two paramedian lines.

The more medial line passes first through XIV 14 at the median line, below the seventh cervical vertebra, then travels down in line with the lateral edge of the transverse processes, 2 ACI from the median line, and then at $2\frac{1}{2}$ ACI from the median line in the lumbar region. Between the second and third lumbar vertebrae, at III 23, a deep branch penetrates to the kidney and thence to the bladder itself. The superficial inner line continues down paramedially, over the sacrum, to the level of the fourth sacral foramen. It then rises medially to enter the first sacral foramen and returns down through each of the foramina to a point just lateral to the coccyx, III 35. The pathway crosses the gluteus maximus to the fold of the buttock, at III 50, and travels obliquely laterally down the posterior surface of the thigh to the lateral side of the popliteal region, and then to meet the other line in the centre of the popliteal fossa.

The more lateral line travels down the back in line with the medial border of the scapula, 4 ACI from the median line, and at $4\frac{1}{2}$ ACI from the median line in the lumbar region to the level of the fourth sacral foramen, III 49. It turns laterally into the gluteus maximus, to VII 30, posterior to the greater trochanter, from where it runs obliquely medially down the posterior surface of the thigh to meet the other line at the centre of the popliteal fossa, at III 54. The single superficial meridian now passes over the posterior surface of the gastrocnemius to the inferior edge of the belly, where it moves laterally and then inferiorly to pass posterior to the lateral malleolus, over the calcaneus and along the edge of the fifth metatarsal bone. It ends at the lateral nail point of the little toe, the exit point, III 67. From here it connects with the kidney meridian.

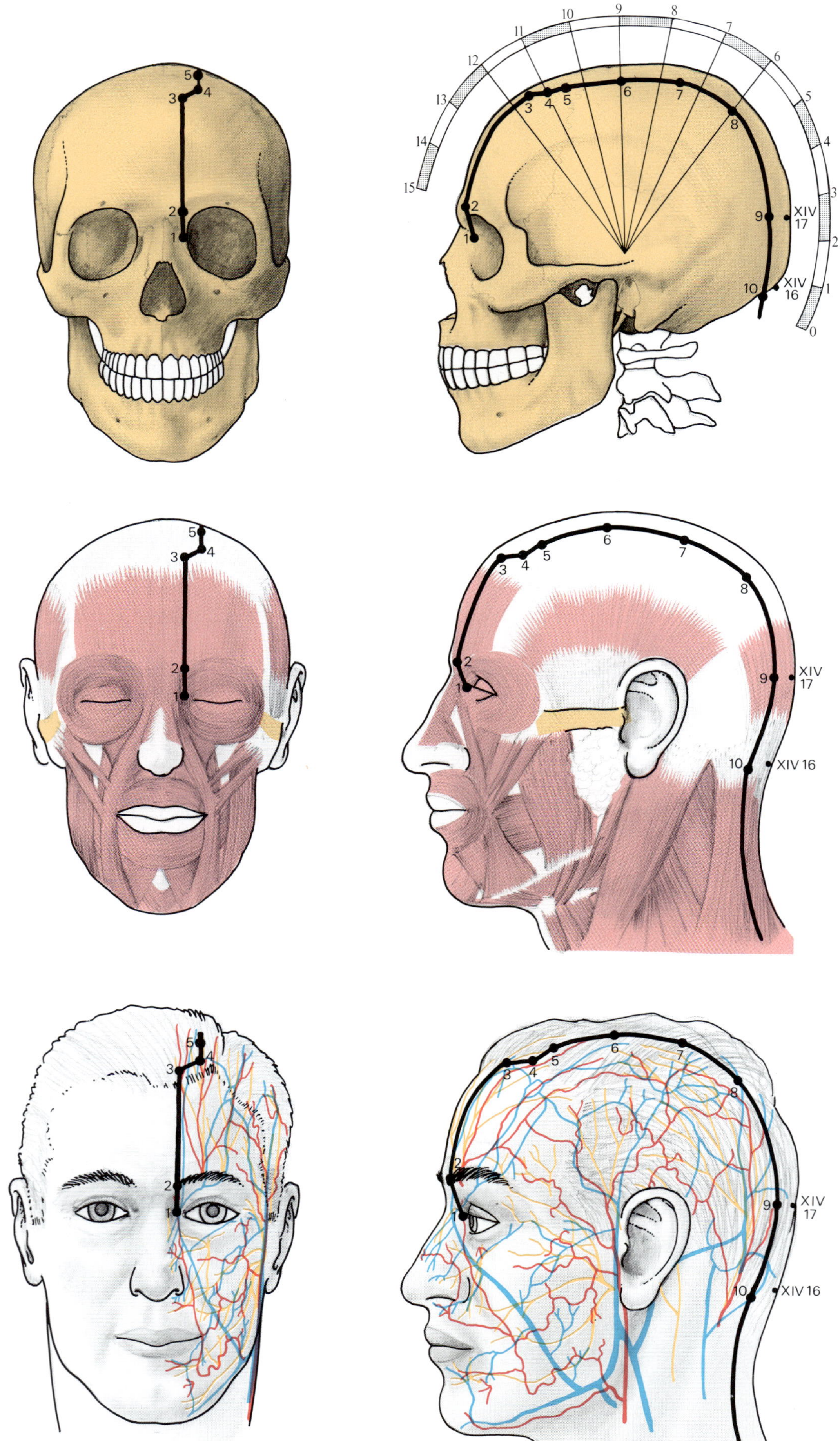
1
2
3
4
5
6
7
8
9
10
XIV 17
XIV 16
0
11
12
13
14
15

III	1	1 fen superior and medial to the medial canthus of the eye, between the two veins.
III	2	In the depression at the medial end of the eyebrow, directly superior to the medial canthus of the eye.
III	3	On the head, $\frac{1}{2}$ ACI superior to the natural hair line, $3\frac{1}{2}$ ACI directly superior to III 2.
III	4	1.3 ACI lateral to the median line of the head, $\frac{1}{2}$ ACI superior to the natural hair line, $\frac{1}{2}$ ACI lateral to III 3.
III	5	1.3 ACI lateral to the median line of the head, $\frac{1}{2}$ ACI superior to III 4.
III	6	1.3 ACI lateral to the median line of the head, $1\frac{1}{2}$ ACI posterior to III 5.
III	7	1.3 ACI lateral to the median line of the head, $1\frac{1}{2}$ ACI posterior to III 6.
III	8	1.3 ACI lateral to the median line of the head, $1\frac{1}{2}$ ACI inferior to III 7.
III	9	1.3 ACI lateral to the median line of the head, on the occipital bone, at the level of XIV 17.
III	10	On the neck, 1.3 ACI lateral to the posterior median line, at the base of the occipital bone, on the trapezius, at the level of XIV 16.

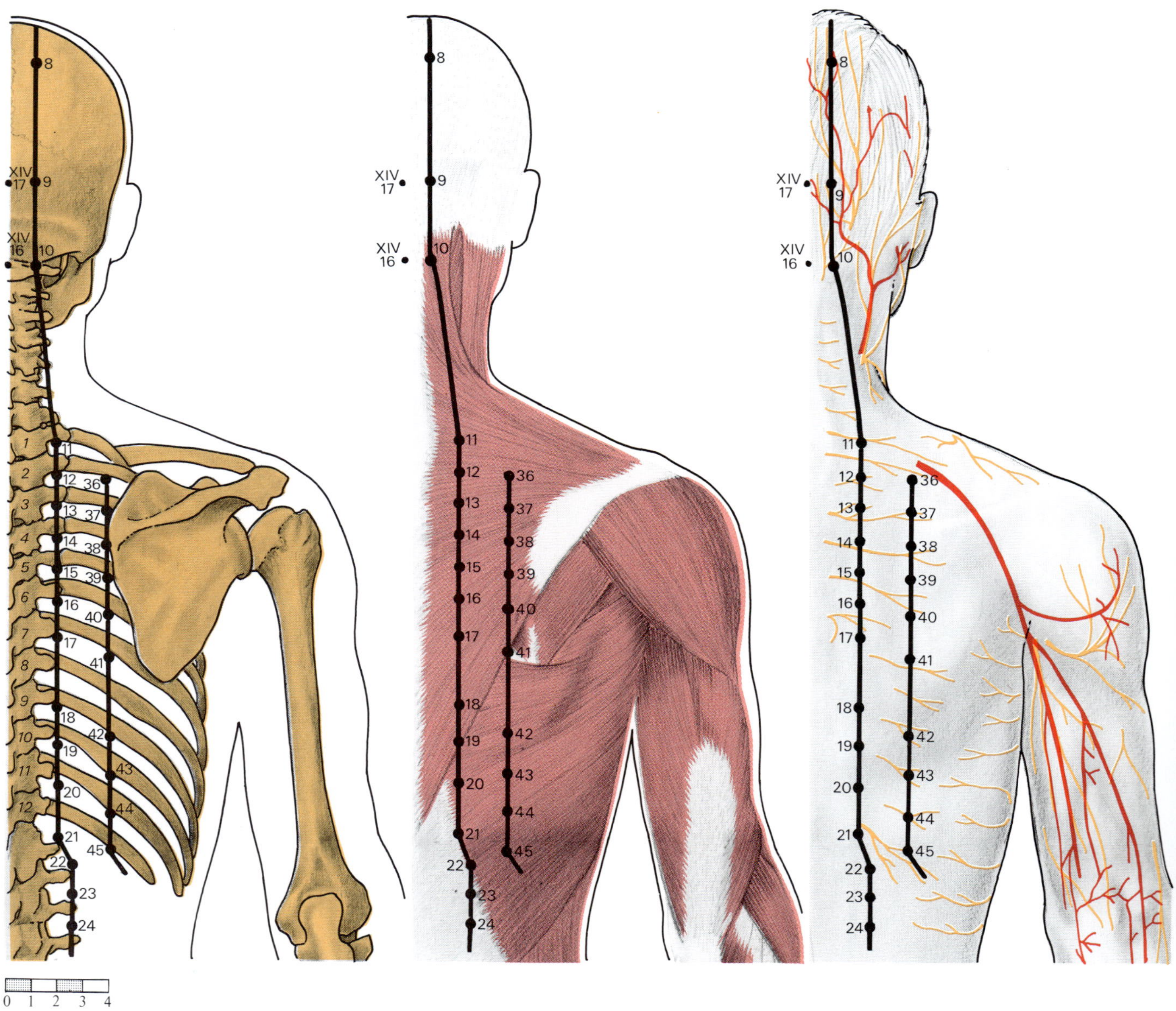

Author's Note: These drawings are done in error. Please note that the inner and outer bladder line points are exactly level with each other and with the intervertebral space. Therefore, for example, XIV 12, III 13 and III 37 are on an exact level line.

III 11 On the back, 2 ACI lateral to the median line, between the transverse processes of the first and second thoracic vertebrae.

III 12 On the back, 2 ACI lateral to the median line, between the transverse processes of the second and third thoracic vertebrae.

III 13 On the back, 2 ACI lateral to the median line, between the transverse processes of the third and fourth thoracic vertebrae.

III 14 On the back, 2 ACI lateral to the median line, between the transverse processes of the fourth and fifth thoracic vertebrae.

III 15 On the back, 2 ACI lateral to the median line, between the transverse processes of the fifth and sixth thoracic vertebrae.

III 16 On the back, 2 ACI lateral to the median line, between the transverse processes of the sixth and seventh thoracic vertebrae.

III 17 On the back, 2 ACI lateral to the median line, between the transverse processes of the seventh and eighth thoracic vertebrae.

III 18 On the back, 2 ACI lateral to the median line, between the transverse processes of the ninth and tenth thoracic vertebrae.

III 19 On the back, 2 ACI lateral to the median line, between the transverse processes of the tenth and eleventh thoracic vertebrae.

III 20 On the back, 2 ACI lateral to the median line, between the transverse processes of the eleventh and twelfth thoracic vertebrae.

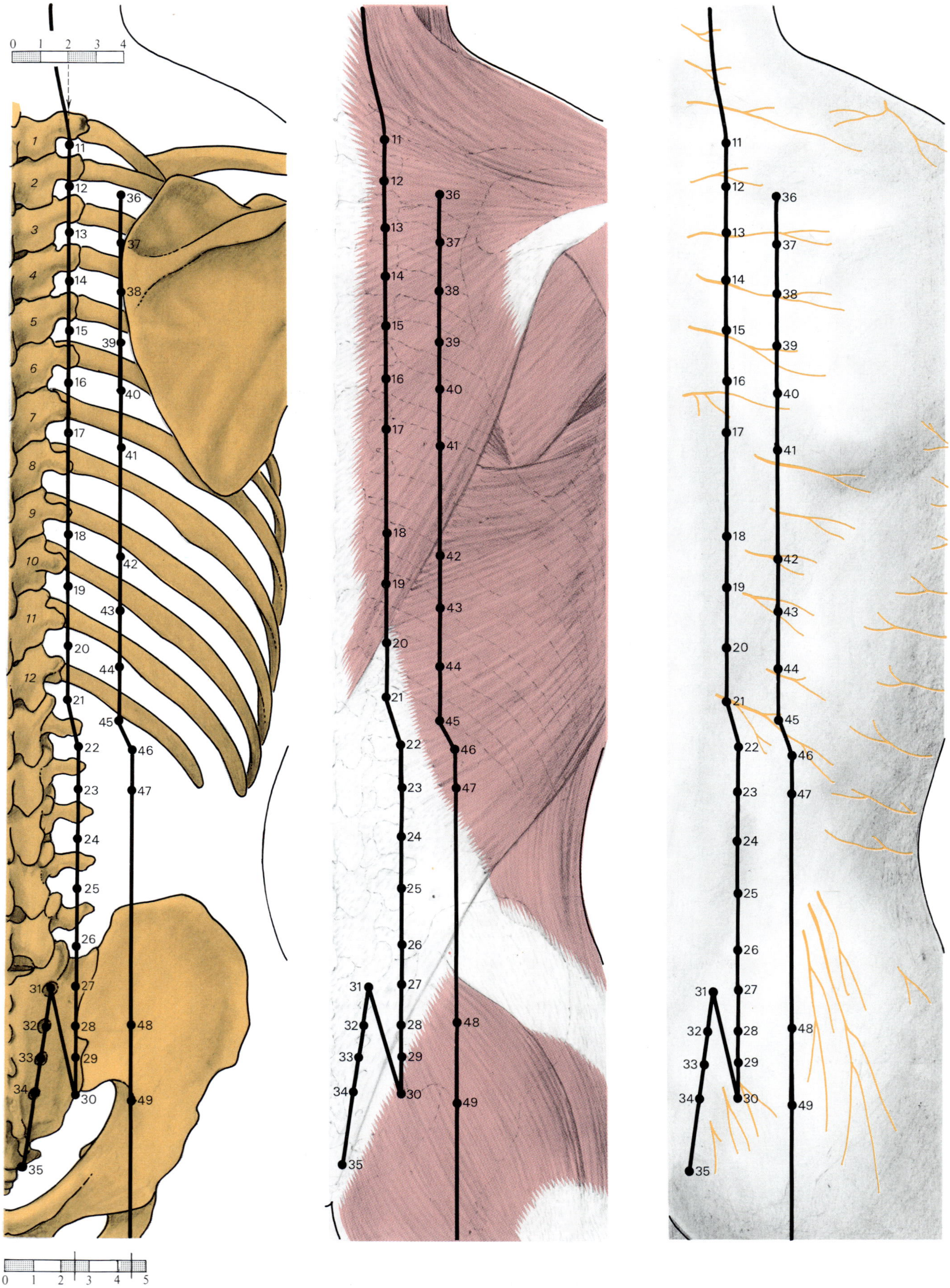
0 1 2 3 4
1 2 3 4 5 6 7 8 9 10 11 12
11 12 13 14 15 16 17 18 19 20 21 22 23 24 25 26 27 28 29 30
31 32 33 34 35
36 37 38 39 40 41 42 43 44 45 46 47 48 49
0 1 2 3 4 5

III	21	On the back, 2 ACI lateral to the median line, between the transverse processes of the twelfth thoracic and the first lumbar vertebrae.
III	22	On the back, $2\frac{1}{2}$ ACI lateral to the median line, at the level of the depression between the first and second lumbar vertebrae.
III	23	On the back, $2\frac{1}{2}$ ACI lateral to the median line, at the level of the depression between the second and third lumbar vertebrae.
III	24	On the back, $2\frac{1}{2}$ ACI lateral to the median line, at the level of the depression between the third and fourth lumbar vertebrae.
III	25	On the back, $2\frac{1}{2}$ ACI lateral to the median line, at the level of the depression between the fourth and fifth lumbar vertebrae.
III	26	On the back, $2\frac{1}{2}$ ACI lateral to the median line, at the level of the depression between the fifth lumbar and the first sacral vertebrae.
III	27	On the sacrum, $2\frac{1}{2}$ ACI lateral to the median line, at the level of the first sacral foramen.
III	28	On the sacrum, $2\frac{1}{2}$ ACI lateral to the median line, at the level of the second sacral foramen.
III	29	On the sacrum, $2\frac{1}{2}$ ACI lateral to the median line, at the level of the third sacral foramen.
III	30	On the sacrum, $2\frac{1}{2}$ ACI lateral to the median line, at the level of the fourth sacral foramen.
III	31	On the sacrum, in the first sacral foramen.
III	32	On the sacrum, in the second sacral foramen.
III	33	On the sacrum, in the third sacral foramen.
III	34	On the sacrum, in the fourth sacral foramen.
III	35	On the buttock, lateral to the sacrococcygeal articulation, $\frac{1}{2}$ ACI lateral to the median line.

Author's Note: These drawings are done in error. Please note that the inner and outer bladder line points are exactly level with each other and with the intervertebral space. Therefore, for example, XIV 12, III 13 and III 37 are on an exact level line.

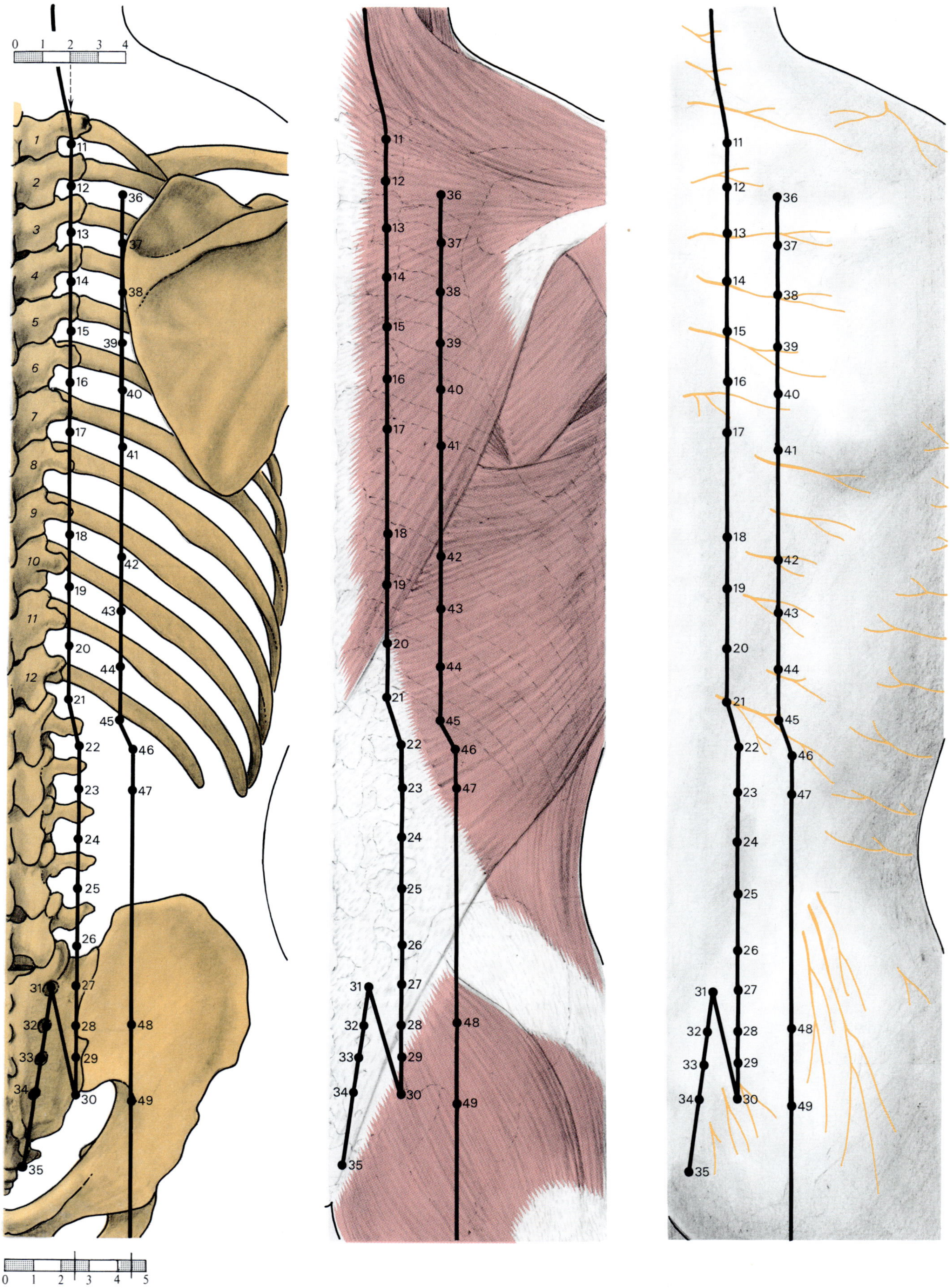
0 1 2 3 4
1
2
3
4
5
6
7
8
9
10
11
12
11
12
13
14
15
16
17
18
19
20
21
22
23
24
25
26
27
28
29
30
31
32
33
34
35
36
37
38
39
40
41
42
43
44
45
46
47
48
49
0 1 2 3 4 5

III 36 On the back, 4 ACI lateral to the median line, between the second and third ribs, about on a level with the tip of the spinous process of the second thoracic vertebra.

III 37 On the back, 4 ACI lateral to the median line, between the third and fourth ribs, about on a level with the tip of the spinous process of the third thoracic vertebra.

III 38 On the back, 4 ACI lateral to the median line, between the fourth and fifth ribs, about on a level with the tip of the spinous process of the fourth thoracic vertebra.

III 39 On the back, 4 ACI lateral to the median line, between the fifth and sixth ribs, about on a level with the tip of the spinous process of the fifth thoracic vertebra.

III 40 On the back, 4 ACI lateral to the median line, between the sixth and seventh ribs, about on a level with the tip of the spinous process of the sixth thoracic vertebra.

III 41 On the back, 4 ACI lateral to the median line, between the seventh and eighth ribs, about on a level with the tip of the spinous process of the seventh thoracic vertebra.

III 42 On the back, 4 ACI lateral to the median line, between the ninth and tenth ribs, about on a level with the tip of the spinous process of the ninth thoracic vertebra.

III 43 On the back, 4 ACI lateral to the median line, between the tenth and eleventh ribs, about on a level with the tip of the spinous process of the tenth thoracic vertebra.

III 44 On the back, 4 ACI lateral to the median line, between the eleventh and twelfth ribs, about on a level with the tip of the spinous process of the eleventh thoracic vertebra.

III 45 On the back, 4 ACI lateral to the median line, about on a level with the tip of the spinous process of the twelfth thoracic vertebra.

III 46 On the back, $4\frac{1}{2}$ ACI lateral to the median line, at the level of the depression between the first and second lumbar vertebrae.

III 47 On the back, $4\frac{1}{2}$ ACI lateral to the median line, at the level of the depression between the second and third lumbar vertebrae.

III 48 Lateral to the sacro-iliac joint, $4\frac{1}{2}$ ACI lateral to the median line, at the level of the second sacral foramen.

III 49 On the buttock, $4\frac{1}{2}$ ACI lateral to the median line, slightly inferior to the level of the fourth sacral foramen.

Author's Note: These drawings are done in error. Please note that the inner and outer bladder line points are exactly level with each other and with the intervertebral space. Therefore, for example, XIV 12, III 13 and III 37 are on an exact level line.

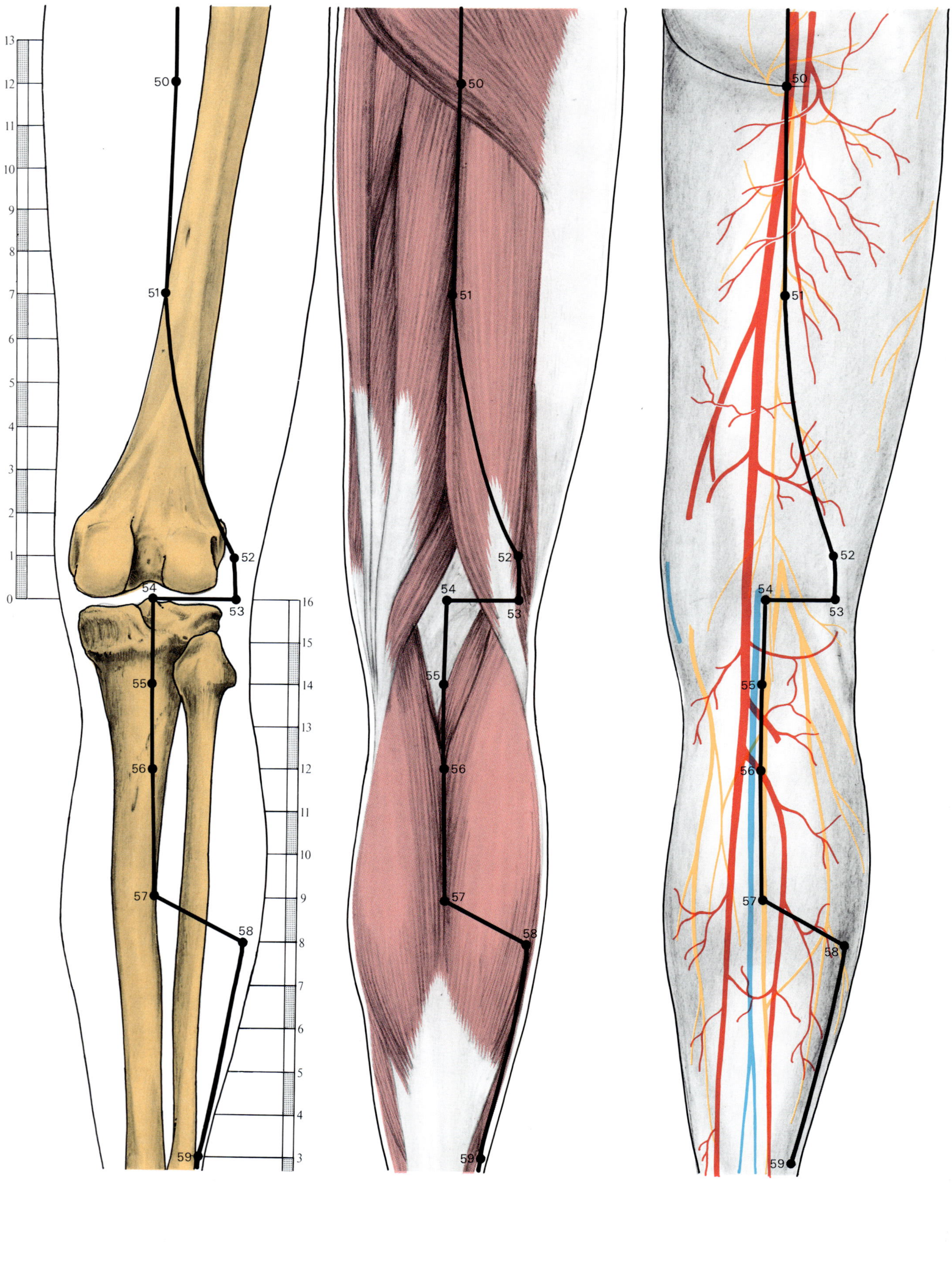
50
51
52
53
54
55
56
57
58
59
0 1 2 3 4 5 6 7 8 9 10 11 12 13
3 4 5 6 7 8 9 10 11 12 13 14 15 16

III 50 At the mid-point of the gluteal fold, directly distal to III 49, between the biceps femoris and the semitendinosus.

III 51 On the posterior surface of the thigh, at the mid-point between the biceps femoris and the semitendinosus, 7 ACI proximal to the knee crease.

III 52 On the posterior surface of the thigh, 1 ACI proximal to the lateral end of the knee crease, medial to the tendon of the biceps femoris.

III 53 On the lateral side of the knee crease, medial to the tendon of the biceps femoris.

III 54 On the posterior surface of the leg, in the centre of the knee crease.

III 55 On the posterior surface of the leg, 14 ACI proximal to the level of the prominence of the lateral malleolus, between the lateral and medial heads of the gastrocnemius.

III 56 On the posterior surface of the leg, 12 ACI proximal to the level of the prominence of the lateral malleolus, between the lateral and medial heads of the gastrocnemius.

III 57 On the posterior surface of the leg, 9 ACI proximal to the level of the prominence of the lateral malleolus, between the lateral and medial heads of the gastrocnemius.

III 58 On the posterolateral surface of the leg, 8 ACI proximal to the level of the prominence of the lateral malleolus, between the gastrocnemius and the soleus.

III 59 On the posterolateral surface of the leg, 3 ACI proximal to the level of the prominence of the lateral malleolus, posterior to the peroneus longus, directly proximal to III 60.

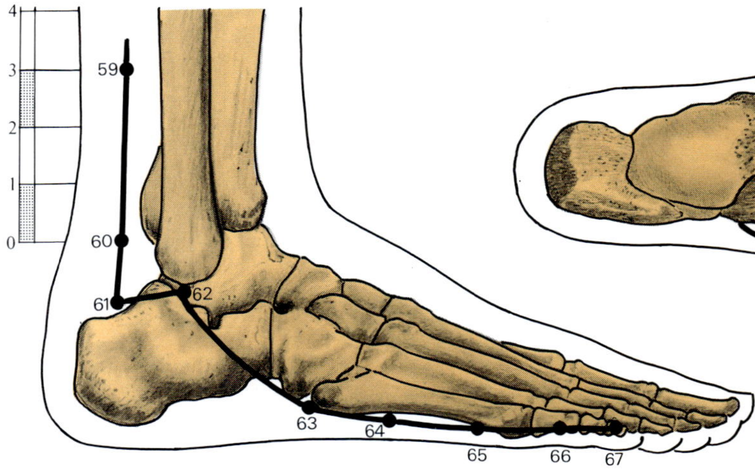
0
1
2
3
4
59
60
61
62
63
64
65
66
67

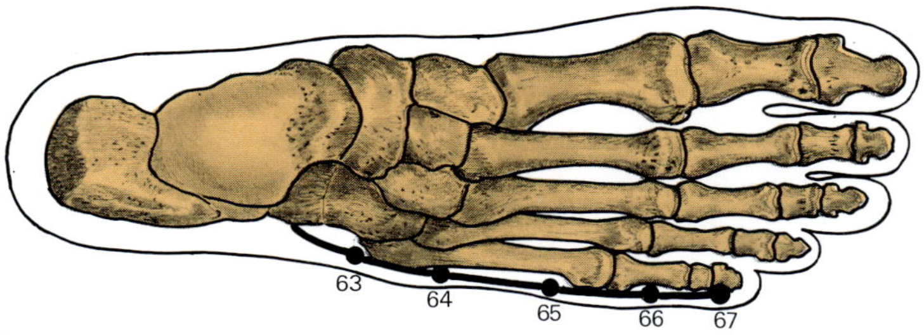
63
64
65
66
67

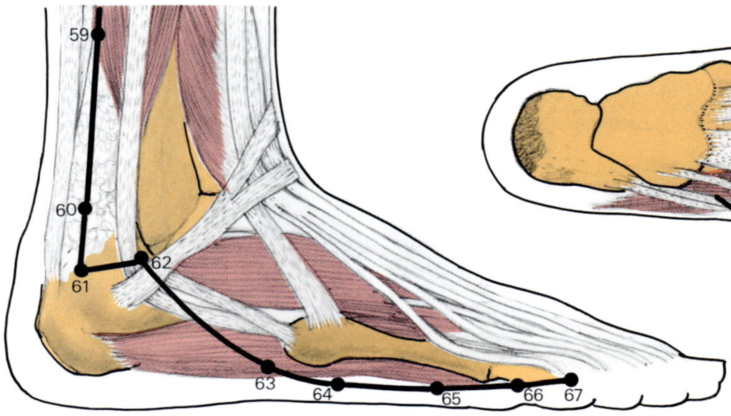
59
60
61
62
63
64
65
66
67

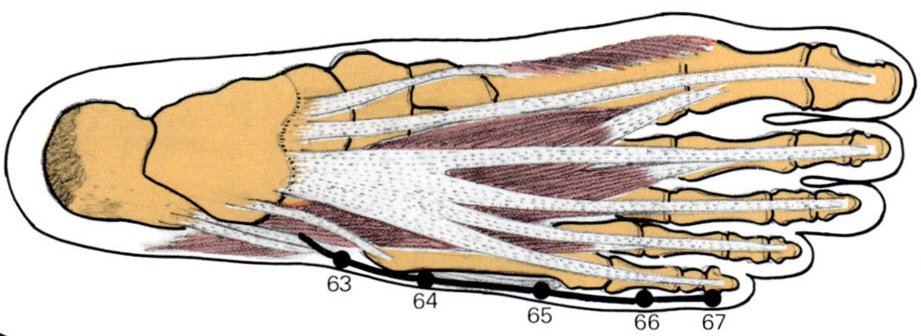
63
64
65
66
67

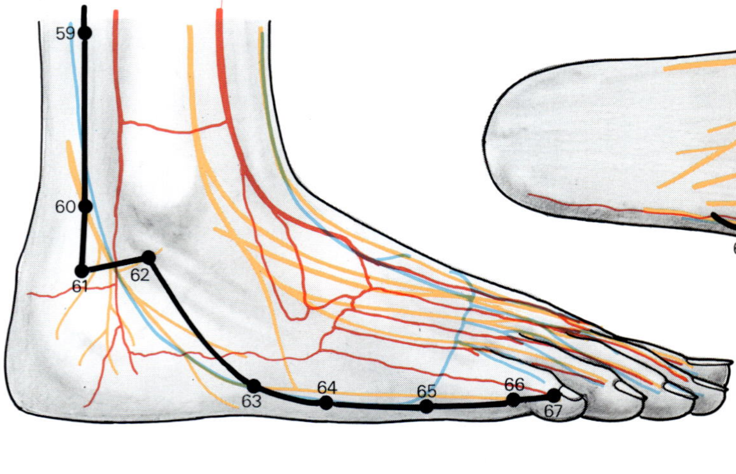
59
60
61
62
63
64
65
66
67

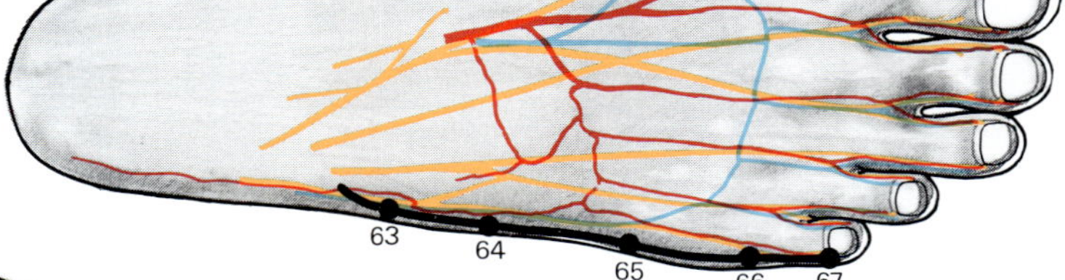
63
64
65
66
67

III	59	On the posterolateral surface of the leg, 3 ACI proximal to the level of the prominence of the lateral malleolus, posterior to the peroneus longus, directly proximal to III 60.
III	60	Mid-way between the prominence of the lateral malleolus and the Achilles tendon, on the peroneal artery.
III	61	On the superior edge of the lateral surface of the calcaneus, directly inferior to III 60.
III	62	One half ACI distal to the tip of the lateral malleolus, between the tendons of the peroneus longus and the peroneus brevis.
III	63	On the lateral border of the foot, just proximal to the tubercle of the fifth metatarsal bone.
III	64	On the lateral border of the foot, distal to the tubercle of the fifth metatarsal bone.
III	65	On the lateral border of the foot, just proximal to the head of the fifth metatarsal bone.
III	66	On the lateral border of the foot, just distal to the base of the proximal phalanx of the little toe.
III	67	Lateral nail point of the little toe.

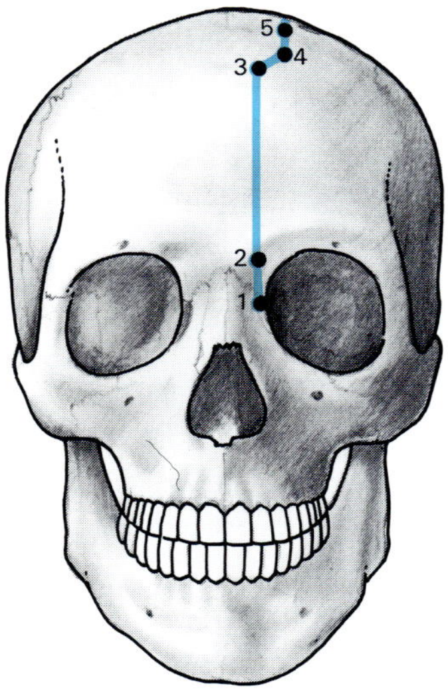
5
4
3
2
1

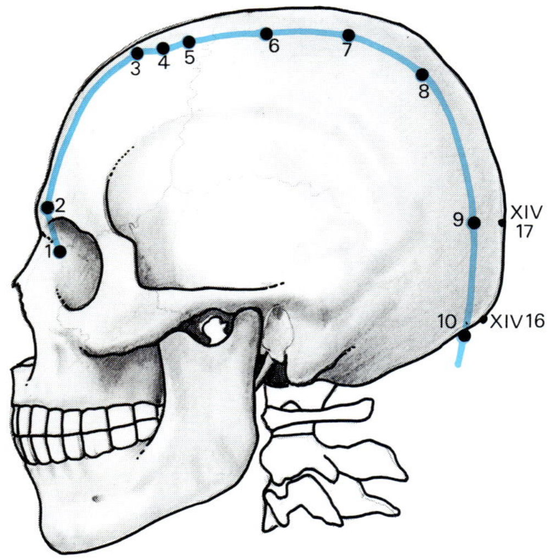
3
4
5
6
7
8
2
1
9
XIV
17
10
XIV 16

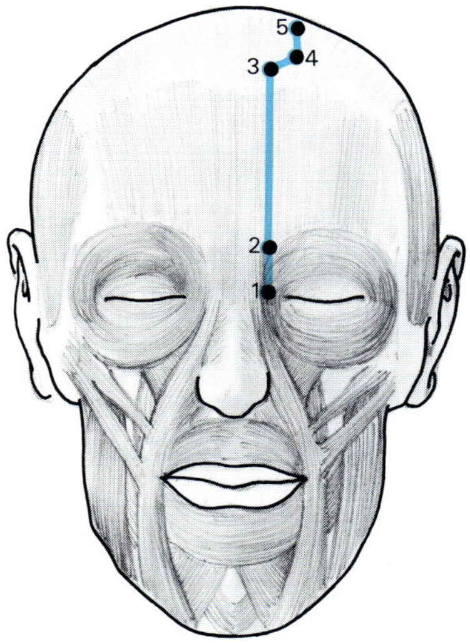
5
4
3
2
1

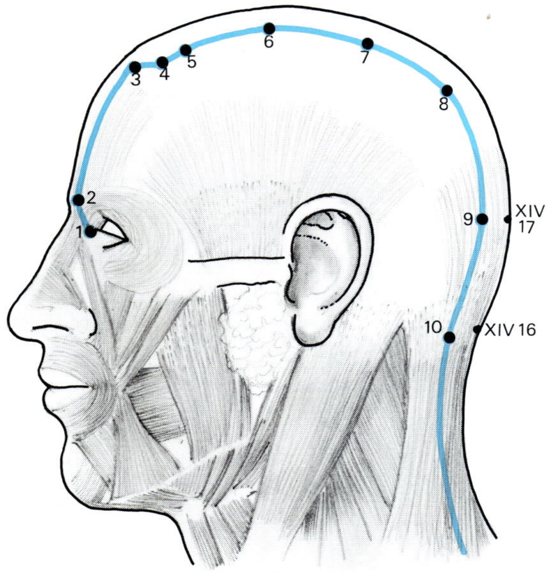
3
4
5
6
7
8
2
1
9
XIV
17
10
XIV 16

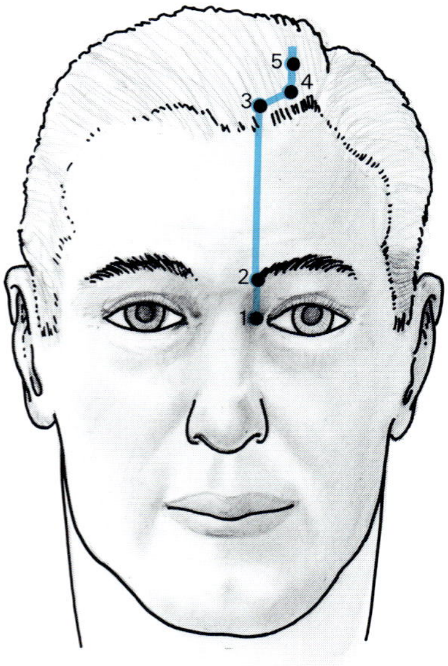
5
4
3
2
1

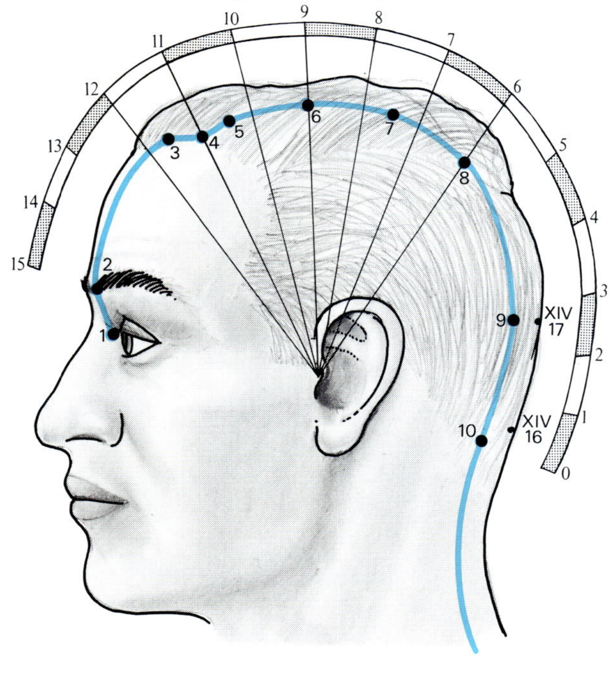
15
14
13
12
11
10
9
8
7
6
5
4
3
2
1
0
3
4
5
6
7
8
2
1
9
XIV
17
10
XIV
16

III **1** **Eyes Bright** (Chingming)

⊥ 3 Entry
△ X

1 fen superior and medial to the medial canthus of the eye, between the two veins.

Supplementary reinforcement for the Eight Extra Meridians
Point of Yang Qiao Mo
Point of Yin Qiao Mo

III **2** **Collect Bamboo** (Tsanchu)

⊥ 2
△ X

In the depression at the medial end of the eyebrow, directly superior to the medial canthus of the eye.

III **3** **Eyebrows Rushing** (Meichung)

⊥ 3
△ 3

On the head, $\frac{1}{2}$ ACI superior to the natural hair line, $3\frac{1}{2}$ ACI directly superior to III 2.

III **4** **Crooked Servant** (Chucha)

⊥ 2
△ 3–5

1.3 ACI lateral to the median line of the head, $\frac{1}{2}$ ACI superior to the natural hair line, $\frac{1}{2}$ ACI lateral to III 3.

III **5** **Five Places** (Wuchu)

⊥ 3
△ X

1.3 ACI lateral to the median line of the head, $\frac{1}{2}$ ACI superior to III 4.

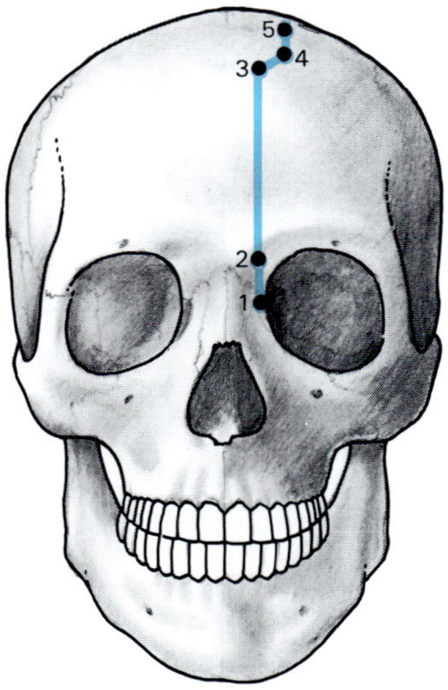
5
4
3
2
1

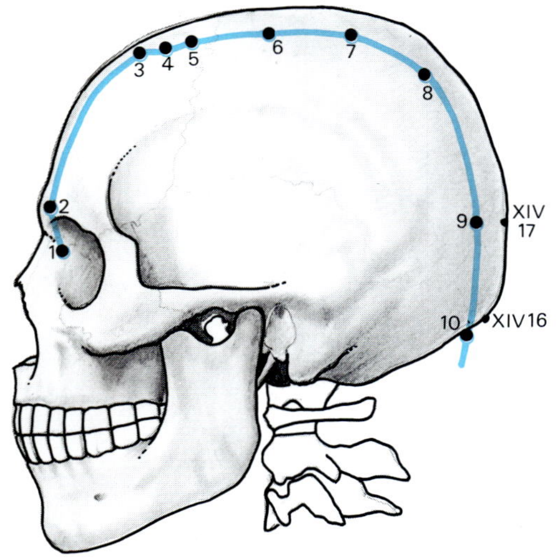
3 4 5 6 7
8
2
1
9
XIV 17
10
XIV 16

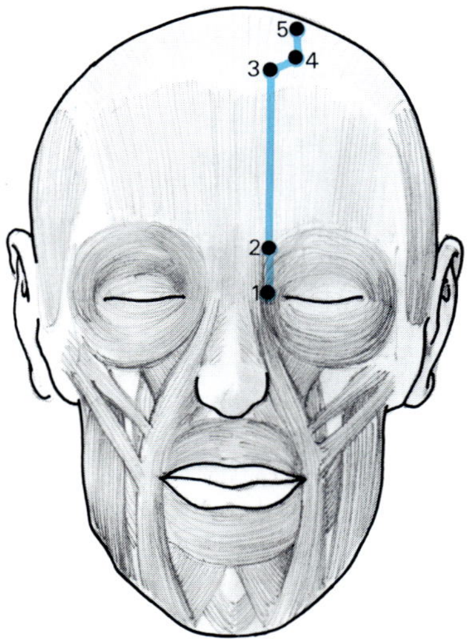
5
4
3
2
1

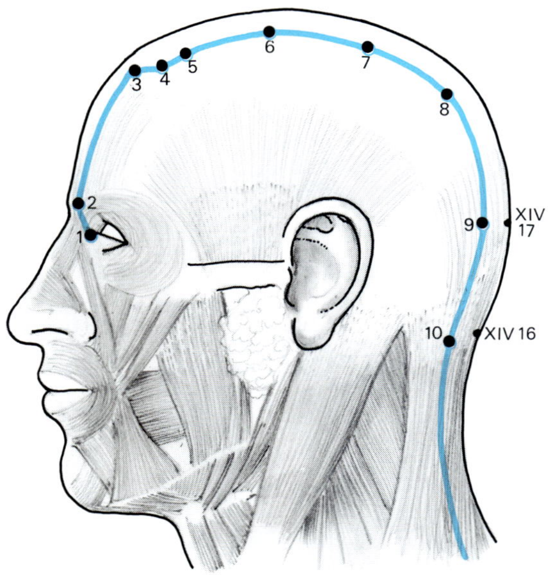
3 4 5 6 7
8
2
1
9
XIV 17
10
XIV 16

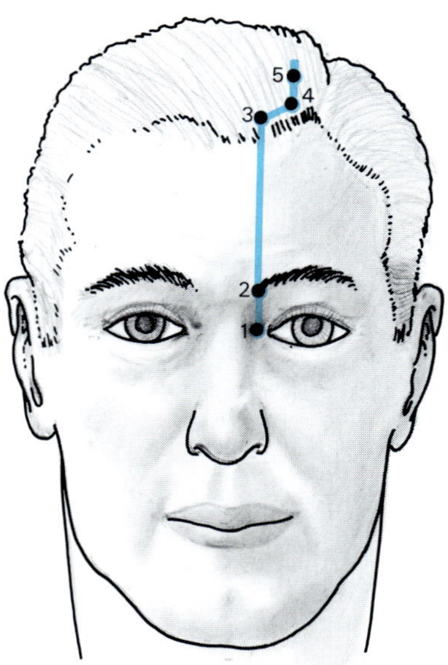
5
4
3
2
1

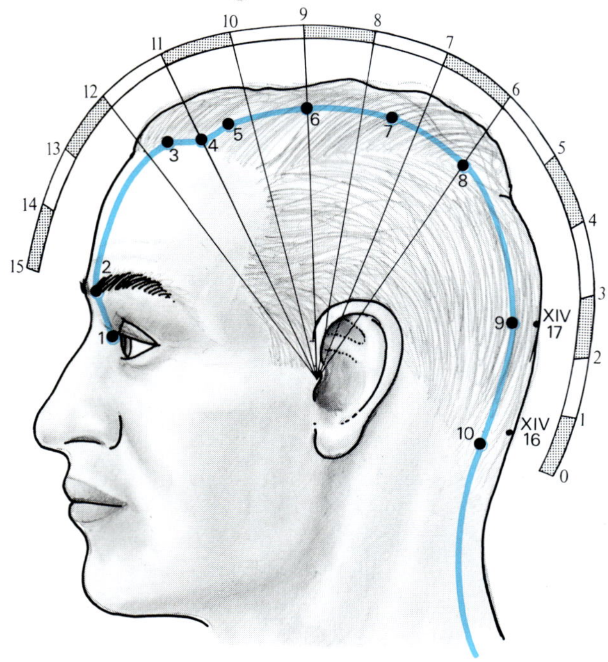
15 14 13 12 11 10 9 8 7 6 5 4 3 2 1 0
3 4 5 6 7
8
2
1
9
XIV 17
10
XIV 16

III **6** **Receive Light** (Chengkuang)

⊥ 3
△ X

1.3 ACI lateral to the median line of the head, $1\frac{1}{2}$ ACI posterior to III 5.

III **7** **Penetrate Heaven** (Tungtien)

⊥ 3
△ 3–5

1.3 ACI lateral to the median line of the head, $1\frac{1}{2}$ ACI posterior to III 6.

III **8** **Lou End** (Lochueh)

⊥ 3
△ 3–5

1.3 ACI lateral to the median line of the head, $1\frac{1}{2}$ ACI inferior to III 7.

III **9** **Jade Pillow** (Yuchen)

⊥ 3
△ 3–5

1.3 ACI lateral to the median line of the head, on the occipital bone, at the level of XIV 17.

III **10** **Heavenly Pillar** (Tienchu)

⊥ 3–5
△ 3

On the neck, 1.3 ACI lateral to the posterior median line, at the base of the occipital bone, on the trapezius, at the level of XIV 16.

Sea of Energy
Window of the Sky

III Bladder Meridian

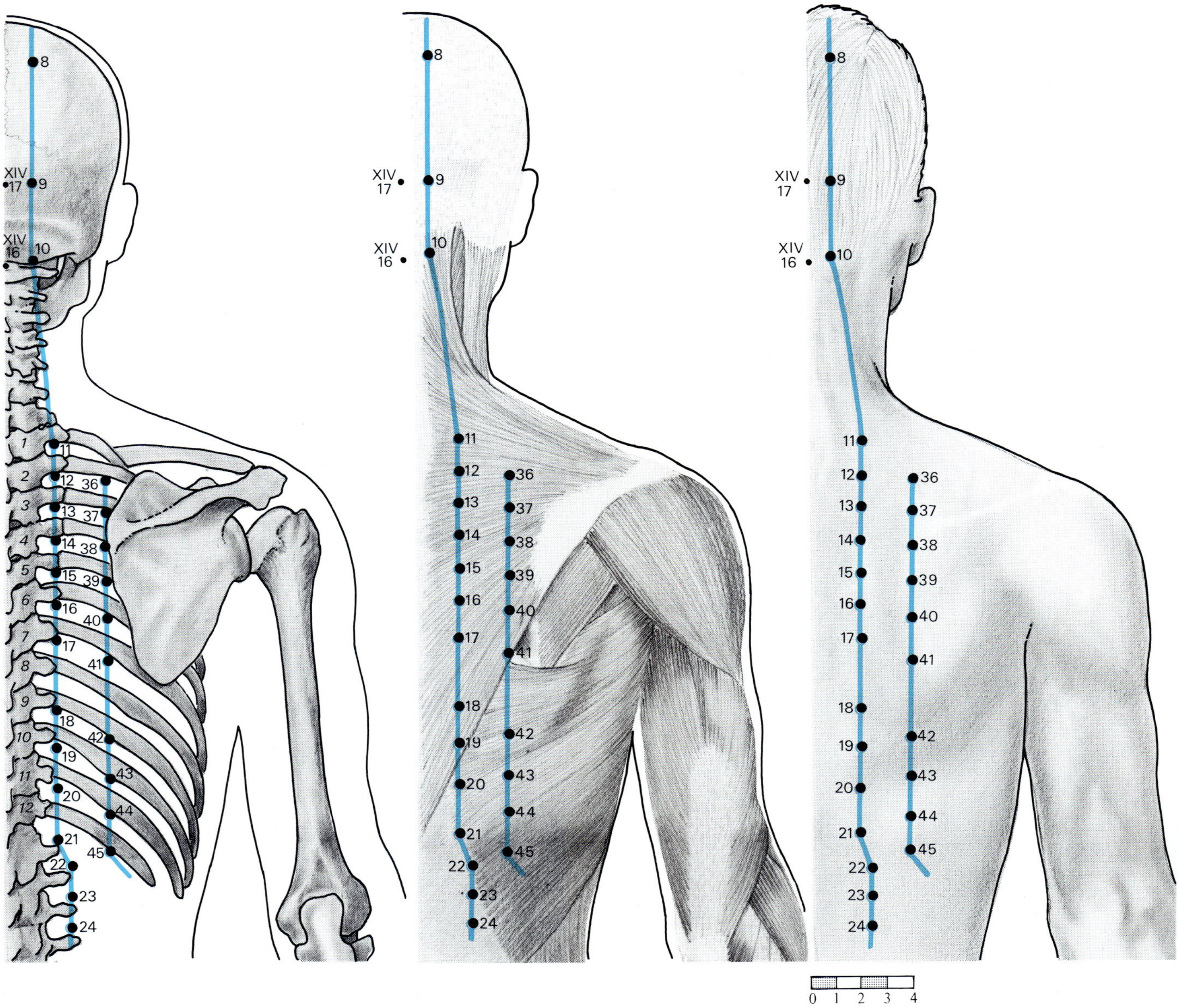

Author's Note: These drawings are done in error. Please note that the inner and outer bladder line points are exactly level with each other and with the intervertebral space. Therefore, for example, XIV 12, III 13 and III 37 are on an exact level line.

III **11** **Great Shuttle** (Tachu)

⊥ 3
△ 7

On the back, 2 ACI lateral to the median line, between the transverse processes of the first and second thoracic vertebrae.

Sea of Blood
A point of the pattern to release the 7 Dragons on the 7 External Demons
Assembling Point for bones
First Aid: fractures, sprains

III **12** **Wind Gate** (Fengmen)

⊥ 5
△ 5–10

On the back, 2 ACI lateral to the median line, between the transverse processes of the second and third thoracic vertebrae.

III **13** **Lungs Correspondence** (Feishu)

⊥ 3–5 Associated Effect Point of IX
△ 7–20

On the back, 2 ACI lateral to the median line, between the transverse processes of the third and fourth thoracic vertebrae.

III **14** **Circulation-Sex Correspondence** (Chuehyinshu)

⊥ 3 Associated Effect Point of V
△ 7

On the back, 2 ACI lateral to the median line, between the transverse processes of the fourth and fifth thoracic vertebrae.

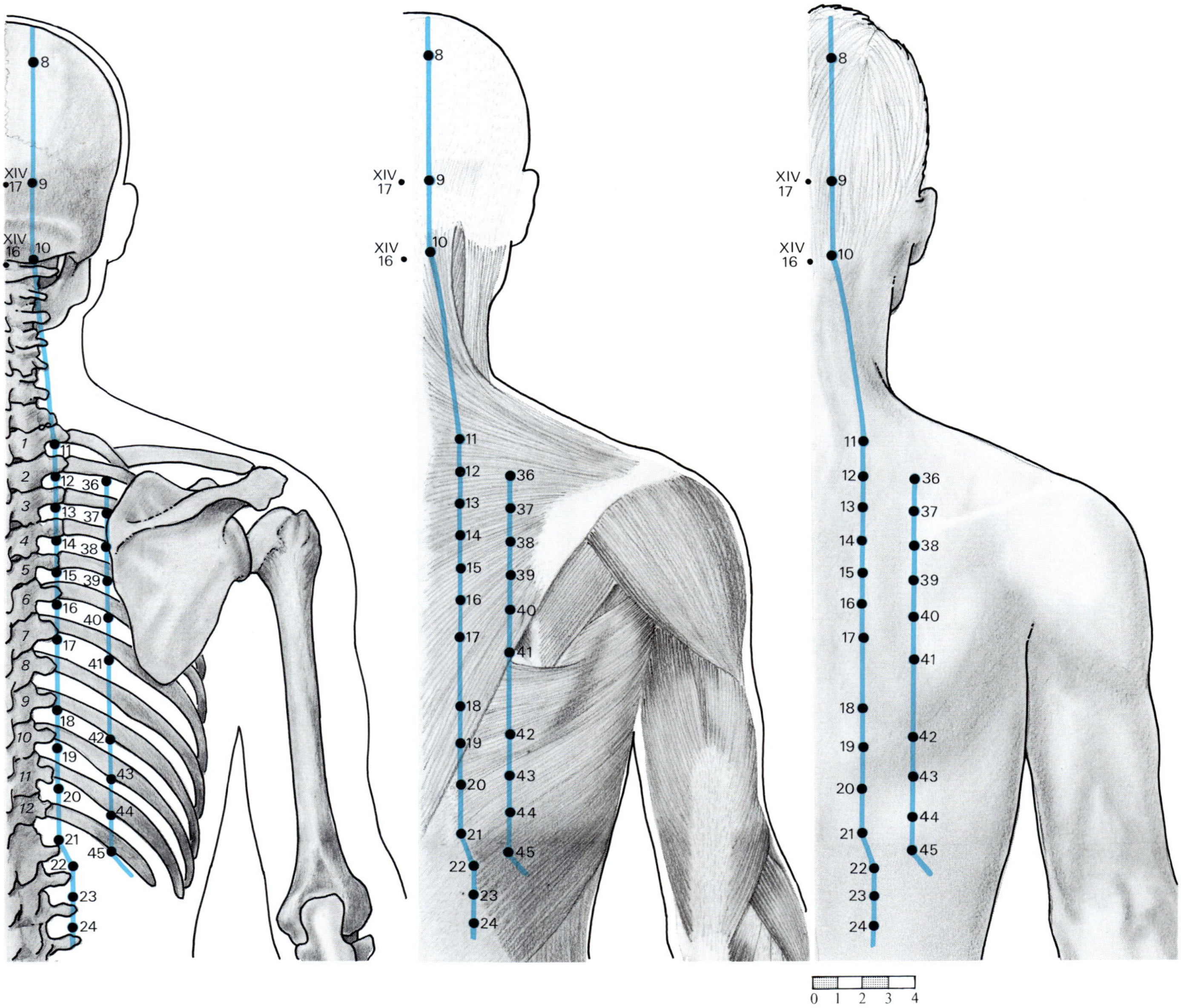

Author's Note: These drawings are done in error. Please note that the inner and outer bladder line points are exactly level with each other and with the intervertebral space. Therefore, for example, XIV 12, III 13 and III 37 are on an exact level line.

III **15** **Heart Correspondence** (Hsinshu)

⊥ 3 Associated Effect Point of I
△ 3

On the back, 2 ACI lateral to the median line, between the transverse processes of the fifth and sixth thoracic vertebrae.

First Aid: heart failure

III **16** **Governor Correspondence** (Tushu)

⊥ X Associated Effect Point of XIV
△ 3

On the back, 2 ACI lateral to the median line, between the transverse processes of the sixth and seventh thoracic vertebrae.

III **17** **Diaphragm Correspondence** (Keshu)

⊥ 4 Associated Effect Point of Diaphragm
△ 7–20

On the back, 2 ACI lateral to the median line, between the transverse processes of the seventh and eighth thoracic vertebrae.

Assembling Point for blood
First Aid: hiccups, numbness

III **18** **Liver Correspondence** (Kanshu)

⊥ 3 Associated Effect Point of VIII
△ 7–20

On the back, 2 ACI lateral to the median line, between the transverse processes of the ninth and tenth thoracic vertebrae.

III **19** **Gall Bladder Correspondence** (Tanshu)

⊥ 3–5 Associated Effect Point of VII
△ 3–15

On the back, 2 ACI lateral to the median line, between the transverse processes of the tenth and eleventh thoracic vertebrae.

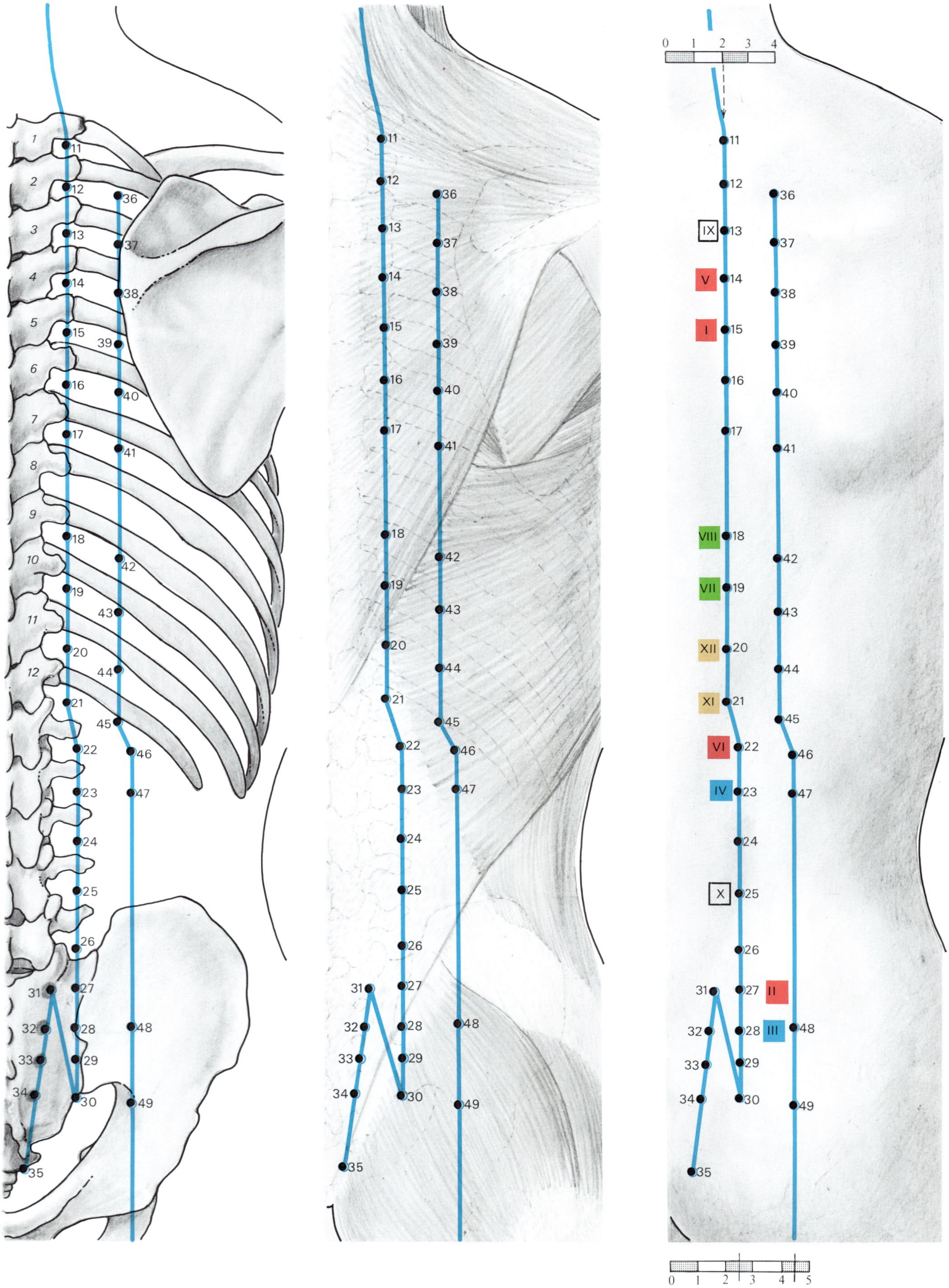

Author's Note: These drawings are done in error. Please note that the inner and outer bladder line points are exactly level with each other and with the intervertebral space. Therefore, for example, XIV 12, III 13 and III 37 are on an exact level line.

III **20** **Spleen Correspondence** (Pishu)

⊥ 3–5 Associated Effect Point of XII
△ 7–20

On the back, 2 ACI lateral to the median line, between the transverse processes of the eleventh and twelfth thoracic vertebrae.

III **21** **Stomach Correspondence** (Weishu)

⊥ 3–5 Associated Effect Point of XI
△ 7–21

On the back, 2 ACI lateral to the median line, between the transverse processes of the twelfth thoracic and the first lumbar vertebrae.

III **22** **Three Heater Correspondence** (Sanchiaoshu)

⊥ 3–5 Associated Effect Point of VI
△ 7–20

On the back, $2\frac{1}{2}$ ACI lateral to the median line, at the level of the depression between the first and second lumbar vertebrae.

III **23** **Kidneys Correspondence** (Shenshu)

⊥ 5–8 Associated Effect Point of IV
△ 3–15

On the back, $2\frac{1}{2}$ ACI lateral to the median line, at the level of the depression between the second and third lumbar vertebrae.

Point of Dai Mo
A point of the pattern to release the 7 Dragons on the 7 External Demons

III **24** **Sea of Ch'i Correspondence** (Chihaishu)

⊥ 5
△ 3–5

On the back, $2\frac{1}{2}$ ACI lateral to the median line, at the level of the depression between the third and fourth lumbar vertebrae.

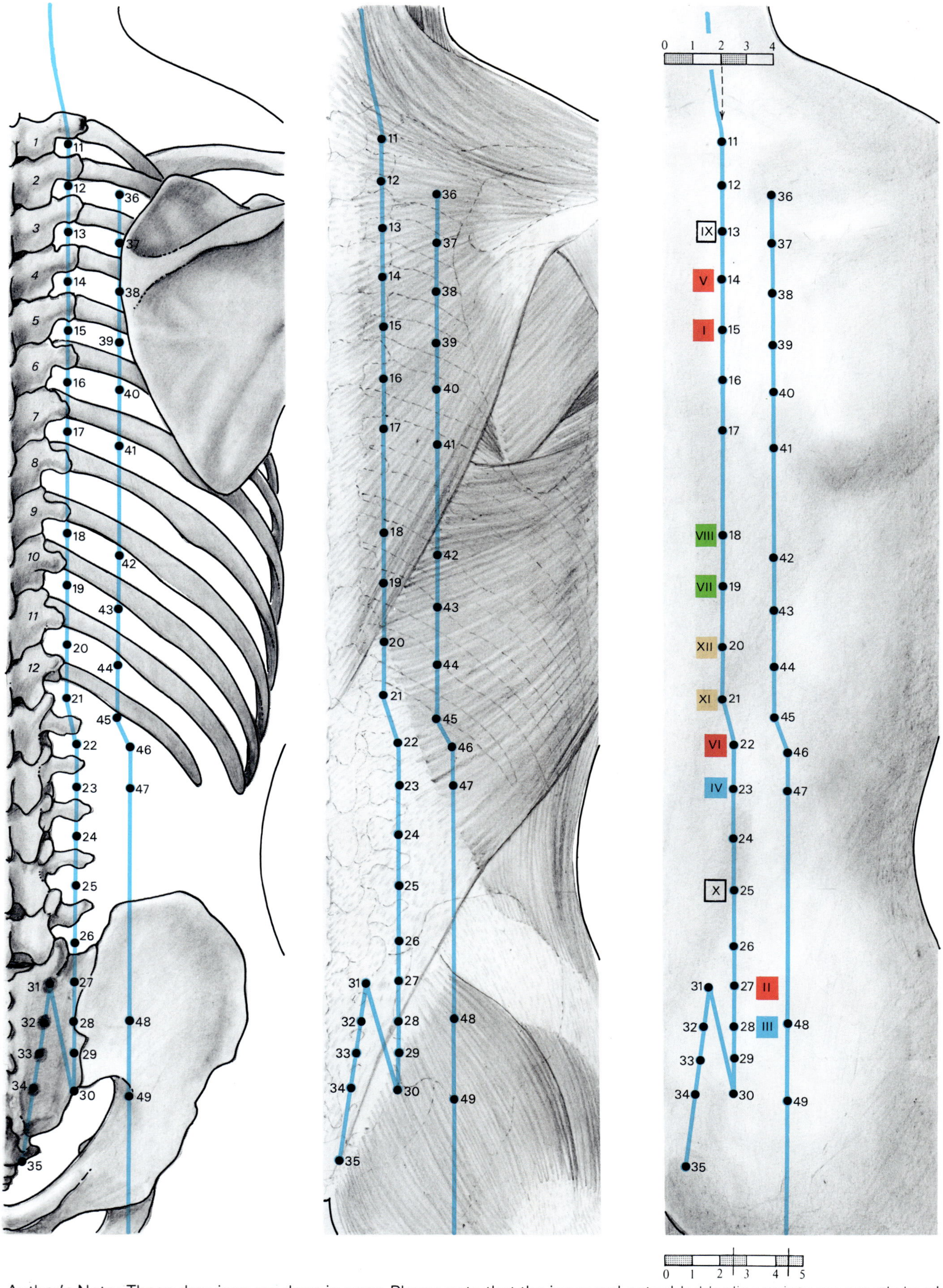

Author's Note: These drawings are done in error. Please note that the inner and outer bladder line points are exactly level with each other and with the intervertebral space. Therefore, for example, XIV 12, III 13 and III 37 are on an exact level line.

III **25** **Large Intestine Correspondence** (Tachangshu)

⊥ 8–10 Associated Effect Point of X
△ 7–20

On the back, $2\frac{1}{2}$ ACI lateral to the median line, at the level of the depression between the fourth and fifth lumbar vertebrae.

First Aid: haemorrhage

III **26** **First Gate Correspondence** (Kuanyuanshu)

⊥ 10
△ 3

On the back, $2\frac{1}{2}$ ACI lateral to the median line, at the level of the depression between the fifth lumbar and the first sacral vertebrae.

III **27** **Small Intestine Correspondence** (Hsiaochangshu)

⊥ 8–10 Associated Effect Point of II
△ 7–20

On the sacrum, $2\frac{1}{2}$ ACI lateral to the median line, at the level of the first sacral foramen.

III **28** **Bladder Correspondence** (Pangkuangshu)

⊥ 8–10 Associated Effect Point of III
△ 7–15

On the sacrum, $2\frac{1}{2}$ ACI lateral to the median line, at the level of the second sacral foramen.

III **29** **Middle Of The Backbone Correspondence** (Chunglushu)

⊥ 5
△ 7–15

On the sacrum, $2\frac{1}{2}$ ACI lateral to the median line, at the level of the third sacral foramen.

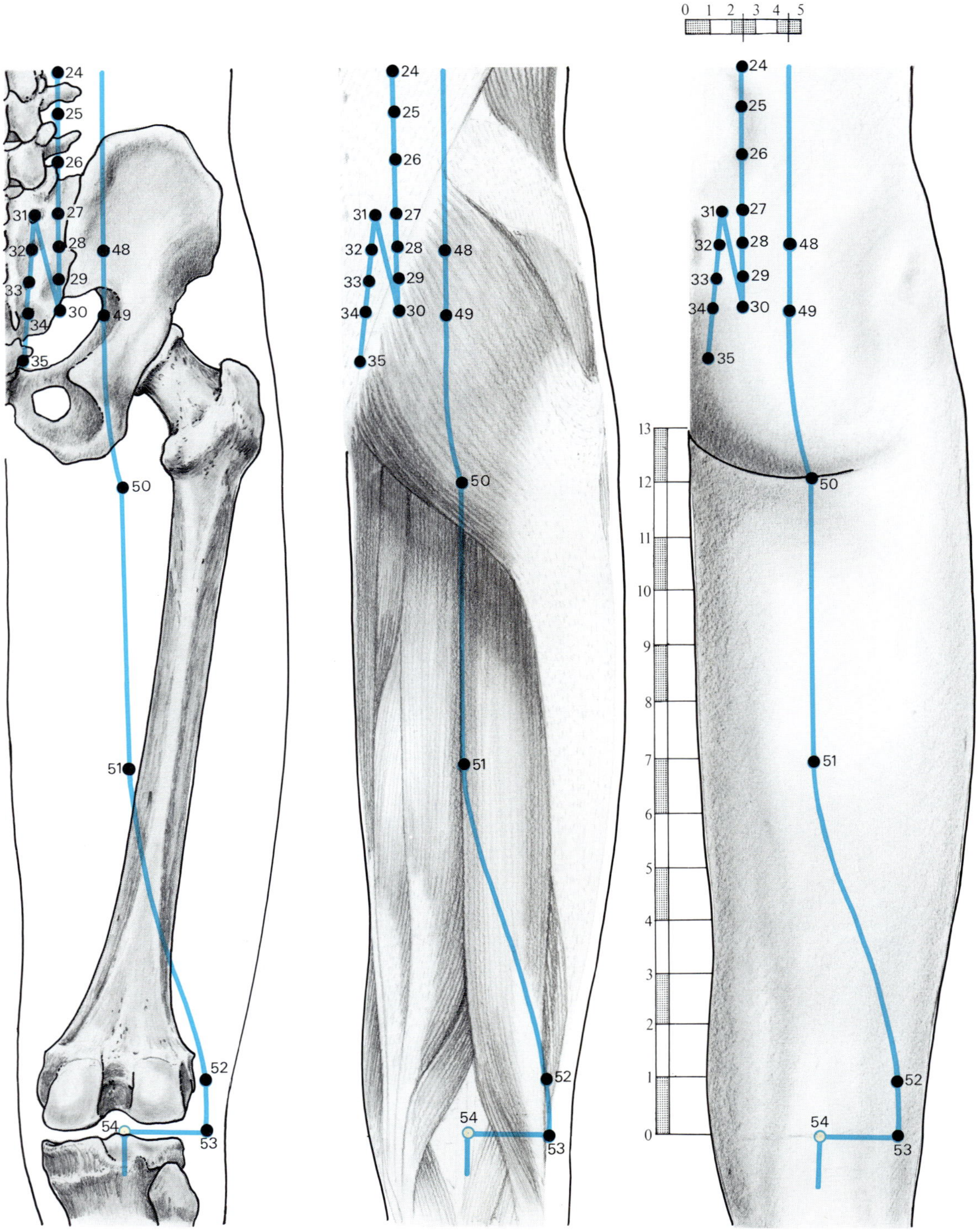
24
25
26
27
28
29
30
31
32
33
34
35
48
49
50
51
52
53
54
24
25
26
27
28
29
30
31
32
33
34
35
48
49
50
51
52
53
54
0 1 2 3 4 5
24
25
26
27
28
29
30
31
32
33
34
35
48
49
50
51
52
53
54
13
12
11
10
9
8
7
6
5
4
3
2
1
0

III **30** **White Ring Correspondence** (Paihuanshu)

⊥ 3–5
△ X

On the sacrum, $2\frac{1}{2}$ ACI lateral to the median line, at the level of the fourth sacral foramen.

III **31** **Upper Sacral Bone** (Shangliao)

⊥ 8–10
△ 7–15

On the sacrum; in the first sacral foramen.

First Aid: apoplexy, concussion, insensibility, snake bites

III **32** **Second Sacral Bone** (Tzuliao)

⊥ 8–10
△ 7–15

On the sacrum, in the second sacral foramen.

III **33** **Middle Sacral Bone** (Chungliao)

⊥ 8–10
△ 7–15

On the sacrum, in the third sacral foramen.

III **34** **Lower Sacral Bone** (Hsialiao)

⊥ 6–8
△ 7–15

On the sacrum, in the fourth sacral foramen.

III **35** **Meeting Of Yang** (Huiyang)

⊥ 4
△ 5

On the buttock, lateral to the sacrococcygeal articulation, $\frac{1}{2}$ ACI lateral to the median line.

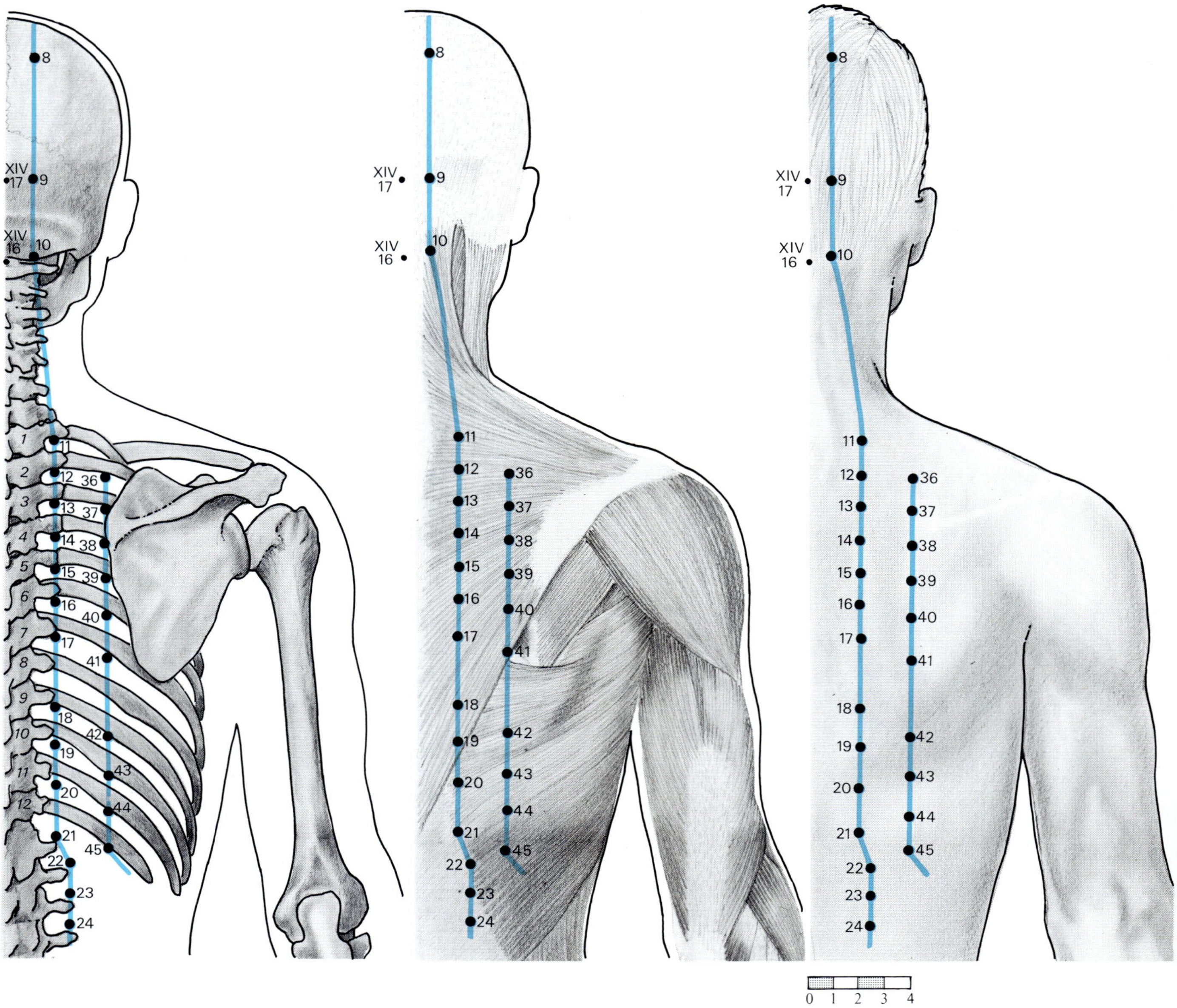

Author's Note: These drawings are done in error. Please note that the inner and outer bladder line points are exactly level with each other and with the intervertebral space. Therefore, for example, XIV 12, III 13 and III 37 are on an exact level line.

III **36** **Near Division** (Fufen)

⊥ 4
△ 7

On the back, 4 ACI lateral to the median line, between the second and third ribs, about on a level with the tip of the spinous process of the second thoracic vertebra.

III **37** **Soul Door** (Pohu)

⊥ 5
△ 7–15

On the back, 4 ACI lateral to the median line, between the third and fourth ribs, about on a level with the tip of the spinous process of the third thoracic vertebra.

III **38** **Rich For The Vitals Correspondence** (Kaohuang)

⊥ 3
△ 7–50

On the back, 4 ACI lateral to the median line, between the fourth and fifth ribs, about on a level with the tip of the spinous process of the fourth thoracic vertebra.

III **39** **Spirit Hall** (Shentang)

⊥ 3
△ 5

On the back, 4 ACI lateral to the median line, between the fifth and sixth ribs, about on a level with the tip of the spinous process of the fifth thoracic vertebra.

III **40** **Wail Of Grief** (Yihsi)

⊥ 3
△ 5–15

On the back, 4 ACI lateral to the median line, between the sixth and seventh ribs, about on a level with the tip of the spinous process of the sixth thoracic vertebra.

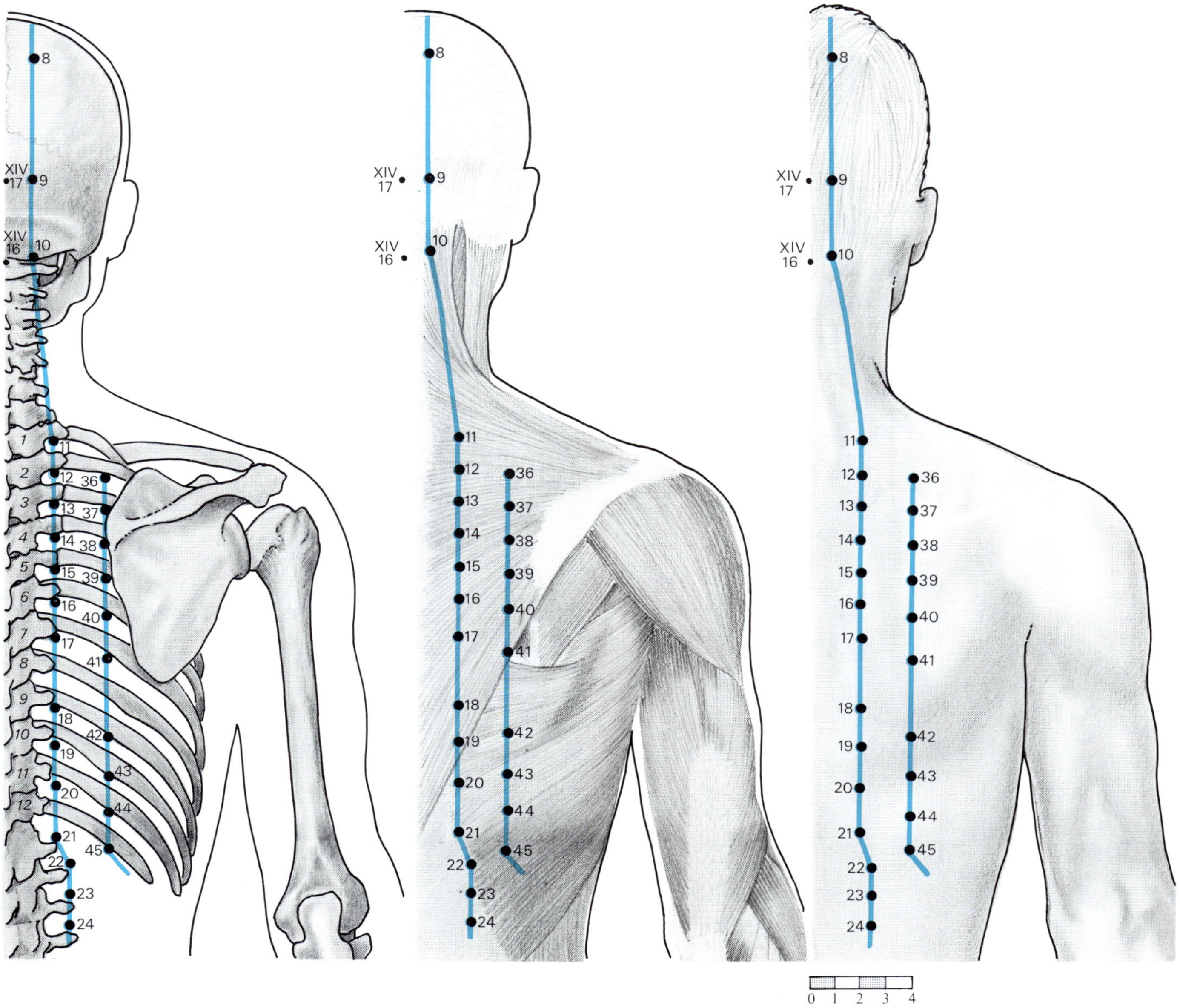

Author's Note: These drawings are done in error. Please note that the inner and outer bladder line points are exactly level with each other and with the intervertebral space. Therefore, for example, XIV 12, III 13 and III 37 are on an exact level line.

III **41** **Diaphragm Border** (Kekuan)

⊥ 5
△ 3–15

On the back, 4 ACI lateral to the median line, between the seventh and eighth ribs, about on a level with the tip of the spinous process of the seventh thoracic vertebra.

III **42** **Spiritual Soul Gate** (Hunmen)

⊥ 5
△ 3–15

On the back, 4 ACI lateral to the median line, between the ninth and tenth ribs, about on a level with the tip of the spinous process of the ninth thoracic vertebra.

III **43** **Yang Net** (Yangkang)

⊥ 5–7
△ 5

On the back, 4 ACI lateral to the median line, between the tenth and eleventh ribs, about on a level with the tip of the spinous process of the tenth thoracic vertebra.

III **44** **Thought Dwelling** (Yishe)

⊥ 5–7
△ 5–15

On the back, 4 ACI lateral to the median line, between the eleventh and twelfth ribs, about on a level with the tip of the spinous process of the eleventh thoracic vertebra.

III **45** **Stomach Granary** (Weitsang)

⊥ 5–7
△ 5–10

On the back, 4 ACI lateral to the median line, about on a level with the tip of the spinous process of the twelfth thoracic vertebra.

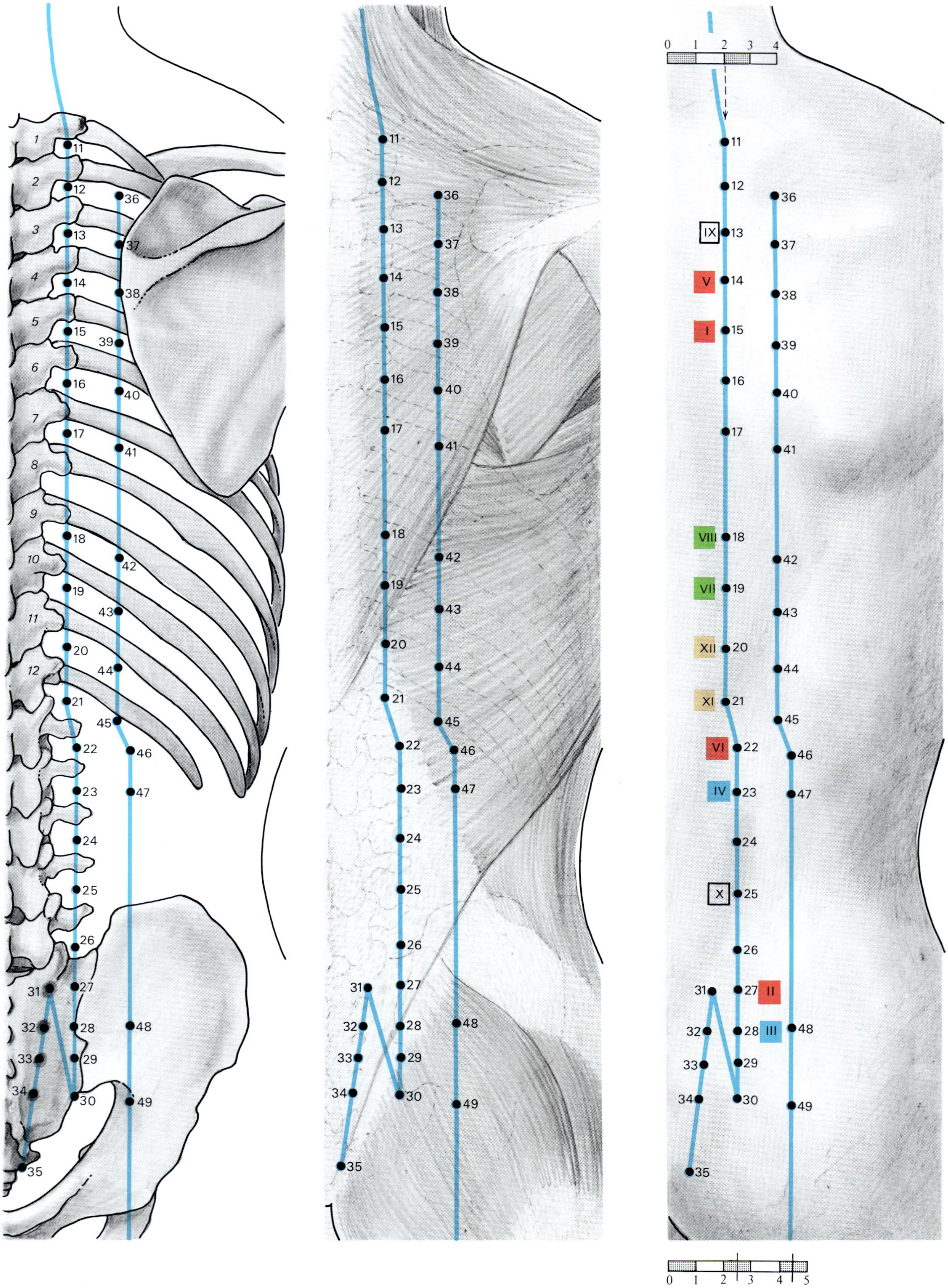

Author's Note: These drawings are done in error. Please note that the inner and outer bladder line points are exactly level with each other and with the intervertebral space. Therefore, for example, XIV 12, III 13 and III 37 are on an exact level line.

III **46** **Diaphragm Gate Of Vitality** (Huangmen)

⊥ 5–7
△ 7–15

On the back, $4\frac{1}{2}$ ACI lateral to the median line, at the level of the depression between the first and second lumbar vertebrae.

III **47** **Ambition Room** (Chihshih)

⊥ 7–9
△ 7–15

On the back, $4\frac{1}{2}$ ACI lateral to the median line, at the level of the depression between the second and third lumbar vertebrae.

III **48** **Womb And Heart Diaphragm** (Paohuang)

⊥ 5–7
△ 5–10

Lateral to the sacro-iliac joint, $4\frac{1}{2}$ ACI lateral to the median line, at the level of the second sacral foramen.

III **49** **Orderly Frontier** (Chihpien)

⊥ 5
△ 7

On the buttock, $4\frac{1}{2}$ ACI lateral to the median line, slightly inferior to the level of the fourth sacral foramen.

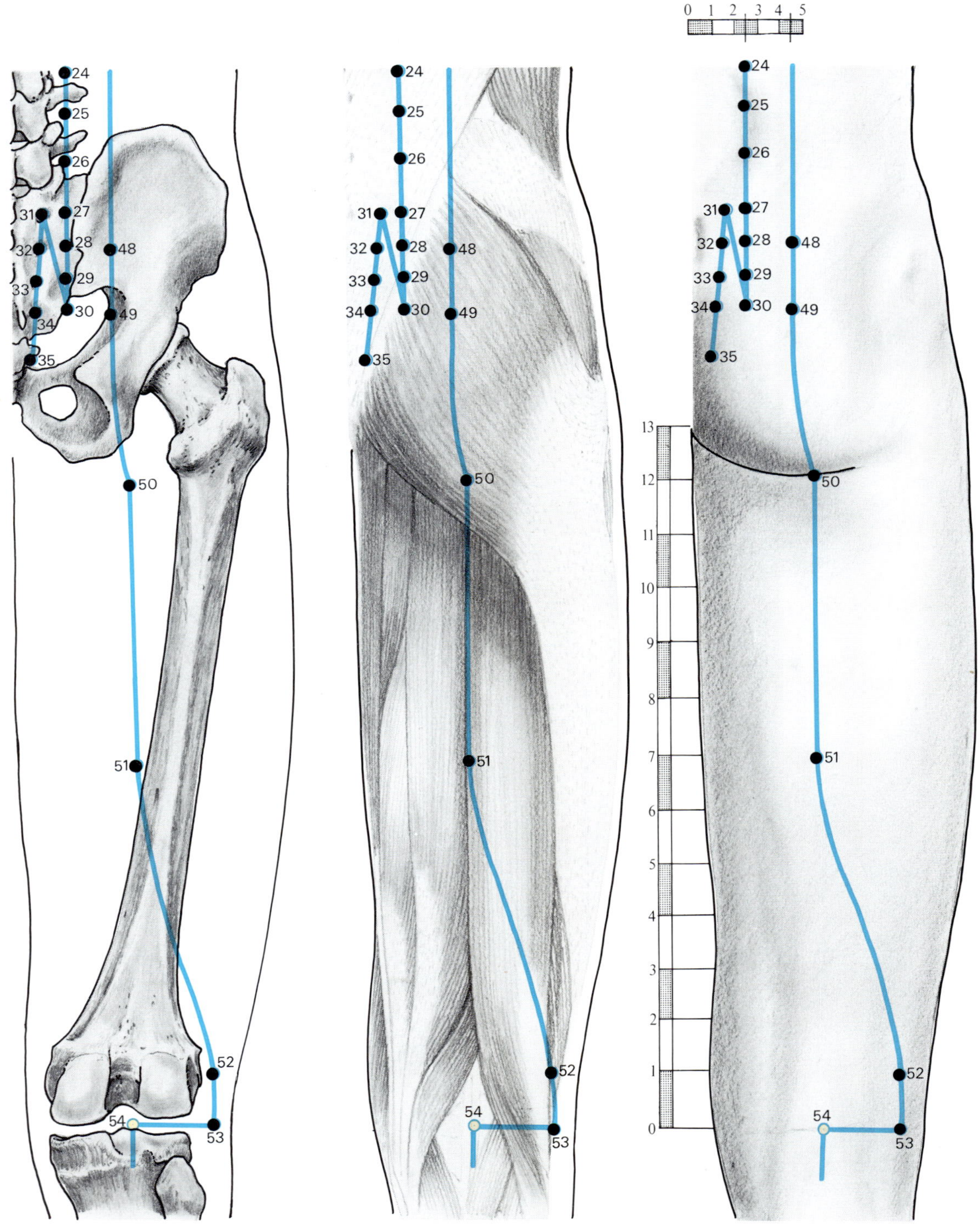
0 1 2 3 4 5
24
25
26
27
28
29
30
31
32
33
34
35
48
49
50
51
52
53
54
13 12 11 10 9 8 7 6 5 4 3 2 1 0

III **50** **Receive And Support** (Chengfu)

⊥ 8
△ X

At the mid-point of the gluteal fold, directly distal to III 49, between the biceps femoris and the semitendinosus.

III **51** **Prosperous Gate** (Yinmen)

⊥ 7
△ X

On the posterior surface of the thigh, at the mid-point between the biceps femoris and the semitendinosus, 7 ACI proximal to the knee crease.

III **52** **Floating Reserve** (Fuhsi)

⊥ 5
△ 3–7

On the posterior surface of the thigh, 1 ACI proximal to the lateral end of the knee crease, medial to the tendon of the biceps femoris.

III **53** **Equilibrium Yang** (Weiyang)

⊥ 7
△ 3–5

On the lateral side of the knee crease, medial to the tendon of the biceps femoris.

III **54** **Equilibrium Middle** (Weichung)

⊥ 5 Earth
△ X

On the posterior surface of the leg, in the centre of the knee crease.

Point of Ho (Autumn)
Greater Assembling Point of the back and vertebrae
First Aid: spinal injury

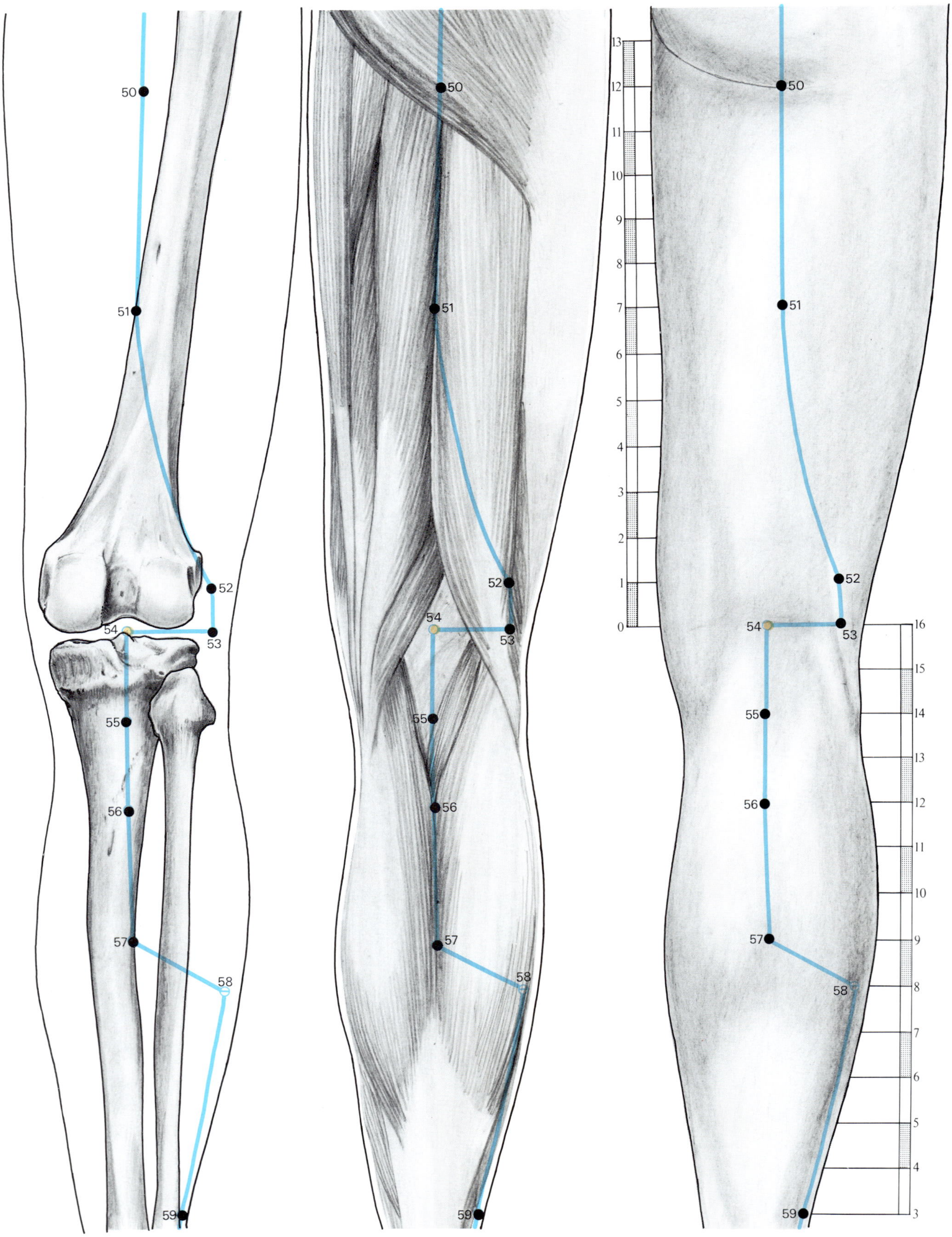
50
51
52
53
54
55
56
57
58
59
50
51
52
53
54
55
56
57
58
59
13
12
11
10
9
8
7
6
5
4
3
2
1
0
50
51
52
53
54
55
56
57
58
59
16
15
14
13
12
11
10
9
8
7
6
5
4
3

III **55** **Uniting Yang** (Hoyang)

⊥ 5
△ 3–7

On the posterior surface of the leg, 14 ACI proximal to the level of the prominence of the lateral malleolus, between the lateral and medial heads of the gastrocnemius.

III **56** **Supporting Muscles** (Chengchin)

⊥ X
△ 3–7

On the posterior surface of the leg, 12 ACI proximal to the level of the prominence of the lateral malleolus, between the lateral and medial heads of the gastrocnemius.

III **57** **Supporting Mountain** (Chengshan)

⊥ 7
△ 5–15

On the posterior surface of the leg, 9 ACI proximal to the level of the prominence of the lateral malleolus, between the lateral and medial heads of the gastrocnemius.

III **58** **Fly And Scatter** (Feiyang)

⊖ ⊥ 5 Junction
△ 3–7

On the posterolateral surface of the leg, 8 ACI proximal to the level of the prominence of the lateral malleolus, between the gastrocnemius and the soleus.

A Centre of Energy

III **59** **Foot Bone Yang** (Fuyang)

⊥ 5
△ 5–7

On the posterolateral surface of the leg, 3 ACI proximal to the level of the prominence of the lateral malleolus, posterior to the peroneus longus, directly proximal to III 60.

Point of Yang Qiao Mo
First Aid: food poisoning

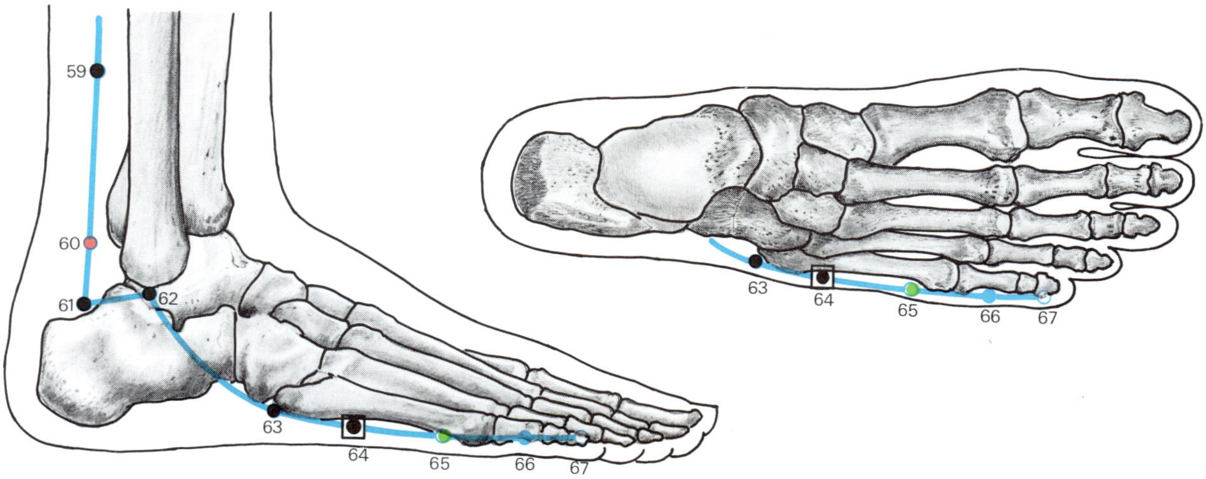

Author's Note: On the above diagram, III 62 is shown too close to the inferior tip of the lateral malleolus. Refer to written location opposite.

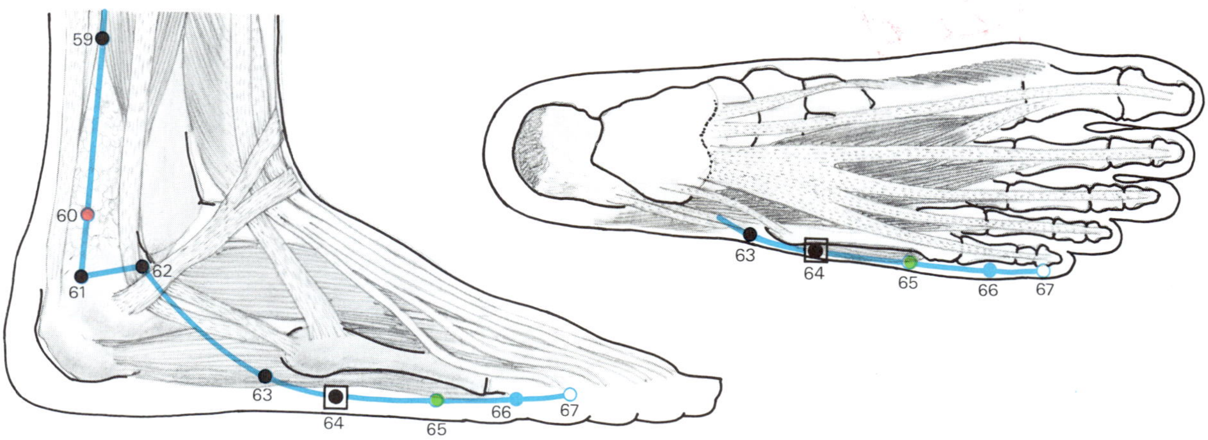

Author's Note: On the above diagram, the line between III 66 and III 63 is shown, in error, as being inferior to the fifth metatarsal bone, rather than along its lateral edge. Refer to written location of these points.

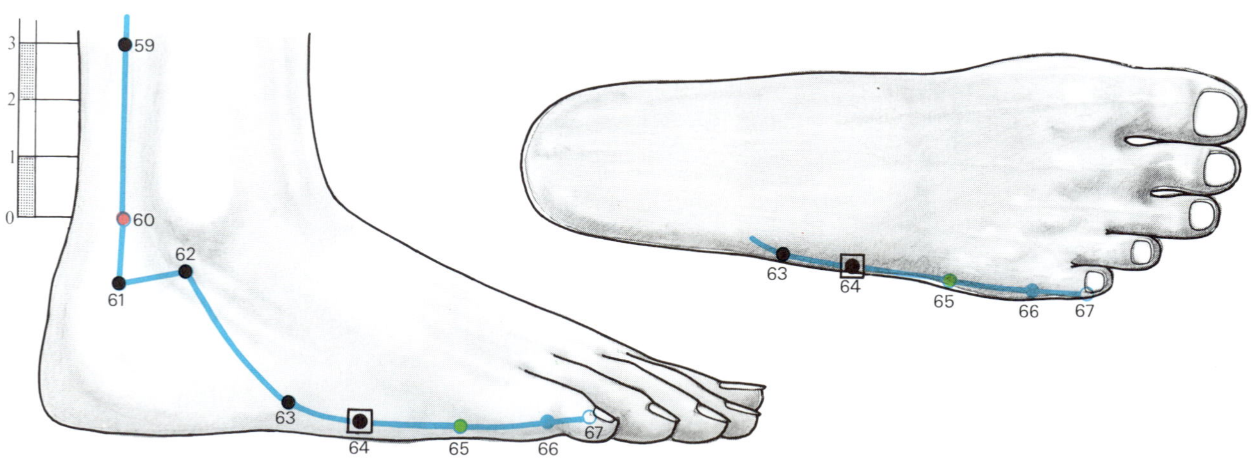

III **60** **Kunlun Mountain** (Kunlun)

⊥ 3–5 Fire
△ 3–7

Mid-way between the prominence of the lateral malleolus and the Achilles tendon, on the peroneal artery.

Point of Ching (late Summer)
First Aid: anxiety, facial neuralgia, fractures, spinal injury, sprains

III **61** **Servant's Aide** (Pushen)

⊥ 3
△ 3–7

On the superior edge of the lateral surface of the calcaneus, directly inferior to III 60.

Point of Yang Qiao Mo
A point of the pattern to release the 7 Dragons on the 7 External Demons

III **62** **Extended Meridian** (Shenmo)

⊥ 3
△ X

One half ACI distal to the tip of the lateral malleolus, between the tendons of the peroneus longus and the peroneus brevis.

Master Point of Yang Qiao Mo
Coupled Point of Du Mo

III **63** **Golden Gate** (Chinmen)

⊥ 3
△ 3–5

On the lateral border of the foot, just proximal to the tubercle of the fifth metatarsal bone.

Point of Yang Wei Mo

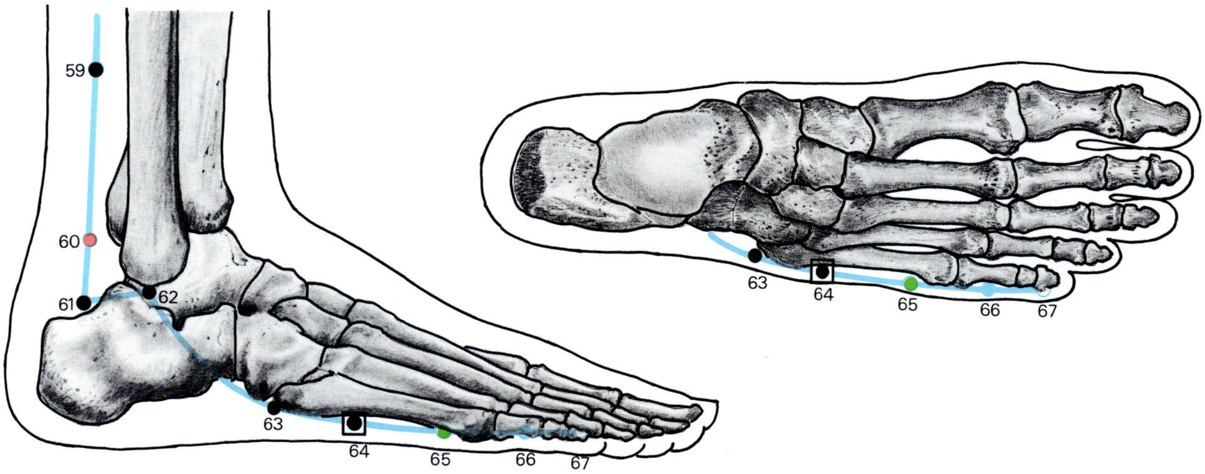

Author's Note: On the above diagram, III 62 is shown too close to the inferior tip of the lateral malleolus. Refer to written location opposite.

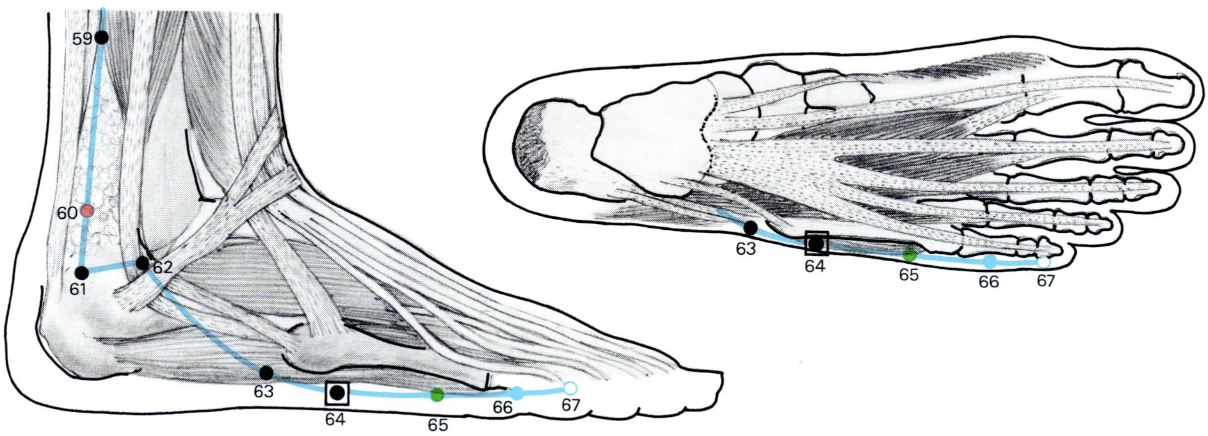

Author's Note: On the above diagram, the line between III 66 and III 63 is shown, in error, as being inferior to the fifth metatarsal bone, rather than along its lateral edge. Refer to written location of these points.

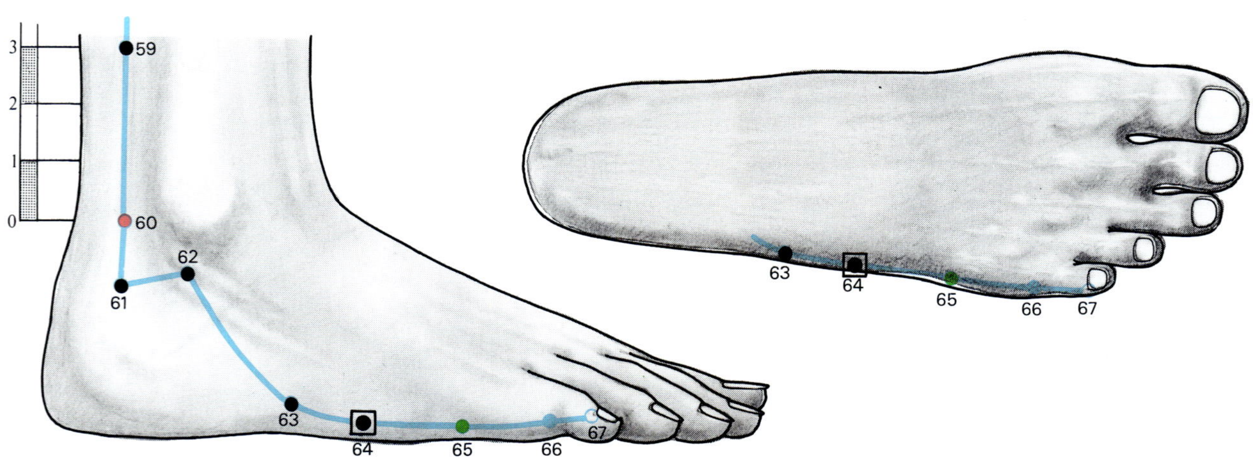

III **64** **Capital Bone** (Chingku)

□ ⊥ 3–5 Source
△ 3–7

On the lateral border of the foot, distal to the tubercle of the fifth metatarsal bone.

First Aid: bee stings

III **65** **Bone Binder** (Shuku)

● ⊥ 3 Wood
△ 3–5 Sedation

On the lateral border of the foot, just proximal to the head of the fifth metatarsal bone.

Point of Yu (Summer)
First Aid: burns, cystitis, food poisoning, insect bites, poison, scalds, sunburn, urine retention

III **66** **Penetrating Valley** (Tsu tungku)

● ⊥ 2 Water
△ 3–5 Horary 3 p.m.–5 p.m.

On the lateral border of the foot, just distal to the base of the proximal phalanx of the little toe.

Point of Yung (Spring)

III **67** **Extremity Of Yin** (Chihyin)

○ ⊥ 2 Metal
△ 3 Tonification
Exit

Lateral nail point of the little toe.

Point of Cheng (Winter)

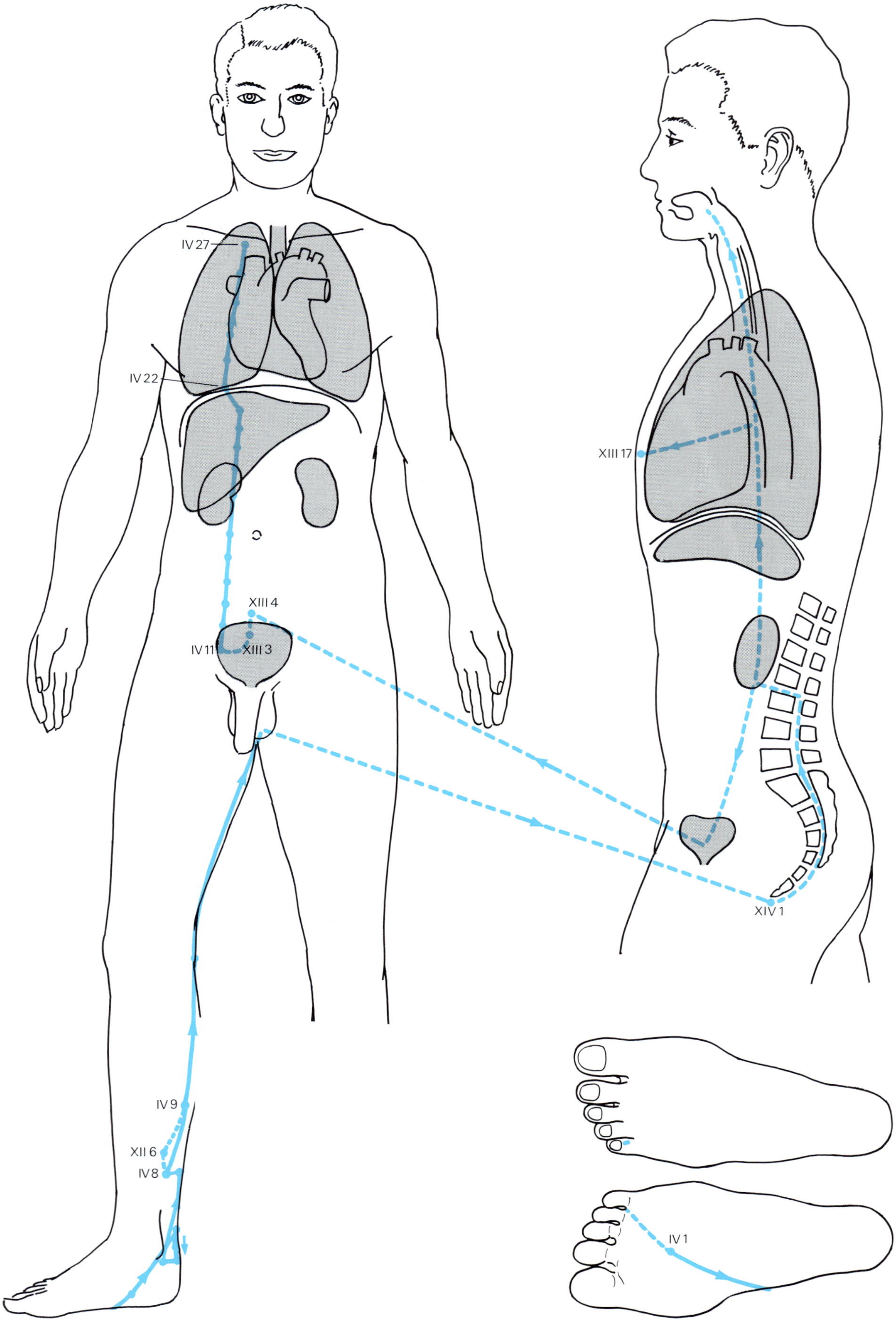
IV 27
IV 22
XIII 17
XIII 4
IV 11
XIII 3
XIV 1
IV 9
XII 6
IV 8
IV 1

The kidney meridian begins at a deep level on the plantar surface of the little toe and travels deep, to become superficial at the entry point IV 1 between the second and third metatarsal bones, posterior to the metatarsal heads, on the sole of the foot. It then runs medially below the navicular bone, ascends over the medial malleolus to the line of the posterior tibial artery and then loops down anterior to the Achilles tendon, to the calcaneus and the inferior tip of the medial malleolus.

The meridian then ascends the posteromedial surface of the leg, then continues up the gastrocnemius to the medial border of the popliteal fossa. A deep branch travels from IV 8 to XII 6, and rejoins the superficial meridian at IV 9. From the knee it runs over the posterior medial surface of the thigh and the adductor muscles to the groin. The pathway becomes deep at the groin, as it joins to the tip of the coccyx, at XIV 1, and continues up the spine to the space between the second and third lumbar vertebrae. Then it enters the kidney.

A branch leaves the kidney to enter the bladder. From the bladder the pathway joins the median line, at XIII 4, descends to XIII 3 and then goes $1\frac{1}{2}$ ACI laterally on a level with the superior edge of the pubic symphysis, to IV 11. The meridian now becomes superficial and travels up the abdomen through the rectus abdominis muscles, paramedially. When it reaches the thorax at the fifth intercostal space it ascends at 2 ACI lateral to the medial line, to the exit point IV 22, to end just below the clavicle at its last point, IV 27.

A second deep branch from the kidney ascends the abdomen to enter the liver, penetrates the diaphragm and enters the lungs. It then proceeds up the trachea and larynx to the root of the tongue.

A branch leaves the deep pathway from the lungs, connects with the heart and travels to the median line of the chest at the level of the nipples, XIII 17. Here it connects with the circulation-sex meridian.

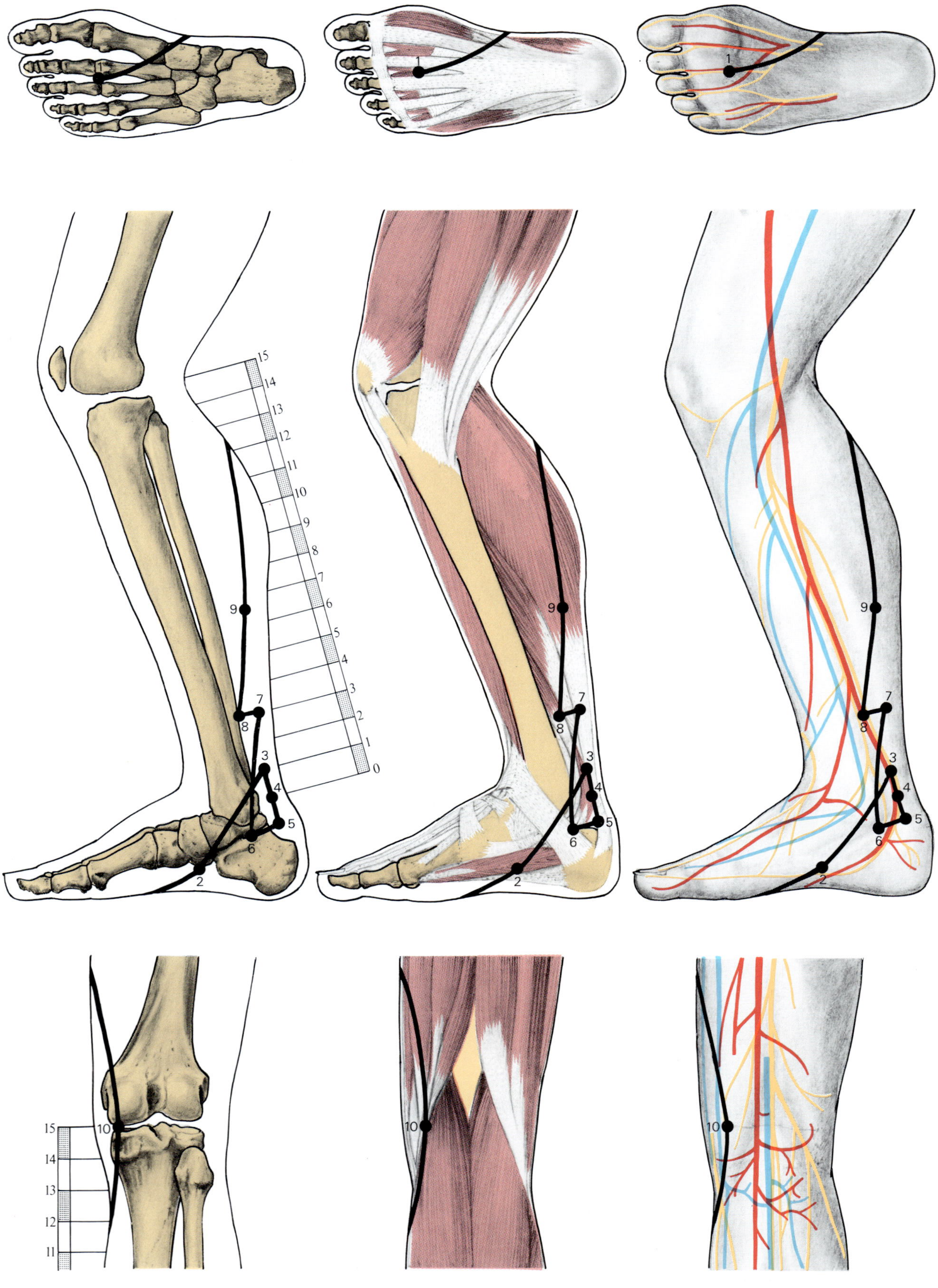
1
2
3
4
5
6
7
8
9
10

IV	1	On the plantar surface of the foot, between the second and third metatarsal bones, in the crease formed when the toes are flexed.
IV	2	On the medial surface of the foot, inferior to the tuberosity of the navicular bone.
IV	3	On the medial surface of the leg, 1 ACI proximal to the prominence of the medial malleolus, upon the posterior tibial artery.
IV	4	On the medial surface of the ankle, posterior to the prominence of the medial malleolus, upon the posterior tibial artery, 1 ACI distal to IV 3.
IV	5	On the medial surface of the ankle, 1 ACI distal to IV 4, on the superior edge of the calcaneus.
IV	6	On the medial surface of the ankle, 4 fen distal to the inferior border of the medial malleolus.
IV	7	On the medial surface of the leg, 3 ACI proximal to the level of the prominence of the medial malleolus, posterior to the flexor digitorum longus.
IV	8	On the medial surface of the leg, 3 ACI proximal to the prominence of the medial malleolus, $\frac{1}{2}$ ACI anterior to IV 7, and anterior to the flexor digitorum longus.
IV	9	On the medial surface of the leg, $6\frac{1}{2}$ ACI proximal to the level of the prominence of the medial malleolus, on the medial edge of the tendon of the gastrocnemius, directly proximal to IV 7.
IV	10	At the medial extremity of the knee crease between the tendons of the semimembranosus and the semitendinosus, when the knee is slightly flexed.

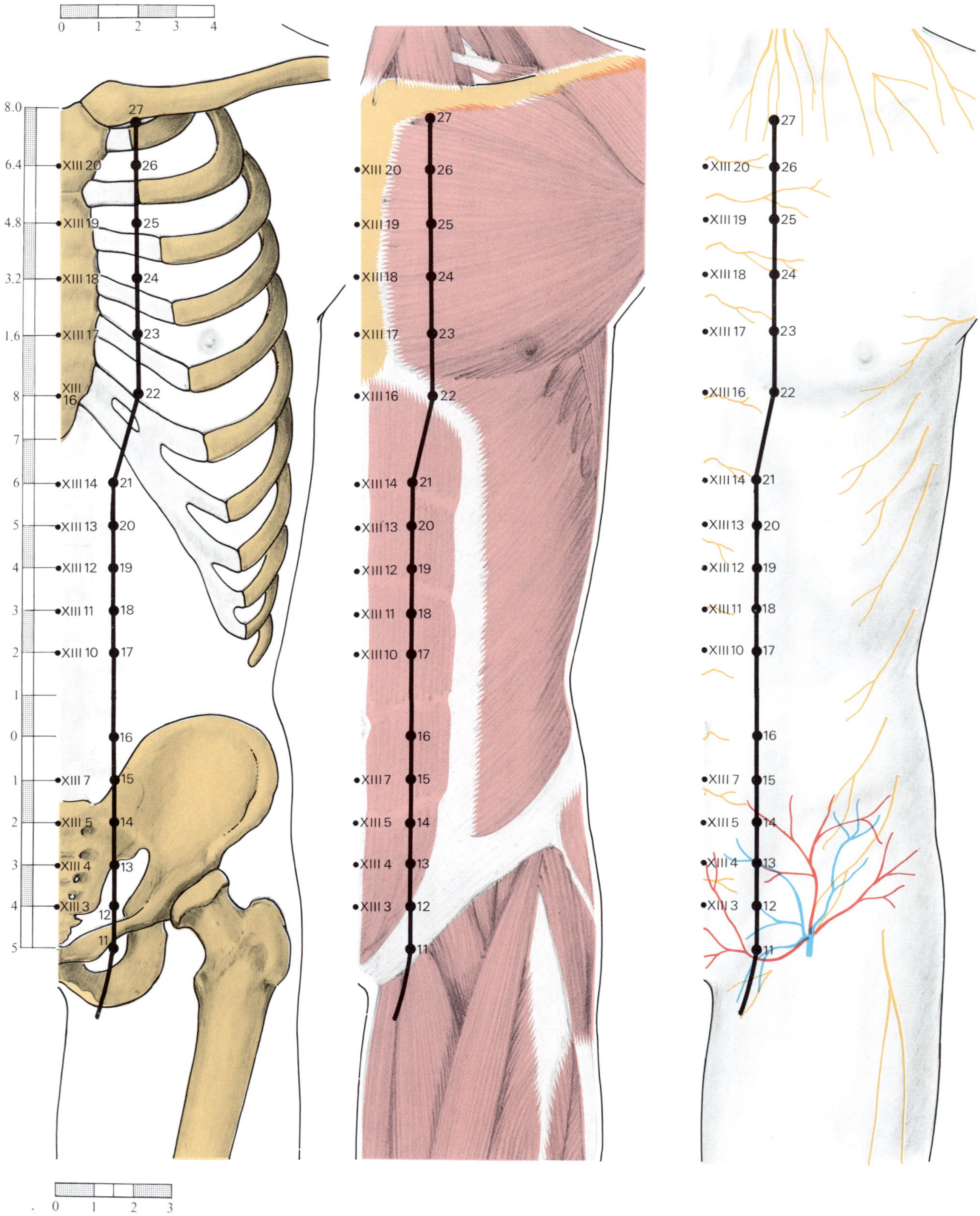
27
26
25
24
23
22
21
20
19
18
17
16
15
14
13
12
11
XIII 20
XIII 19
XIII 18
XIII 17
XIII 16
XIII 14
XIII 13
XIII 12
XIII 11
XIII 10
XIII 7
XIII 5
XIII 4
XIII 3
8.0
6.4
4.8
3.2
1.6
0 1 2 3 4

IV	11	On the abdomen, $1\frac{1}{2}$ ACI lateral to the median line, at the level of the superior edge of the pubic symphysis, 5 ACI inferior to the level of the umbilicus.
IV	12	On the abdomen, $1\frac{1}{2}$ ACI lateral to the median line, 4 ACI inferior to the level of the umbilicus, at the level of XIII 3.
IV	13	On the abdomen, $1\frac{1}{2}$ ACI lateral to the median line, 3 ACI inferior to the level of the umbilicus, at the level of XIII 4.
IV	14	On the abdomen, $1\frac{1}{2}$ ACI lateral to the median line, 2 ACI inferior to the level of the umbilicus, at the level of XIII 5.
IV	15	On the abdomen, $1\frac{1}{2}$ ACI lateral to the median line, 1 ACI inferior to the level of the umbilicus, at the level of XIII 7.
IV	16	On the abdomen, $1\frac{1}{2}$ ACI lateral to the centre of the umbilicus.
IV	17	On the abdomen, $1\frac{1}{2}$ ACI lateral to the median line, 2 ACI superior to the level of the umbilicus, at the level of XIII 10.
IV	18	On the abdomen, $1\frac{1}{2}$ ACI lateral to the median line, 3 ACI superior to the level of the umbilicus, at the level of XIII 11.
IV	19	On the abdomen, $1\frac{1}{2}$ ACI lateral to the median line, 4 ACI superior to the level of the umbilicus, at the level of XIII 12.
IV	20	On the abdomen, $1\frac{1}{2}$ ACI lateral to the median line, 5 ACI superior to the level of the umbilicus, at the level of XIII 13.
IV	21	On the abdomen, $1\frac{1}{2}$ ACI lateral to the median line, 6 ACI superior to the level of the umbilicus, at the level of XIII 14.
IV	22	On the thorax, in the fifth intercostal space, 2 ACI lateral to the median line, on a level with XIII 16.
IV	23	On the thorax, in the fourth intercostal space, 2 ACI lateral to the median line, on a level with XIII 17.
IV	24	On the thorax, in the third intercostal space, 2 ACI lateral to the median line, on a level with XIII 18.
IV	25	On the thorax, in the second intercostal space, 2 ACI lateral to the median line, on a level with XIII 19.
IV	26	On the thorax, in the first intercostal space, 2 ACI lateral to the median line, on a level with XIII 20.
IV	27	In the depression between the first rib and the inferior edge of the clavicle, 2 ACI lateral to the median line.

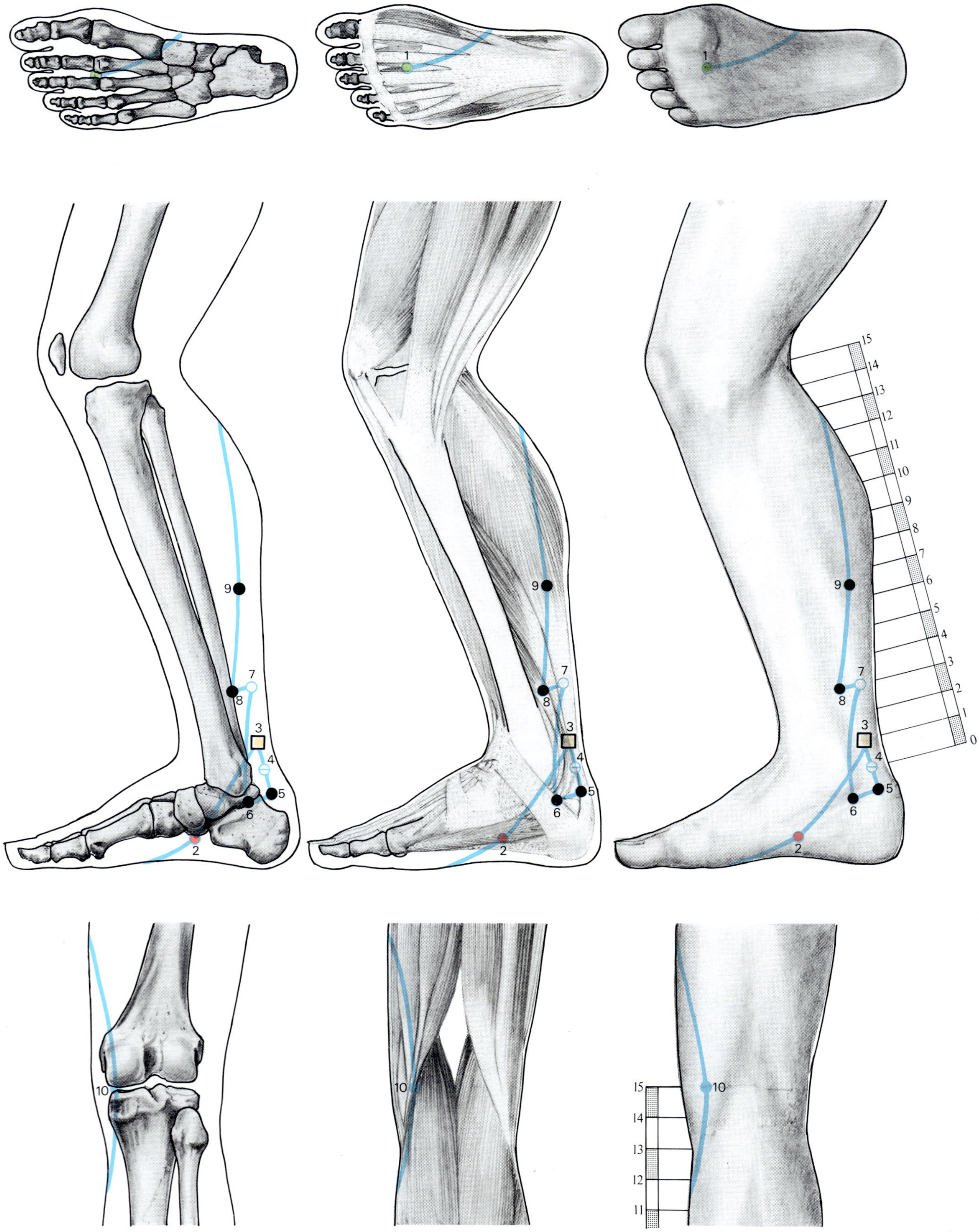
1
2
3
4
5
6
7
8
9
10
0
11
12
13
14
15

IV **1** **Bubbling Spring** (Yungchuan)

● ⊥ 5 Wood
△ 3–7 Sedation
XP8 Entry

On the plantar surface of the foot, between the second and third metatarsal bones, in the crease formed when the toes are flexed.

Point of Cheng (Winter)
First Aid: resuscitation

IV **2** **Blazing Valley** (Janku)

● ⊥ 5 Fire
△ 3–5
XP8

On the medial surface of the foot, inferior to the tuberosity of the navicular bone.

Point of Yung (Spring)
Point of Yin Qiao Mo
First Aid: cystitis, injury to testicles, urine retention

IV **3** **Greater Mountain Stream** (Taihsi)

● ⊥ 3 Earth
□ △ 3–5 Source

On the medial surface of the leg. 1 ACI proximal to the prominence of the medial malleolus, upon the posterior tibial artery.

Point of Yu (Summer)

IV **4** **Great Bell** (Tachung)

⊖ ⊥ 3 Junction
△ 3–7
XP3

On the medial surface of the ankle, posterior to the prominence of the medial malleolus, upon the posterior tibial artery, 1 ACI distal to IV 3.

IV **5** **Water Spring** (Shuichuan)

⊥ 4
△ 5

On the medial surface of the ankle, 1 ACI distal to IV 4, on the superior edge of the calcaneus.

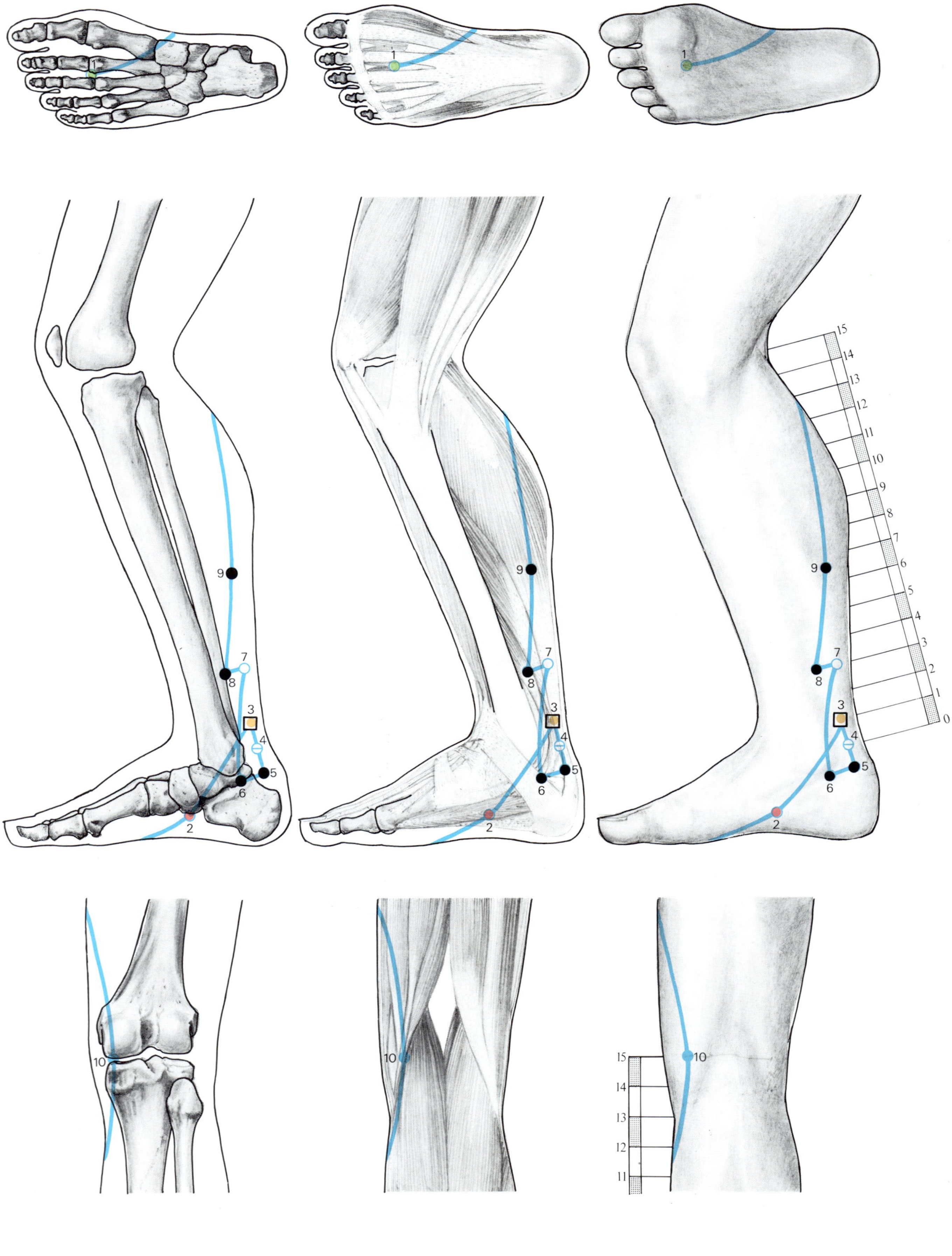

IV **6** **Illuminated Sea** (Chaohai)

⊥ 3
△ 3–5

On the medial surface of the ankle, 4 fen distal to the inferior border of the medial malleolus.

Master Point of Yin Qiao Mo
Coupled Point of Ren Mo
First Aid: apoplexy, bee stings, concussion, haemorrhage, insensibility, snake bites

IV **7** **Returning Current** (Fuliu)

○ ⊥ 4 Metal
△ 3–7 Tonification
XP8

On the medial surface of the leg, 3 ACI proximal to the level of the prominence of the medial malleolus, posterior to the flexor digitorum longus.

Point of Ching (late Summer)

IV **8** **Exchange Pledges** (Chiaohsin)

⊥ 3
△ 5

On the medial surface of the leg, 3 ACI proximal to the prominence of the medial malleolus, $\frac{1}{2}$ ACI anterior to IV 7, and anterior to the flexor digitorum longus.

Point of Yin Qiao Mo

IV **9** **Building Guest** (Chupin)

⊥ 5
△ 3–7

On the medial surface of the leg, $6\frac{1}{2}$ ACI proximal to the level of the prominence of the medial malleolus, on the medial edge of the tendon of the gastrocnemius, directly proximal to IV 7.

Point of Yin Wei Mo

IV **10** **Yin Valley** (Yinku)

● ⊥ 4 Water
△ 3 Horary 5 p.m.–7 p.m.

At the medial extremity of the knee crease between the tendons of the semimembranosus and the semitendinosus, when the knee is slightly flexed.

Point of Ho (Autumn)

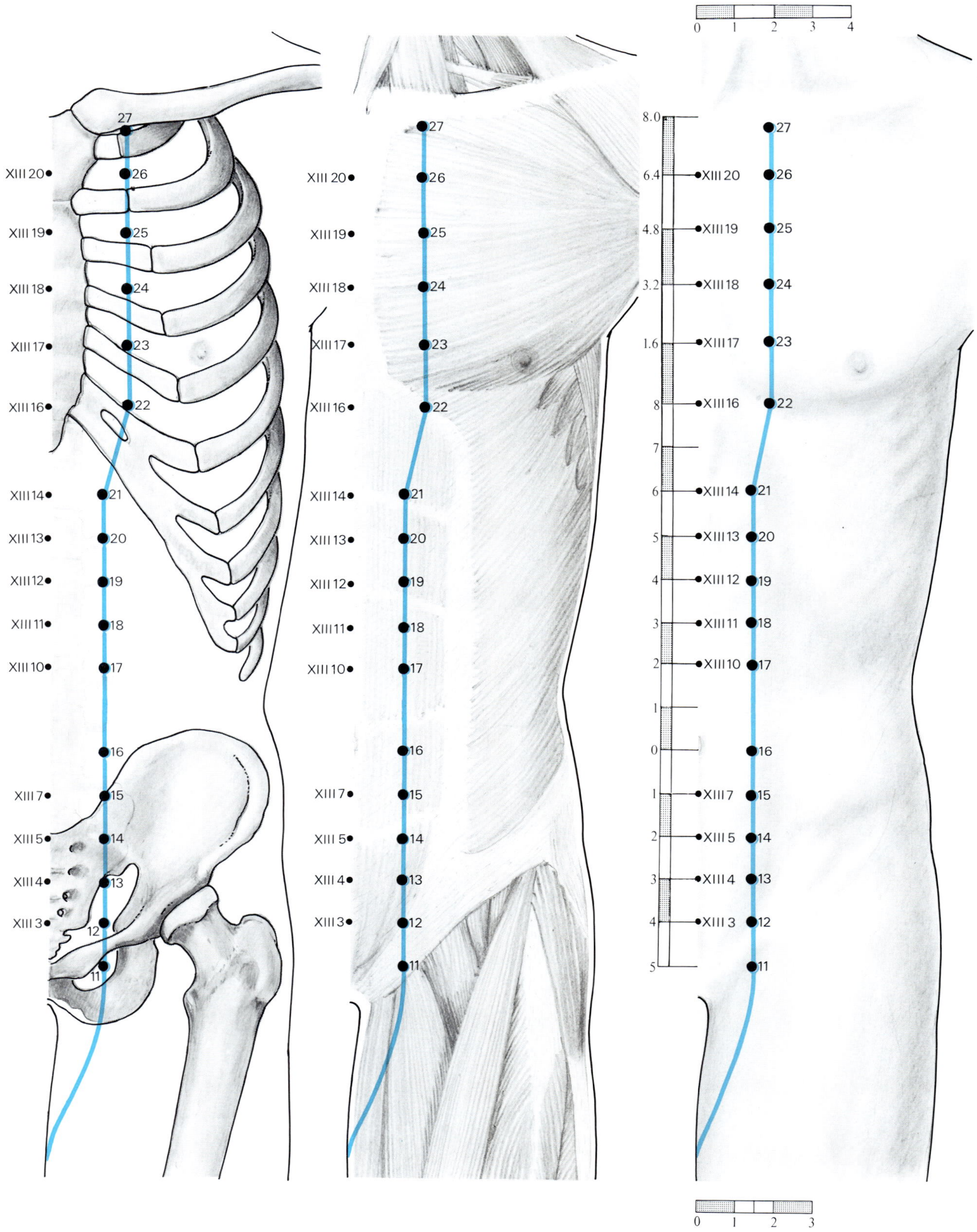
0 1 2 3 4
27
XIII 20
26
XIII 19
25
XIII 18
24
XIII 17
23
XIII 16
22
XIII 14
21
XIII 13
20
XIII 12
19
XIII 11
18
XIII 10
17
16
XIII 7
15
XIII 5
14
XIII 4
13
XIII 3
12
11
8.0
6.4
4.8
3.2
1.6
8
7
6
5
4
3
2
1
0
1
2
3
4
5
0 1 2 3

IV **11** **Transverse Bone** (Hengku)

⊥ X
△ 5–15

On the abdomen, $1\frac{1}{2}$ ACI lateral to the median line, at the level of the superior edge of the pubic symphysis, 5 ACI inferior to the level of the umbilicus.

Point of Chong Mo

IV **12** **Great Brightness** (Taho)

⊥ 5–10
△ 5–10

On the abdomen, $1\frac{1}{2}$ ACI lateral to the median line, 4 ACI inferior to the level of the umbilicus, at the level of XIII 3.

Point of Chong Mo

IV **13** **Door Of Infants** (Tzuhu)

⊥ 5–10
△ 5–10

On the abdomen, $1\frac{1}{2}$ ACI lateral to the median line, 3 ACI inferior to the level of the umbilicus, at the level of XIII 4.

Point of Chong Mo
A Centre of Energy

IV **14** **Four Full** (Szuman)

⊥ 7–10
△ 5–30

On the abdomen, $1\frac{1}{2}$ ACI lateral to the median line, 2 ACI inferior to the level of the umbilicus, at the level of XIII 5.

Point of Chong Mo

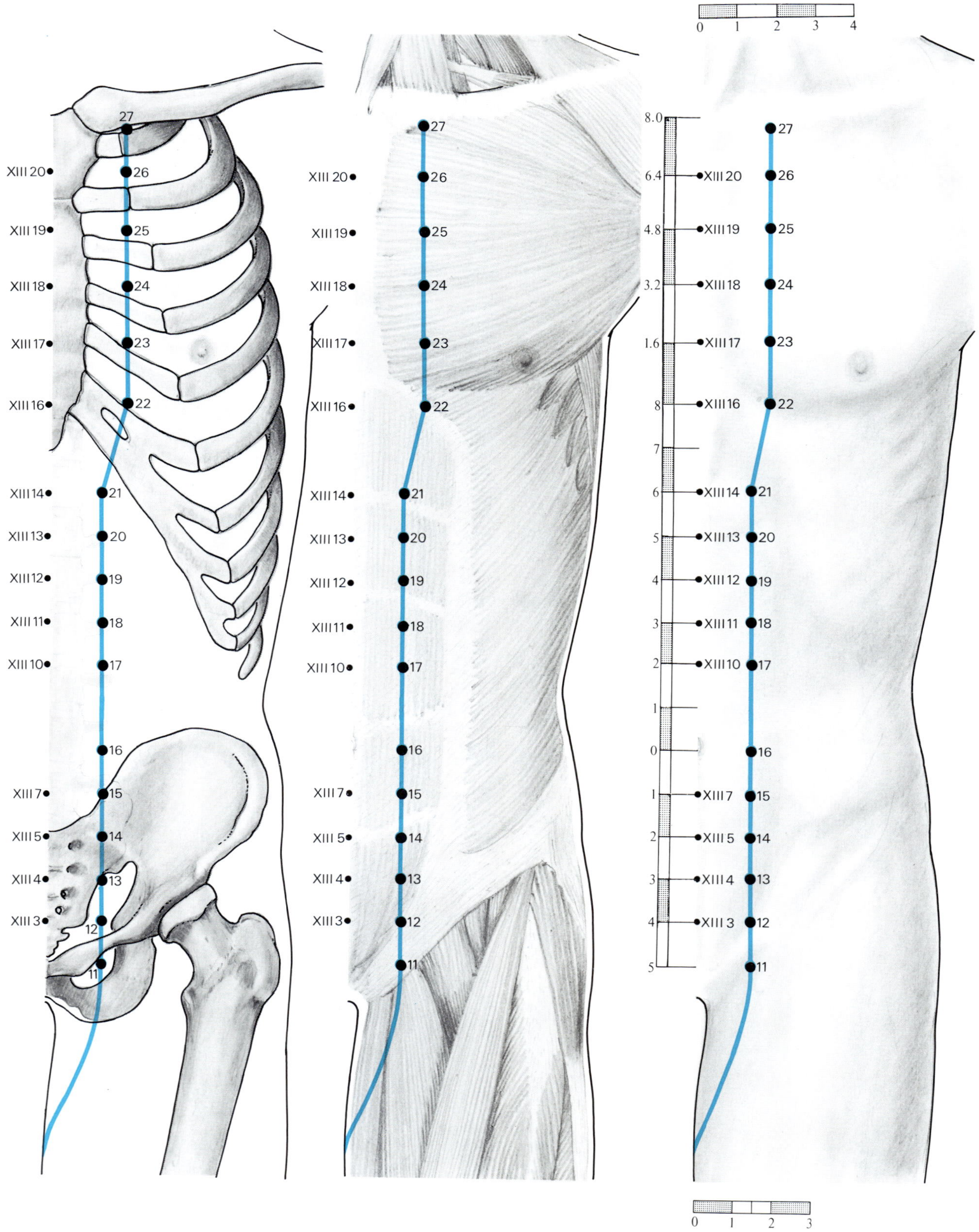
0 1 2 3 4
27
26
25
24
23
22
21
20
19
18
17
16
15
14
13
12
11
XIII 20
XIII 19
XIII 18
XIII 17
XIII 16
XIII 14
XIII 13
XIII 12
XIII 11
XIII 10
XIII 7
XIII 5
XIII 4
XIII 3
8.0
6.4
4.8
3.2
1.6
8
7
6
5
4
3
2
1
0
1
2
3
4
5
0 1 2 3

IV **15** **Middle Flowing Out** (Chungchu)

⊥ 7–10
△ 5–15

On the abdomen, $1\frac{1}{2}$ ACI lateral to the median line, 1 ACI inferior to the level of the umbilicus, at the level of XIII 7.

Point of Chong Mo

IV **16** **Vitals Correspondence** (Huangshu)

⊥ 10
△ 7

On the abdomen, $1\frac{1}{2}$ ACI lateral to the centre of the umbilicus.

Point of Chong Mo

IV **17** **Merchant Crooked** (Shangchu)

⊥ 10
△ 7

On the abdomen, $1\frac{1}{2}$ ACI lateral to the median line, 2 ACI superior to the level of the umbilicus, at the level of XIII 10.

Point of Chong Mo

IV **18** **Stone Border** (Shihkuan)

⊥ 7–10
△ 7

On the abdomen, $1\frac{1}{2}$ ACI lateral to the median line, 3 ACI superior to the level of the umbilicus, at the level of XIII 11.

Point of Chong Mo

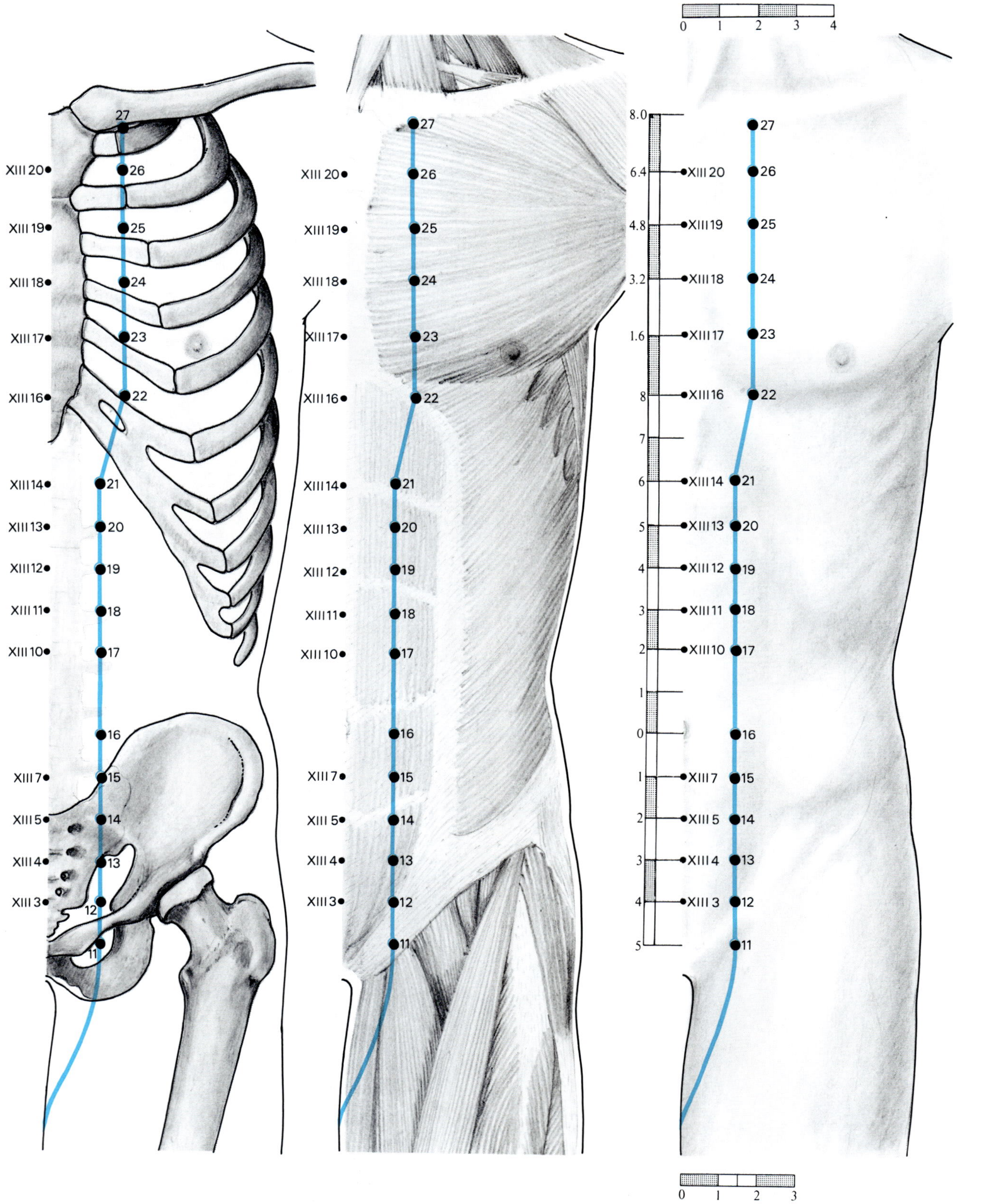

27
XIII 20 26
XIII 19 25
XIII 18 24
XIII 17 23
XIII 16 22
XIII 14 21
XIII 13 20
XIII 12 19
XIII 11 18
XIII 10 17
16
XIII 7 15
XIII 5 14
XIII 4 13
XIII 3 12
11
27
XIII 20 26
XIII 19 25
XIII 18 24
XIII 17 23
XIII 16 22
XIII 14 21
XIII 13 20
XIII 12 19
XIII 11 18
XIII 10 17
16
XIII 7 15
XIII 5 14
XIII 4 13
XIII 3 12
11
0 1 2 3 4
8.0 27
6.4 XIII 20 26
4.8 XIII 19 25
3.2 XIII 18 24
1.6 XIII 17 23
8 XIII 16 22
7
6 XIII 14 21
5 XIII 13 20
4 XIII 12 19
3 XIII 11 18
2 XIII 10 17
1
0 16
1 XIII 7 15
2 XIII 5 14
3 XIII 4 13
4 XIII 3 12
5 11
0 1 2 3

IV **19** **Yin Capital** (Yintu)

⊥ 7–10
△ 7–10

On the abdomen, $1\frac{1}{2}$ ACI lateral to the median line, 4 ACI superior to the level of the umbilicus, at the level of XIII 12.

Point of Chong Mo

IV **20** **Through The Valley** (Fu tungku)

⊥ 5
△ 7–10

On the abdomen, $1\frac{1}{2}$ ACI lateral to the median line, 5 ACI superior to the level of the umbilicus, at the level of XIII 13.

Point of Chong Mo

IV **21** **Dark Gate** (Yumen)

⊥ 5
△ 7–10

On the abdomen, $1\frac{1}{2}$ ACI lateral to the median line, 6 ACI superior to the level of the umbilicus, at the level of XIII 14.

Point of Chong Mo

IV **22** **Walking On The Verandah** (Pulang)

⊥ 3 Exit
△ 5

On the thorax, in the fifth intercostal space, 2 ACI lateral to the median line, on a level with XIII 16.

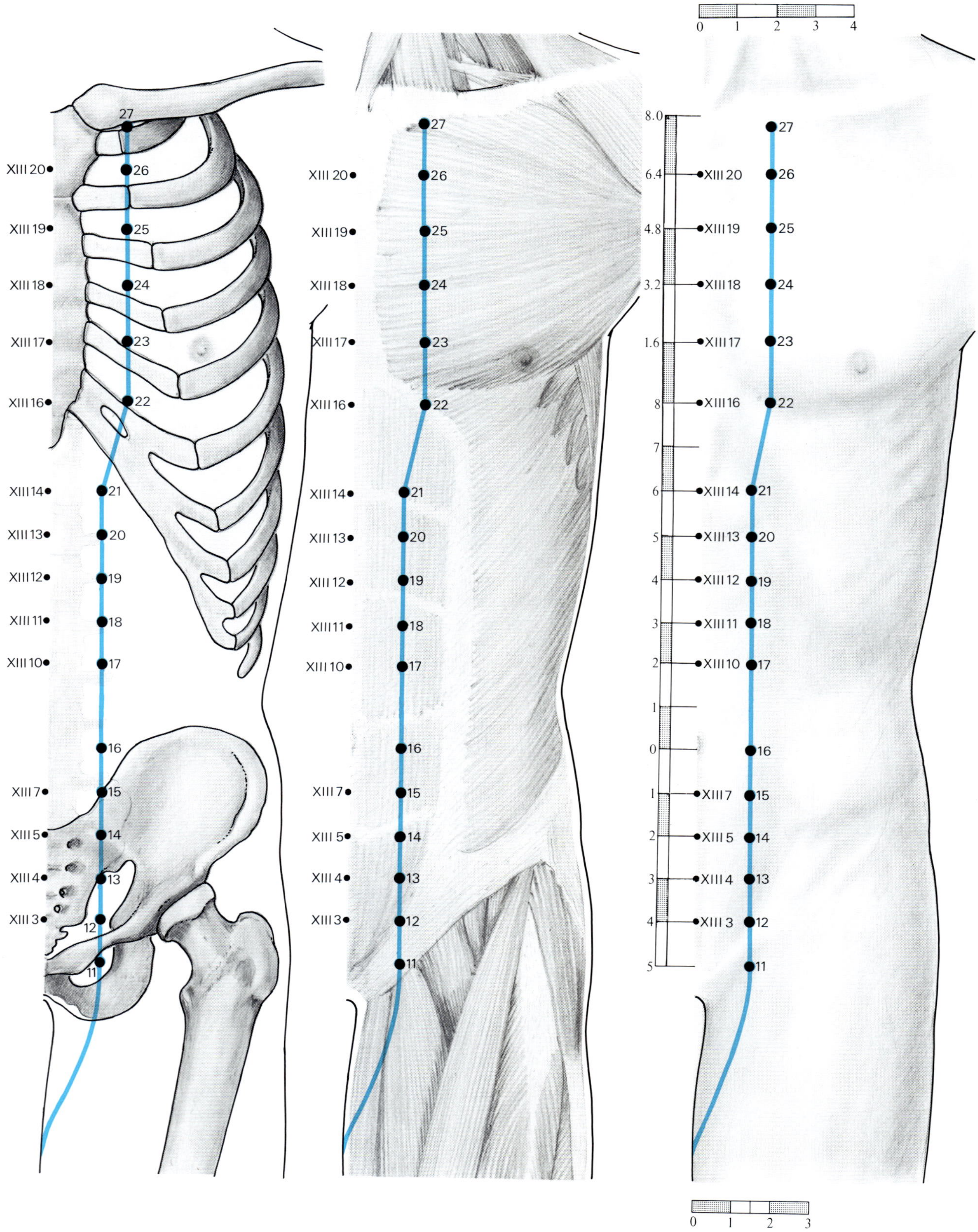
27
XIII 20
26
XIII 19
25
XIII 18
24
XIII 17
23
XIII 16
22
XIII 14
21
XIII 13
20
XIII 12
19
XIII 11
18
XIII 10
17
16
XIII 7
15
XIII 5
14
XIII 4
13
XIII 3
12
11
8.0
6.4
4.8
3.2
1.6
8
7
6
5
4
3
2
1
0
1
2
3
4
5
0 1 2 3 4
0 1 2 3

IV **23** **Spirit Seal** (Shenfeng)

⊥ 3
△ 5

On the thorax, in the fourth intercostal space, 2 ACI lateral to the median line, on a level with XIII 17.

First Aid: sunstroke

IV **24** **Spirit Burial Ground** (Linghsu)

⊥ 3
△ 5

On the thorax, in the third intercostal space, 2 ACI lateral to the median line, on a level with XIII 18.

IV **25** **Spirit Storehouse** (Shentsang)

⊥ 3
△ 5

On the thorax, in the second intercostal space, 2 ACI lateral to the median line, on a level with XIII 19.

IV **26** **Amidst Elegance** (Yuchung)

⊥ 3
△ 5

On the thorax, in the first intercostal space, 2 ACI lateral to the median line, on a level with XIII 20.

IV **27** **Store House** (Shufu)

⊥ 3
△ 5

In the depression between the first rib and the inferior edge of the clavicle, 2 ACI lateral to the median line.

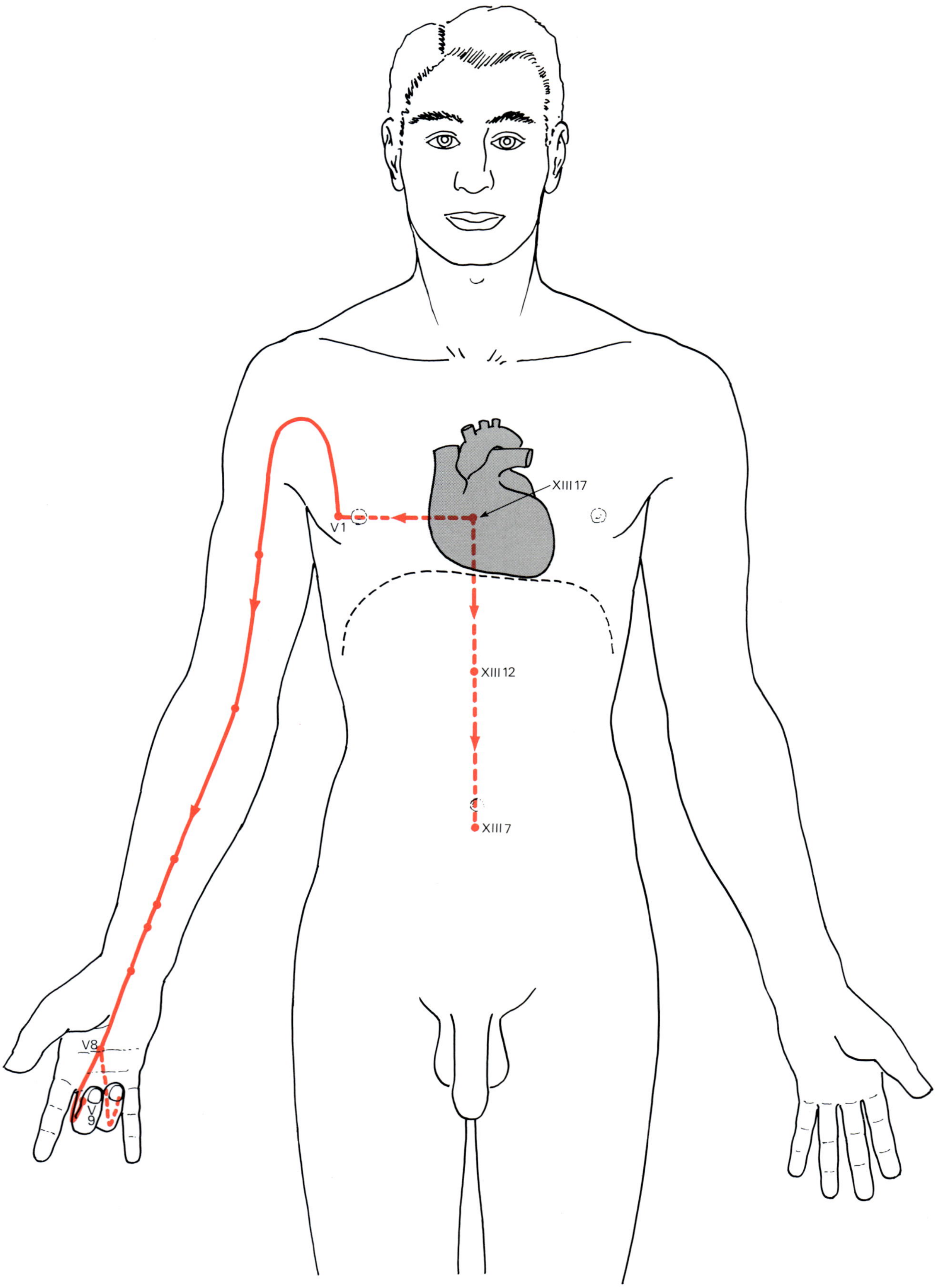
XIII 17
V1
XIII 12
XIII 7
V8
V
9

The circulation-sex meridian begins at a deep level in the thorax, attached to the pericardium. It emerges in the median line at the level of the nipples, at XIII 17, in the region of the Upper Chou, and descends the median line, penetrating the diaphragm, passing XIII 12 in the Middle Chou, down to a point just below the umbilicus, XIII 7, in the Lower Chou.

Another branch runs laterally from the pericardium and emerges just lateral to the nipple, in the fourth intercostal space, to become the superficial pathway at the entry point, V 1. From here it arches over the pectoral muscles to the middle of the anterior surface of the arm, travels down to the hollow medial to the tendon of the biceps, at the flexure of the elbow, then along the anterior surface of the forearm between the palmaris longus and the flexor carpi radialis to the mid-point of the flexure of the wrist. It then traverses the palm between the third and fourth metacarpal bones and runs along the radial side of the middle finger to the radial nail point, its last point, V 9.

A deep branch leaves the meridian from the middle of the palm at the exit point, V 8, and runs down the ring finger to the ulnar nail point, where it connects with the three heater meridian.

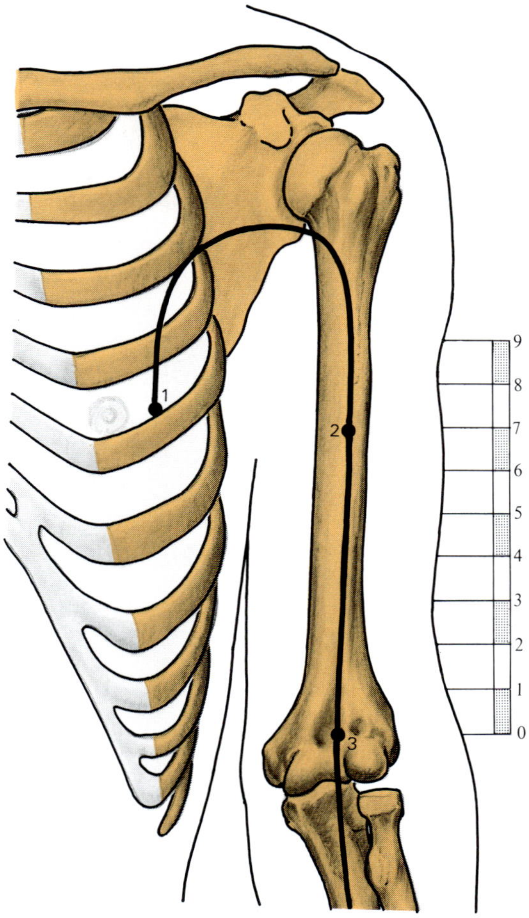
1
2
3
9
8
7
6
5
4
3
2
1
0

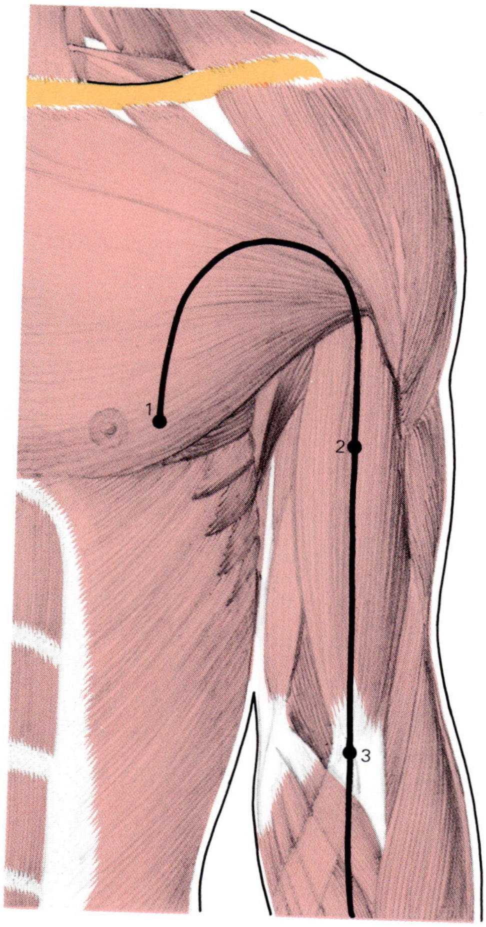
1
2
3

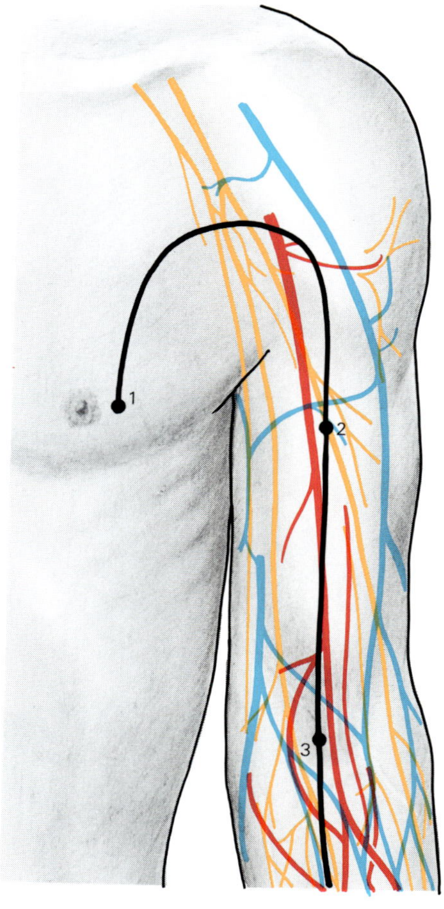
1
2
3

V 1 1 ACI lateral to the centre of the nipple.

V 2 On the anterior surface of the arm, between the heads of the biceps, 7 ACI proximal to the flexure of the elbow.

V 3 On the crease of the elbow, in the major depression which is often lateral to the tendon of the biceps, though on some people this depression may be found medial to the tendon.

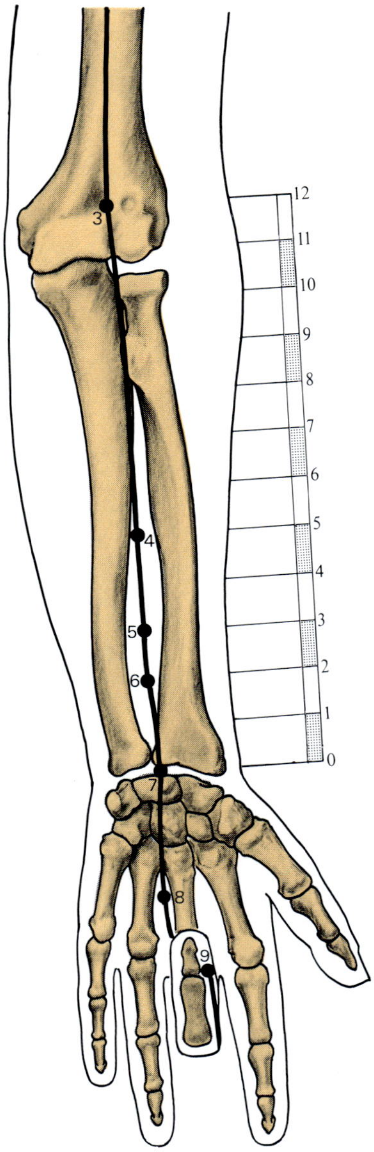
3
4
5
6
7
8
9
12
11
10
9
8
7
6
5
4
3
2
1
0

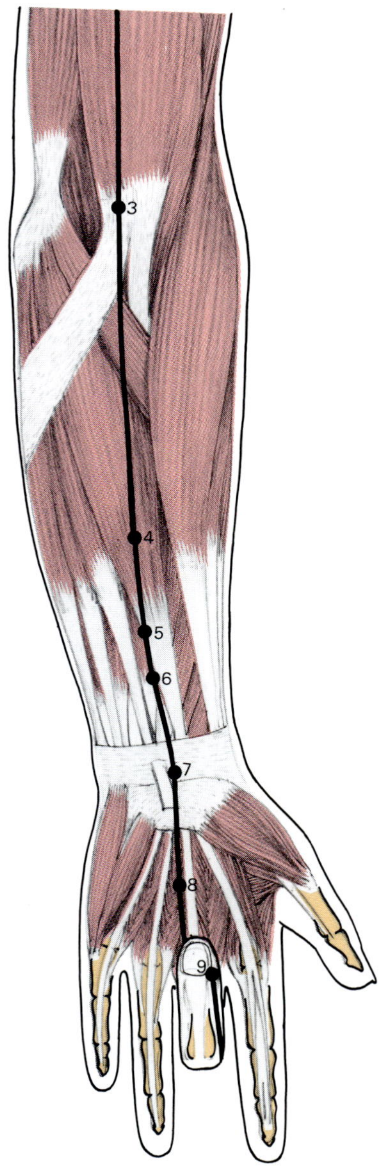
3
4
5
6
7
8
9

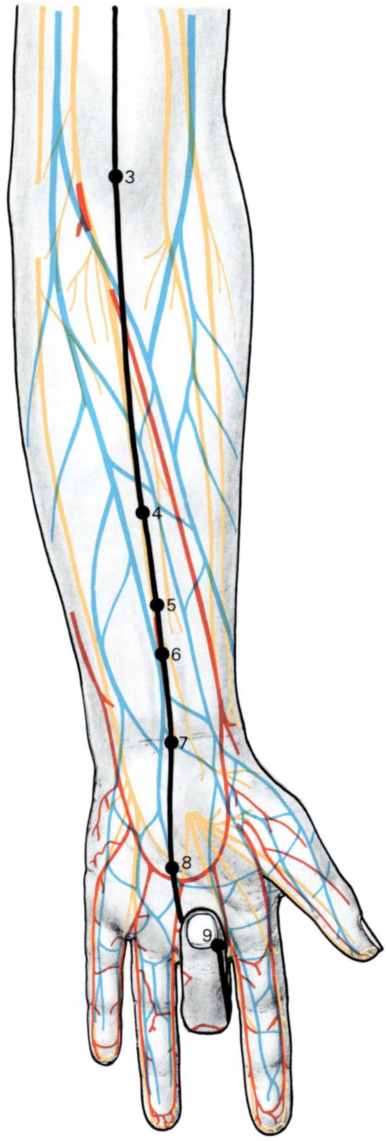
3
4
5
6
7
8
9

V	3	On the crease of the elbow, in the major depression which is often lateral to the tendon of the biceps, though on some people this depression may be found medial to the tendon.
V	4	On the anterior surface of the forearm, between the ulna and the radius, 5 ACI proximal to V 7.
V	5	On the anterior surface of the forearm, between the ulna and the radius, 3 ACI proximal to V 7.
V	6	On the anterior surface of the forearm, between the tendons of the palmaris longus and the flexor carpi radialis, 2 ACI proximal to V 7.
V	7	In the middle of the crease of the wrist, between the tendons of the palmaris longus and the flexor carpi radialis.
V	8	On the palmar surface of the hand, between the third and fourth metacarpal bones, on the proximal transverse crease, or the 'head line' of the hand.
V	9	Radial nail point of the middle finger.

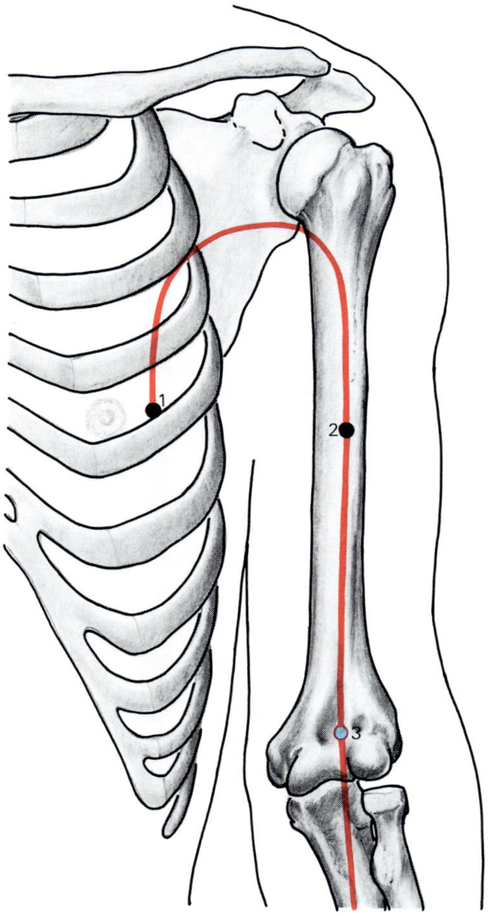
1
2
3

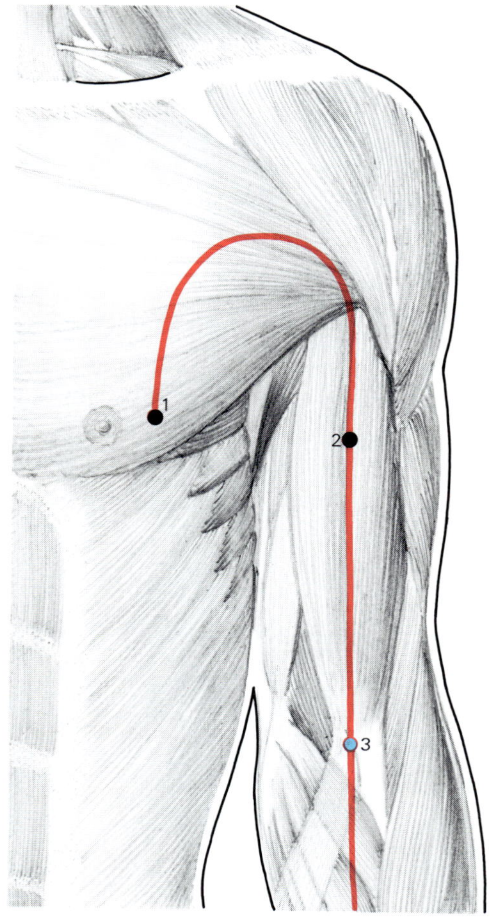
1
2
3

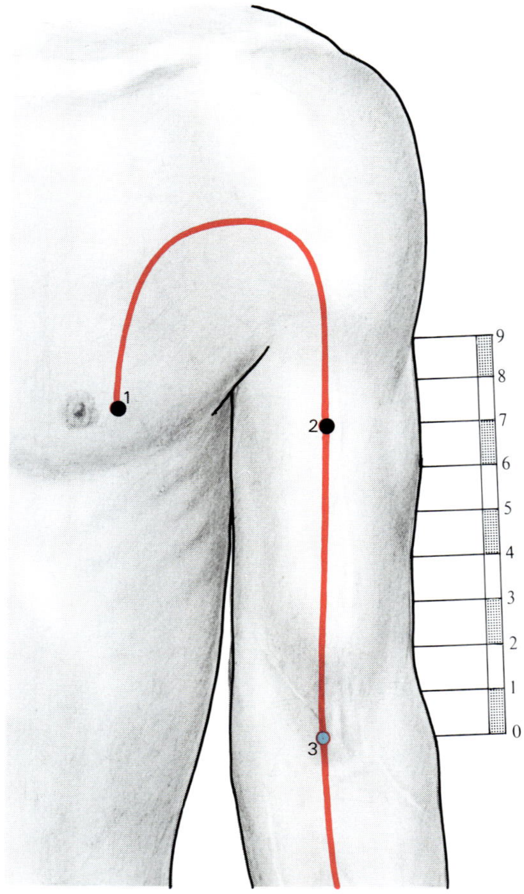
1
2
3
9
8
7
6
5
4
3
2
1
0

V **1** **Heavenly Pond** (Tienchih)

⊥ 3 Entry
△ 3–5
X Women

1 ACI lateral to the centre of the nipple.

Window of the Sky

V **2** **Heavenly Spring** (Tienchuan)

⊥ 5
△ 3

On the anterior surface of the arm, between the heads of the biceps, 7 ACI proximal to the flexure of the elbow.

V **3** **Crooked Marsh** (Chutse)

● ⊥ 3 Water
△ 3–5

On the crease of the elbow, in the major depression which is often lateral to the tendon of the biceps, though on some people this depression may be found medial to the tendon.

Point of Ho (Autumn)

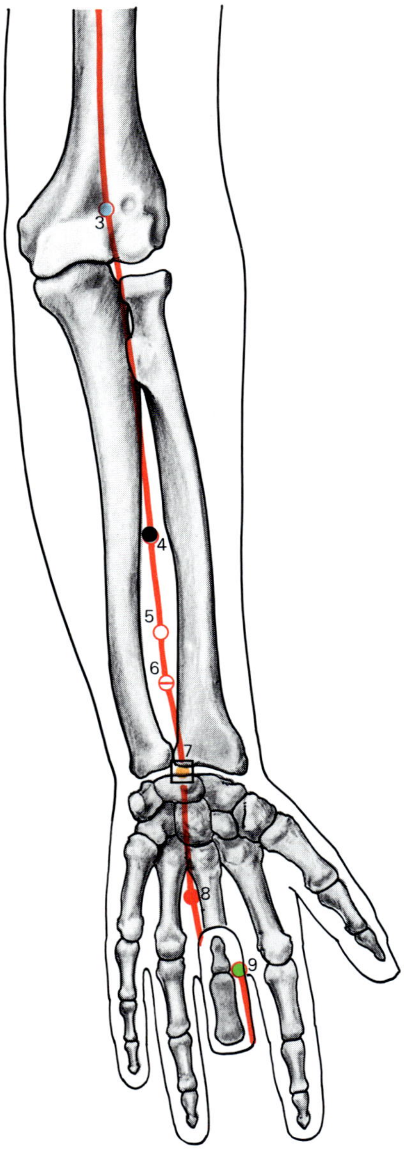
3
4
5
6
7
8
9

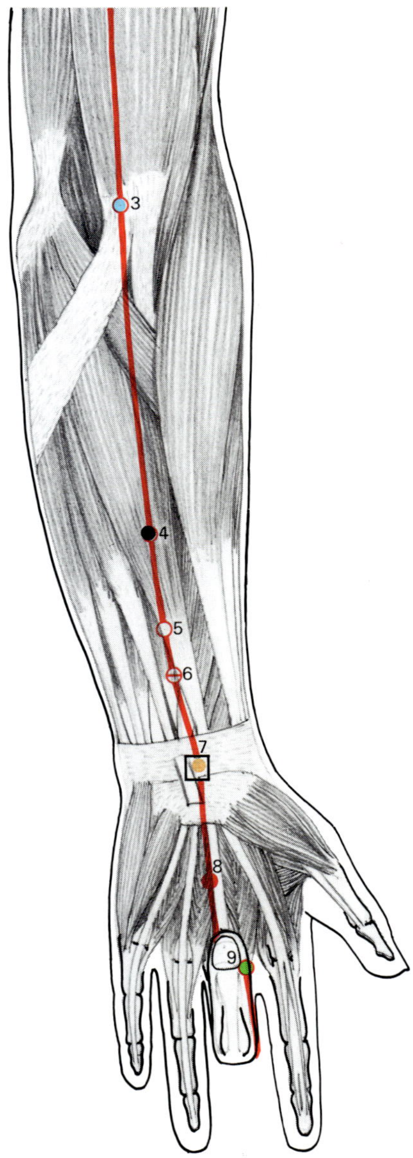
3
4
5
6
7
8
9

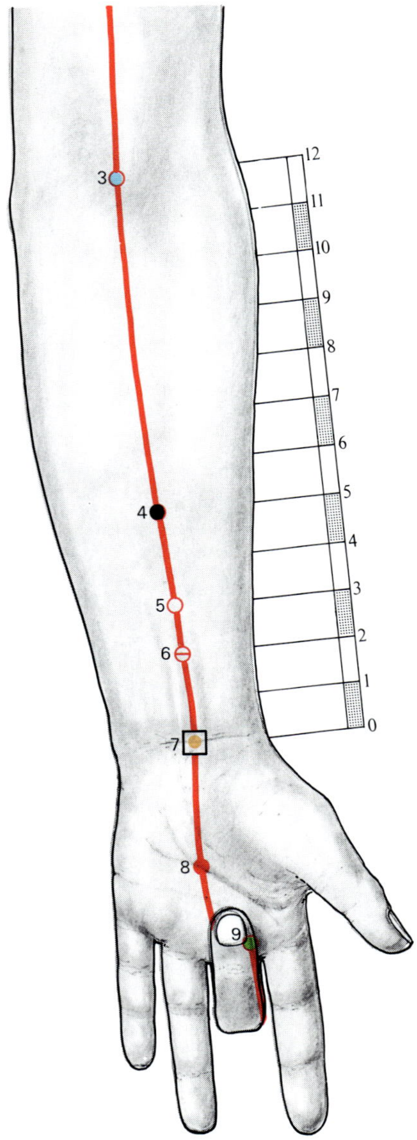
3
4
5
6
7
8
9
12
11
10
9
8
7
6
5
4
3
2
1
0

V **4** **Gate of Ch'i Reserve** (Hsimen)

⊥ 4
△ 5

On the anterior surface of the forearm, between the ulna and the radius, 5 ACI proximal to V 7.

V **5** **The Intermediary** (Chienshih)

○ ⊥ 3 Metal
△ 5

On the anterior surface of the forearm, between the ulna and the radius, 3 ACI proximal to V 7.

Point of Ching (late Summer)
Meeting Point of the three upper Yin meridians (I—V—IX)

V **6** **Inner Frontier Gate** (Neikuan)

⊖ ⊥ 3 Junction
△ 5
XP4

On the anterior surface of the forearm, between the tendons of the palmaris longus and the flexor carpi radialis, 2 ACI proximal to V 7.

Master Point of Yin Wei Mo
Coupled Point of Chong Mo

V **7** **Great Mound** (Taling)

● ⊥ 3 Earth
△ X Sedation
□ Source

In the middle of the crease of the flexure of the wrist, between the tendons of the palmaris longus and the flexor carpi radialis.

Point of Yu (Summer)

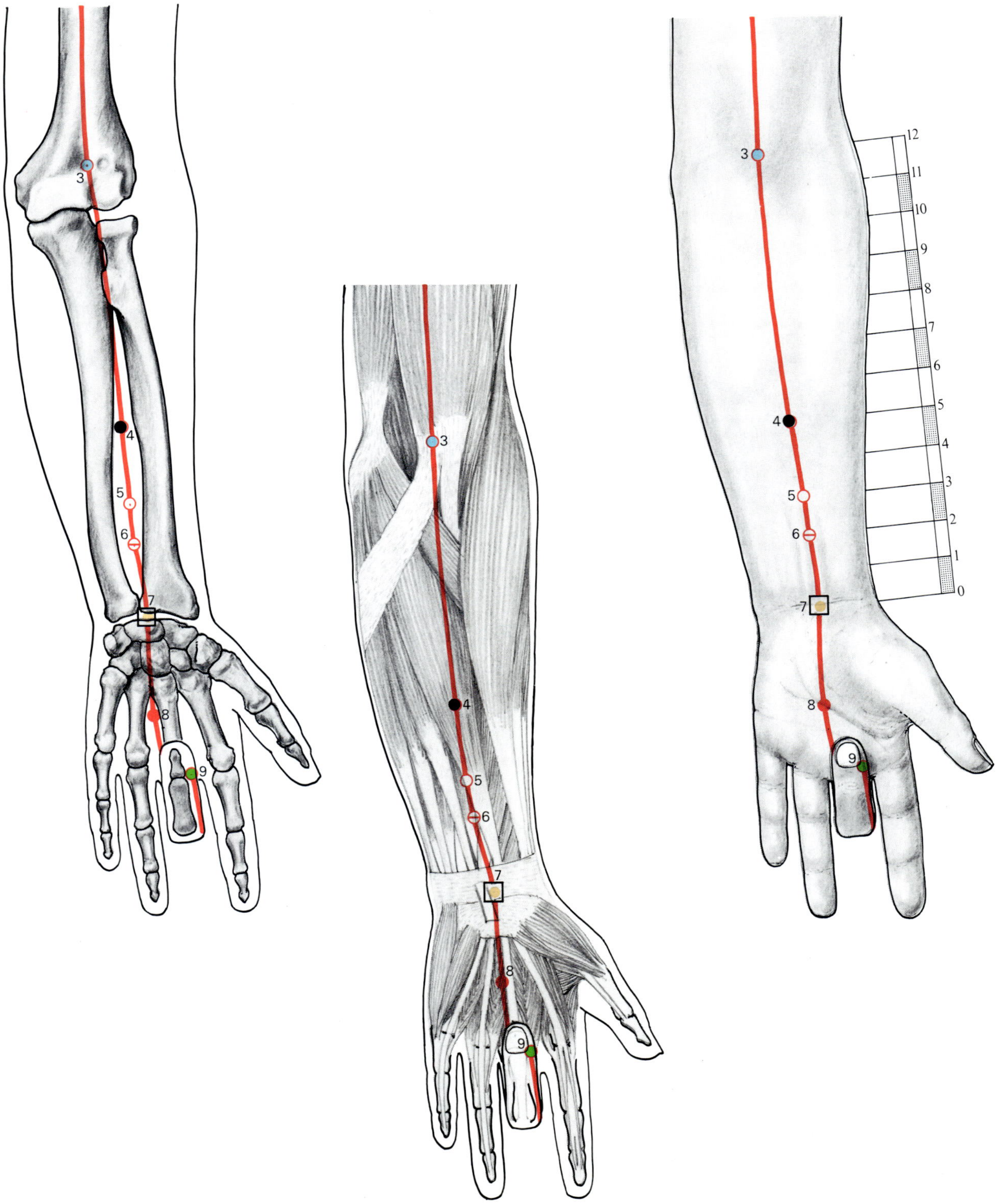
3
4
5
6
7
8
9
3
4
5
6
7
8
9
3
4
5
6
7
8
9
12
11
10
9
8
7
6
5
4
3
2
1
0

	V	**8**	**Palace Of Weariness** (Laokung)
●	⊥	2–3	Fire
	△	3	Horary 7 p.m.–9 p.m.
		XP3	Exit

On the palmar surface of the hand, between the third and fourth metacarpal bones, on the proximal transverse crease, or the 'head line' of the hand.

Point of Yung (Spring)

	V	**9**	**Rushing Into The Middle** (Chungchung)
●	⊥	1	Wood
	△	3	Tonification

Radial nail point of the middle finger.

Point of Cheng (Winter)
First Aid: anxiety, resuscitation

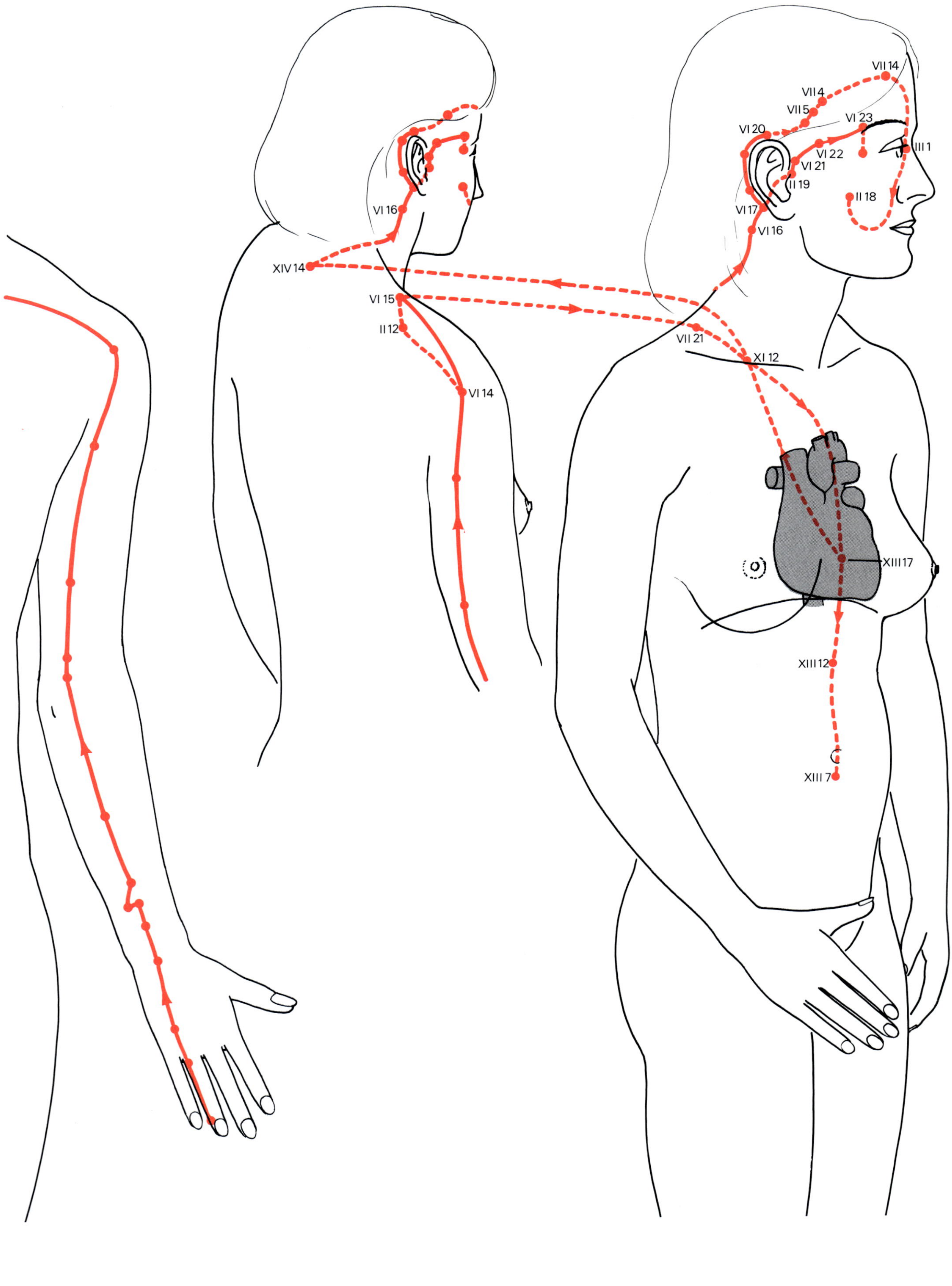
VII 14
VII 4
VII 5
VI 20
VI 23
VI 22
III 1
VI 21
II 19
II 18
VI 17
VI 16
VI 16
XIV 14
VI 15
II 12
VII 21
XI 12
VI 14
XIII 17
XIII 12
XIII 7

The three heater meridian begins as the superficial pathway at the ulnar nail point of the ring finger. It runs along the ulnar side of the ring finger to the dorsal surface of the hand, between the fourth and fifth metacarpal bones, across the wrist to travel up the posterior surface of the forearm between the ulna and the radius, to the elbow. It continues up the middle of the triceps and the posterior portion of the deltoid to the depression which is inferior to the acromion. The meridian then turns medially over the dorsal part of the shoulder to VI 15. From VI 14 a deep branch travels to II 12 and on to connect with VI 15. At VI 15 the deep pathway becomes deep, travels over the shoulder, crossing the gall bladder meridian at VII 21, to the supraclavicular fossa, at XI 12. It continues at a deep level inferiorly and medially through the region of the Upper Chou to reach the median line at XIII 17, and connects with the pericardium. It then penetrates the diaphragm and travels down the median line to the region of the Middle Chou at XIII 12, and from there to the region of the Lower Chou at XIII 7.

From XIII 17 a branch ascends to the supraclavicular fossa, at XI 12, travels posteriorly over the shoulder to the median line, below the seventh cervical vertebra, at XIV 14. The pathway returns to the shoulder where it becomes superficial again just below VI 16. It mounts the neck along the sternocleidomastoid to the mastoid process, and then follows the posterior border of the ear along the hair line to VI 20. Here the pathway again goes deep as it passes to the frontal bone, crossing VII 5 and VII 4, and travels over the forehead by VII 14 to the medial canthus of the eye, at III 1. It continues down the nasolabial groove to the mandible and curves on to the cheek to end at the lower border of the zygomatic arch, at II 18.

A branch leaves the superficial meridian at the mastoid process at VI 17, enters the auditory canal and emerges to become the superficial pathway anterior to the tragus of the ear, at II 19. From here it travels superiorly and medially through VI 21 to the exit point VI 22 and onto the lateral extremity of the eyebrow, the last point, VI 23, and then connects with the gall bladder meridian.

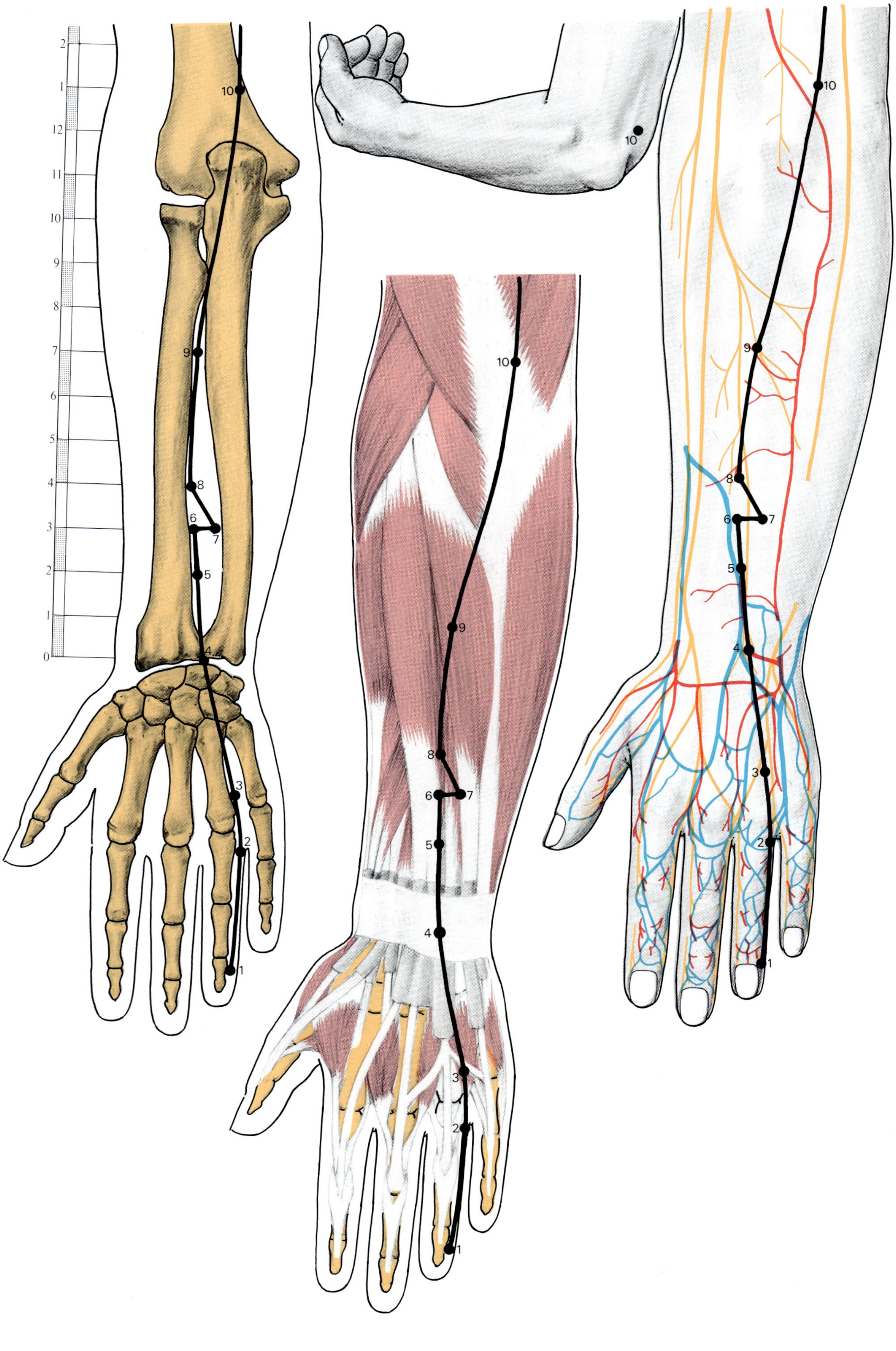

VI	1	Ulnar nail point of the ring finger.
VI	2	On the posteromedial surface of the ring finger, just distal to the base of the proximal phalanx.
VI	3	On the dorsal surface of the hand, immediately proximal to and on the ulnar side of the head of the fourth metacarpal bone.
VI	4	At the dorsal flexure of the wrist, proximal to the fourth metacarpal bone, in the hollow between the bones of the wrist (radius, ulna and lunate).
VI	5	On the posterior surface of the forearm, between the radius and the ulna, 2 ACI proximal to the flexure of the wrist.
VI	6	On the posterior surface of the forearm, between the radius and the ulna, 3 ACI proximal to the flexure of the wrist.
VI	7	On the posterior surface of the forearm, between the radius and the ulna, 3 ACI proximal to the flexure of the wrist, $\frac{1}{2}$ ACI medial to VI 6.
VI	8	On the posterior surface of the forearm, between the radius and the ulna, 4 ACI proximal to the flexure of the wrist.
VI	9	On the posterior surface of the forearm, between the radius and the ulna, 7 ACI proximal to the flexure of the wrist.
VI	10	On the posterior surface of the arm, 1 ACI proximal to the olecranon, slightly medial to the midline, in the depression formed when the elbow is semiflexed.

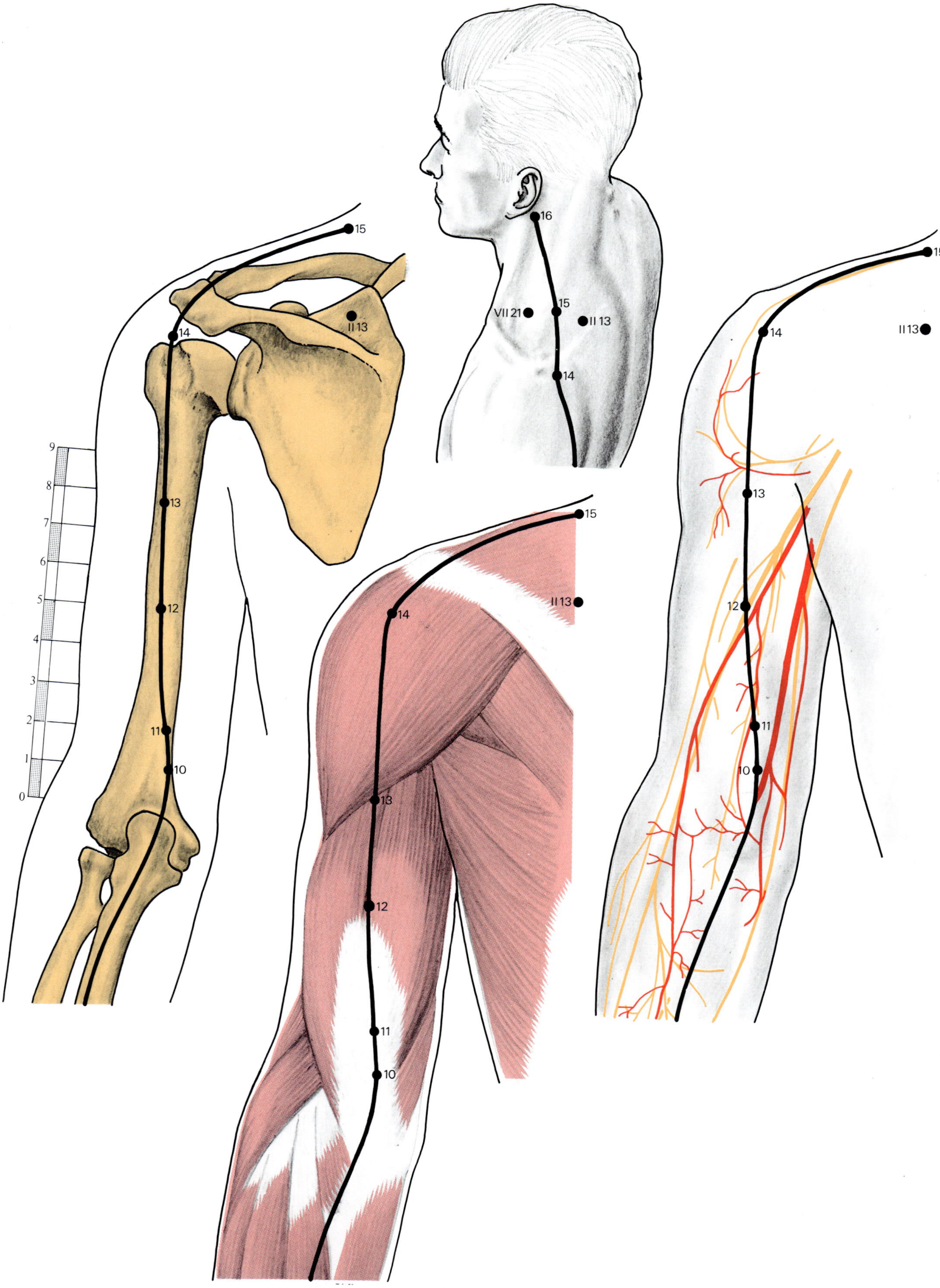
15
II 13
14
13
12
11
10
9
8
7
6
5
4
3
2
1
0
16
VII 21
15
II 13
14
15
14
II 13
13
12
11
10
15
II 13
14
13
12
11
10

VI **10** On the posterior surface of the arm, 1 ACI proximal to the olecranon, slightly medial to the midline, in the depression formed when the elbow is semiflexed.

VI **11** In the centre of the posterior surface of the arm, 2 ACI proximal to the tip of the elbow.

VI **12** In the centre of the posterior surface of the arm, 5 ACI proximal to the tip of the elbow.

VI **13** In the centre of the posterior surface of the arm, on the inferior border of the deltoid, on the triceps.

VI **14** On the posterior surface of the shoulder, posterior and inferior to the acromion, in the concavity formed between the acromion and the greater tubercle of the humerus when the arm is abducted.

VI **15** On the posterior surface of the shoulder, superior to the scapula, mid-way between the spinous process of the seventh cervical vertebra and the tip of the acromion, in line with VII 21 and II 13.

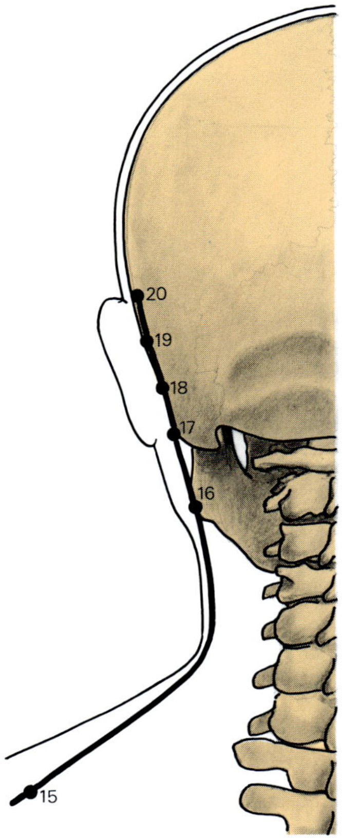
20
19
18
17
16
15

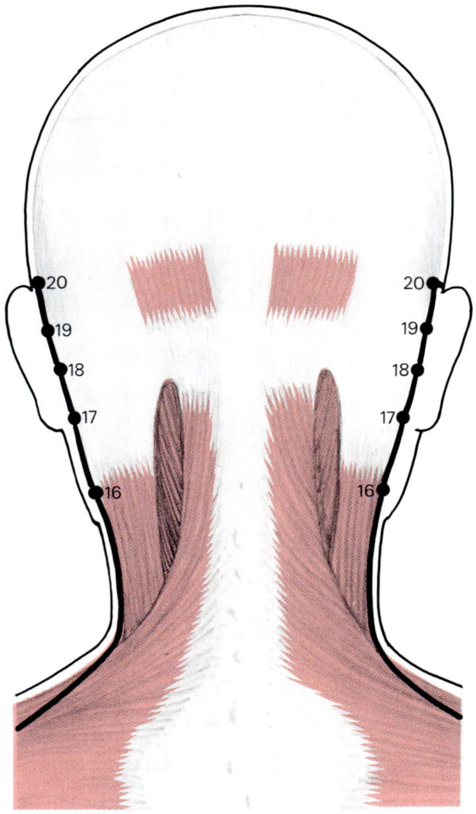
20
19
18
17
16
20
19
18
17
16

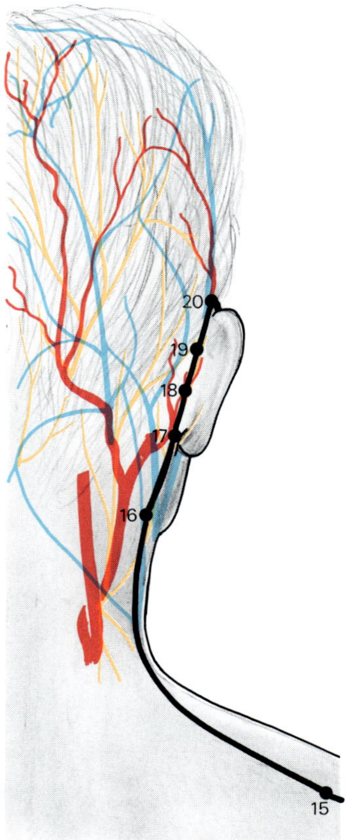
20
19
18
17
16
15

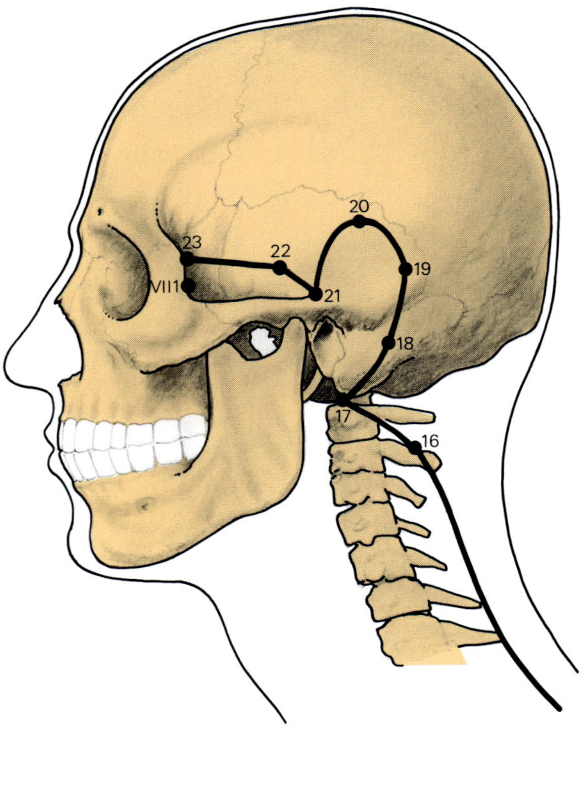
20
23
22
19
VII1
21
18
17
16

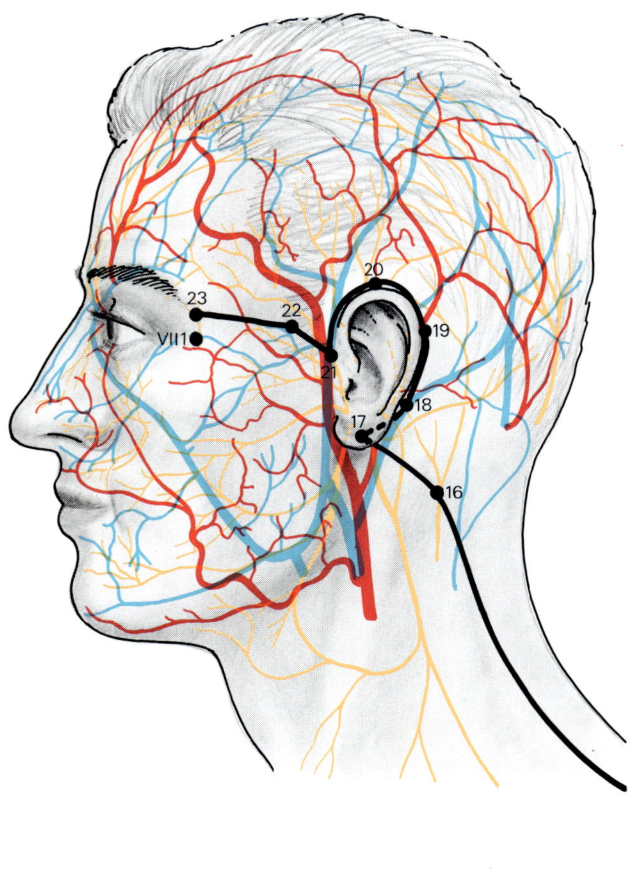
20
23
22
19
VII1
21
18
17
16

VI	**15**	On the posterior surface of the shoulder, superior to the scapula, mid-way between the spinous process of the seventh cervical vertebra and the tip of the acromion, in line with VII 21 and II 13.
VI	**16**	Posterior and inferior to the mastoid process, on the posterior border of the sternocleidomastoid.
VI	**17**	Posterior to the ear lobe, in the depression between the mastoid process and the mandible, adjacent to the cartilage of the external auditory canal.
VI	**18**	On the curve of the hair line, posterior to the ear, one third of the distance from the base to the apex of the pinna.
VI	**19**	On the curve of the hair line, posterior to the ear, two thirds of the distance from the base to the apex of the pinna.
VI	**20**	On the hairline, immediately superior to the level of the apex of the pinna.
VI	**21**	Anterior to the superior edge of the tragus of the ear, in the depression formed when the mouth is open.
VI	**22**	Anterior to the ear, on the hair line, on a level with the superior border of the root of the pinna.
VI	**23**	At the lateral end of the eyebrow, in the depression directly superior to VII 1.

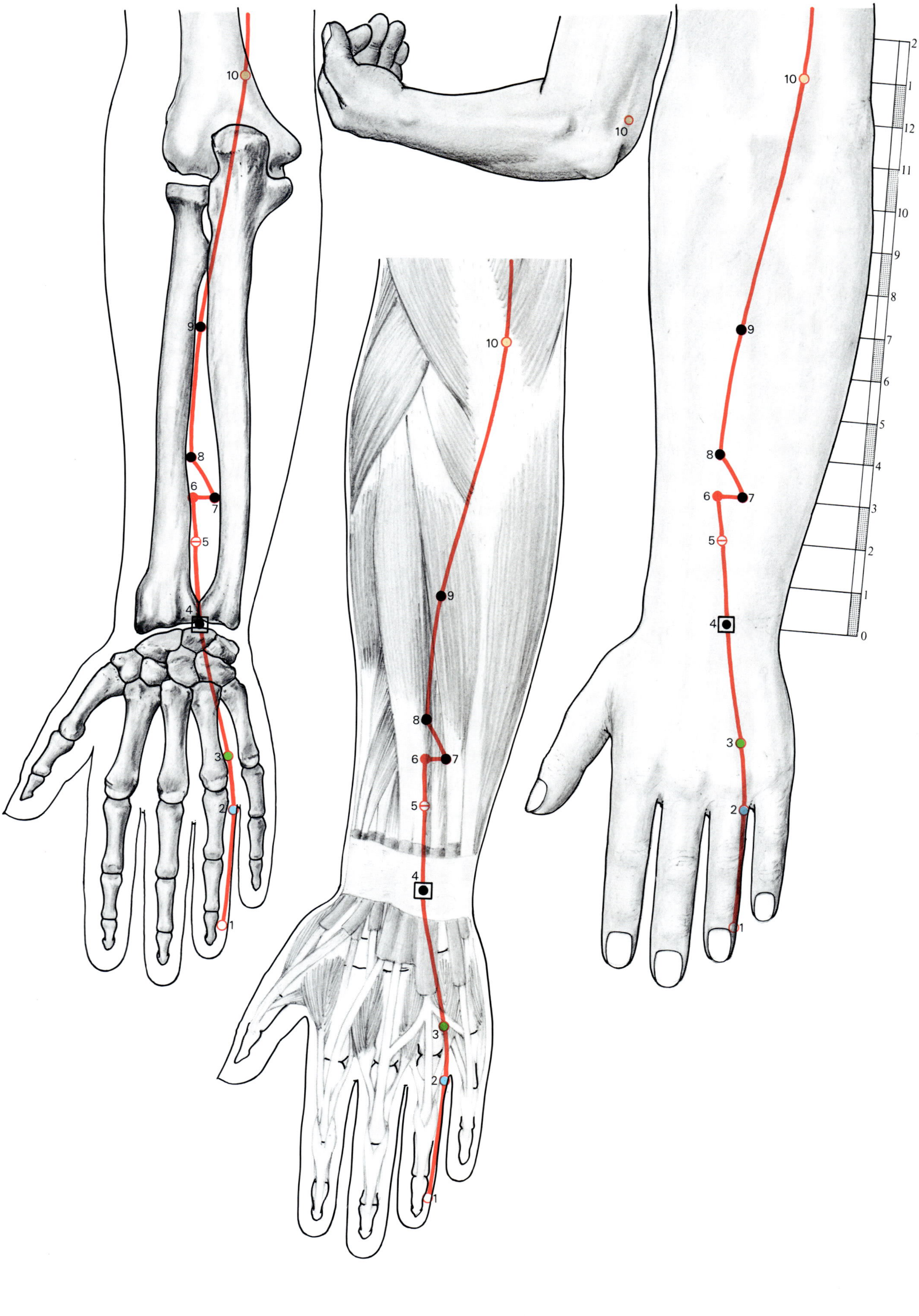

VI **1** **Rushing The Frontier Gate** (Kuanchung)

○ ⊥ 1 Metal
△ 3 Entry

Ulnar nail point of the ring finger

Point of Cheng (Winter)

VI **2** **Fluid Secretion Gate** (Yehmen)

● ⊥ 1 Water
△ 3

On the posteromedial surface of the ring finger, just distal to the base of the proximal phalanx.

Point of Yung (Spring)

VI **3** **Middle Islet** (Chungchu)

● ⊥ 3 Wood
△ 3–5 Tonification

On the dorsal surface of the hand, immediately proximal to and on the ulnar side of the head of the fourth metacarpal bone.

Point of Yu (Summer)
First Aid: exhaustion

VI **4** **Yang Pond** (Yangchih)

□ ⊥ 3 Source
△ X
XP3

At the dorsal flexure of the wrist, proximal to the fourth metacarpal bone, in the hollow between the bones of the wrist (radius, ulna and lunate).

First Aid: earache

VI **5** **Outer Frontier Gate** (Waikuan)

⊖ ⊥ 5 Junction
△ 3–7

On the posterior surface of the forearm, between the radius and the ulna, 2 ACI proximal to the flexure of the wrist.

Master Point of Yang Wei Mo
Coupled Point of Dai Mo

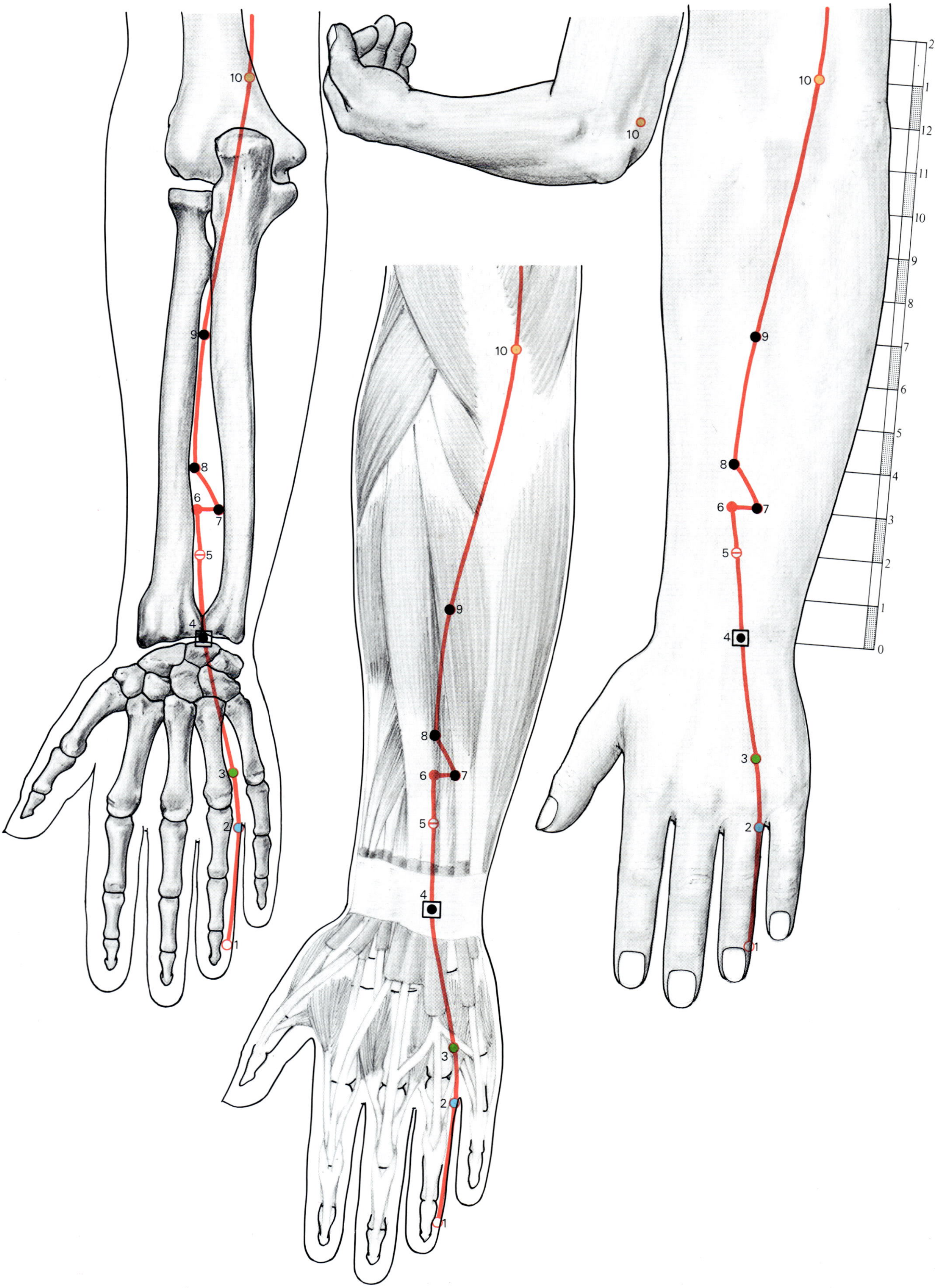
10
9
8
6
7
5
4
3
2
1

VI **6** **Branch Ditch** (Chihkou)

⊥ 5 Fire
△ 5 Horary 9 p.m.–11 p.m.

On the posterior surface of the forearm, between the radius and the ulna, 3 ACI proximal to the flexure of the wrist.

Point of Ching (late Summer)

VI **7** **Assembly Of Ancestors** (Huitsung)

⊥ 3
△ 5–7

On the posterior surface of the forearm, between the radius and the ulna, 3 ACI proximal to the flexure of the wrist. $\frac{1}{2}$ ACI medial to VI 6.

VI **8** **Three Yang Junction** (Sanyanglo)

⊥ X
△ 7

On the posterior surface of the forearm, between the radius and the ulna, 4 ACI proximal to the flexure of the wrist.

Meeting Point of the three upper Yang meridians (II—VI—X)

VI **9** **Fourth Gutter** (Szutu)

⊥ 6
△ 3–7

On the posterior surface of the forearm, between the radius and the ulna, 7 ACI proximal to the flexure of the wrist.

VI **10** **Heavenly Well** (Tienching)

⊥ 3–5 Earth
△ 3–5 Sedation
XP4

On the posterior surface of the arm, 1 ACI proximal to the olecranon, slightly medial to the midline, in the depression formed when the elbow is semiflexed.

Point of Ho (Autumn)

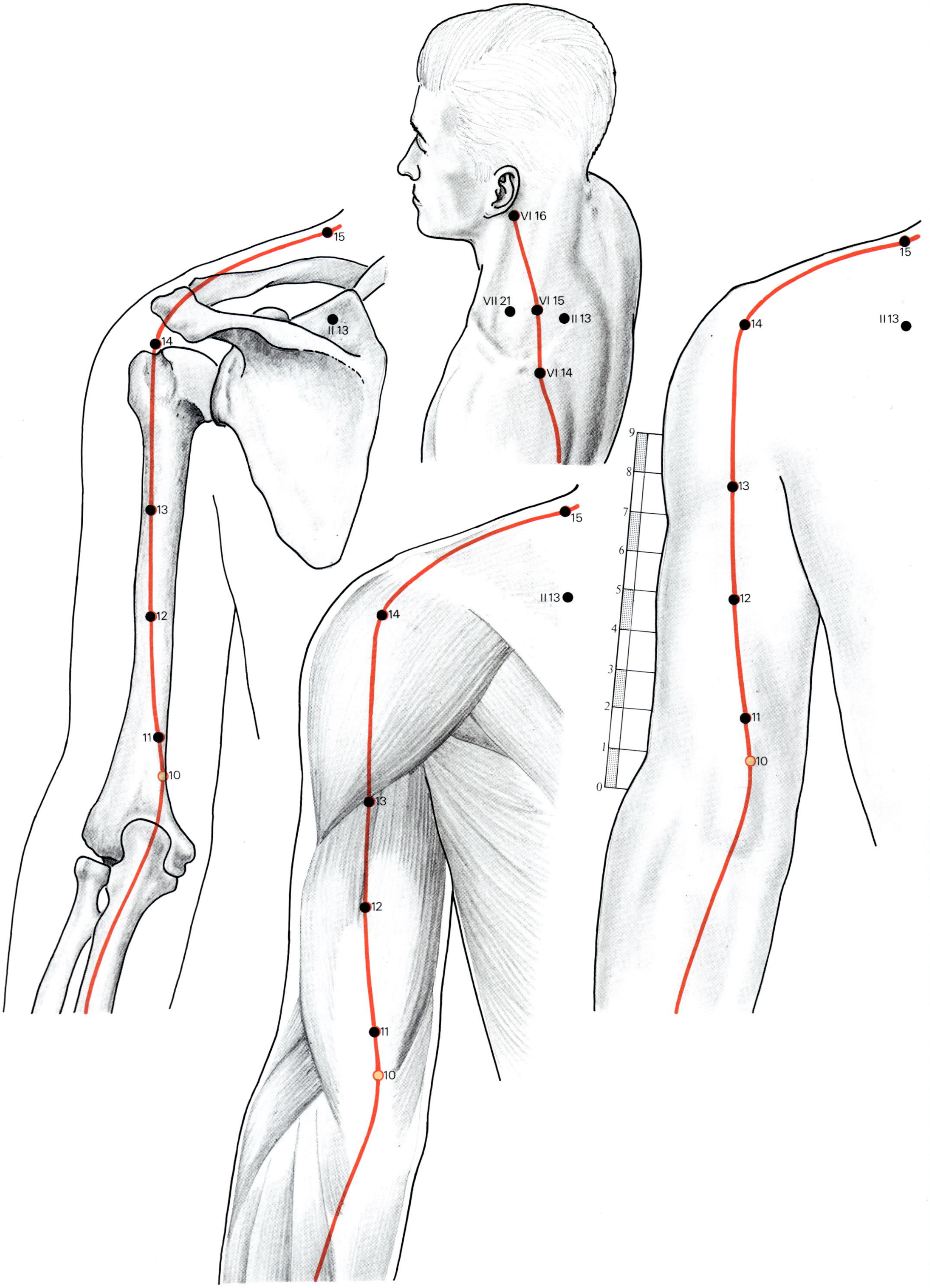
15
II 13
14
13
12
11
10
VI 16
VII 21
VI 15
II 13
VI 14
15
II 13
14
13
12
11
10
9
8
7
6
5
4
3
2
1
0
15
II13
14
13
12
11
10

VI **11** **Pure Cold Abyss** (Chinglengyuan)

⊥ 3
△ 3–7

In the centre of the posterior surface of the arm, 2 ACI proximal to the tip of the elbow.

VI **12** **Relax And Joy** (Hsiaolo)

⊥ 5
△ 3–7

In the centre of the posterior surface of the arm, 5 ACI proximal to the tip of the elbow.

VI **13** **Shoulder Meeting** (Naohui)

⊥ 3–7
△ 5–15

In the centre of the posterior surface of the arm, on the inferior border of the deltoid, on the triceps.

VI **14** **Shoulder Bone** (Chienliao)

⊥ 7
△ 5–7

On the posterior surface of the shoulder, posterior and inferior to the acromion, in the concavity formed between the acromion and the greater tubercle of the humerus when the arm is abducted.

VI **15** **Heavenly Bone** (Tienliao)

⊥ 3–8
△ 5–7

On the posterior surface of the shoulder, superior to the scapula, mid-way between the spinous process of the seventh cervical vertebra and the tip of the acromion, in line with VII 21 and II 13.

Point of Yang Wei Mo
First Aid: colds

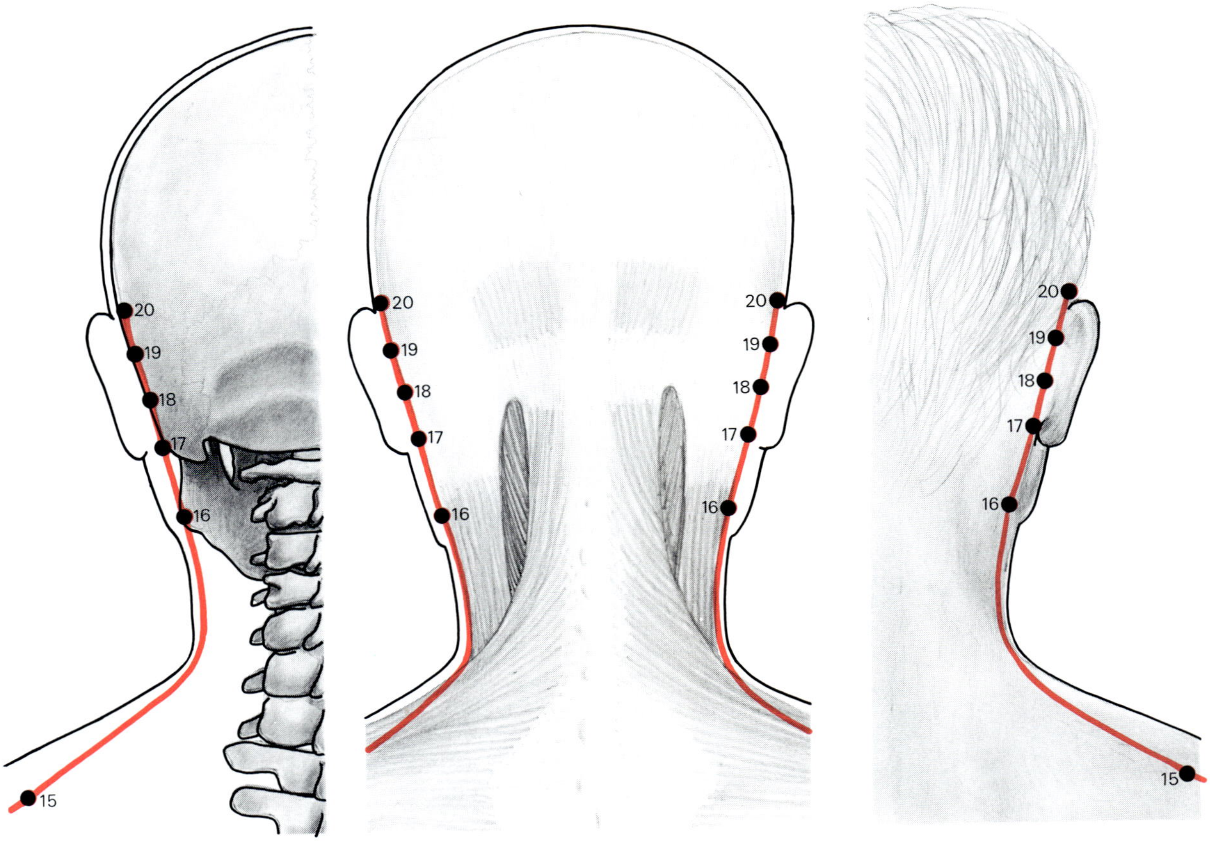
20
19
18
17
16
15
20
19
18
17
16
20
19
18
17
16
20
19
18
17
16
15

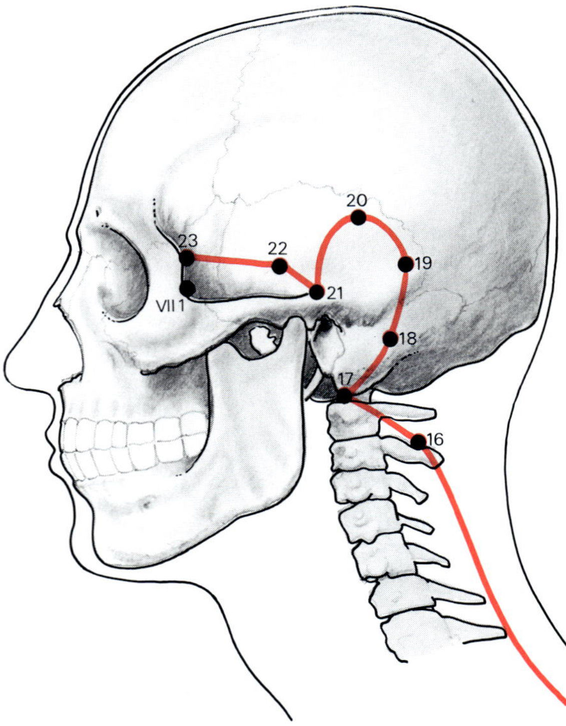
20
23
22
19
21
VII1
18
17
16

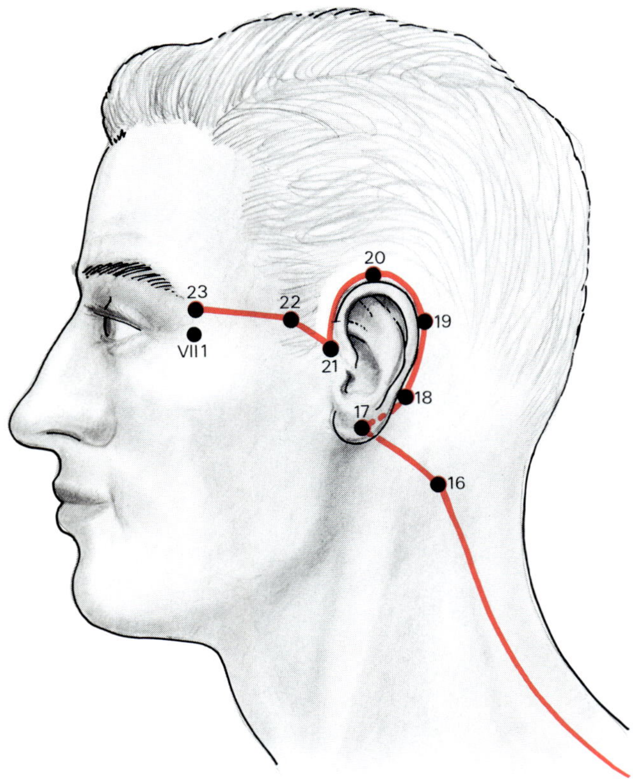
20
23
22
19
VII1
21
18
17
16

VI **16** **Heavenly Window** (Tienyu)

⊥ 3–5
△ X

Posterior and inferior to the mastoid process, on the posterior border of the sternocleidomastoid.

Window of the Sky

VI **17** **Wind Screen** (Yifeng)

⊥ 3
△ 3–7

Posterior to the ear lobe, in the depression between the mastoid process and the mandible, adjacent to the cartilage of the external auditory canal.

VI **18** **Feeding Meridians** (Chimo)

⊥ 1
△ X

On the curve of the hair line, posterior to the ear, one third of the distance from the base to the apex of the pinna.

VI **19** **Skull Breathing** (Luhsi)

⊥ X
△ 3–7

On the curve of the hair line, posterior to the ear, two thirds of the distance from the base to the apex of the pinna.

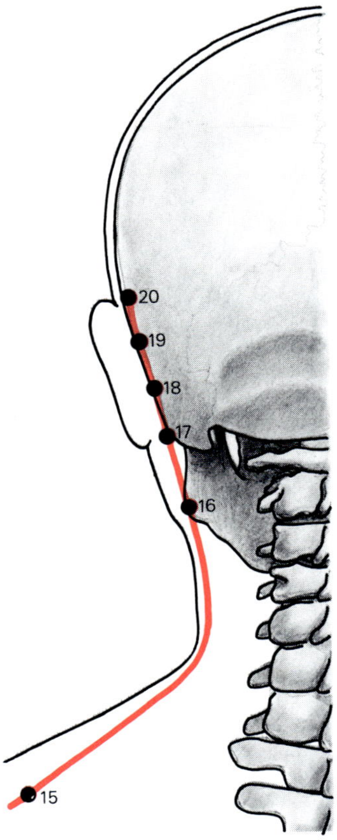
20
19
18
17
16
15

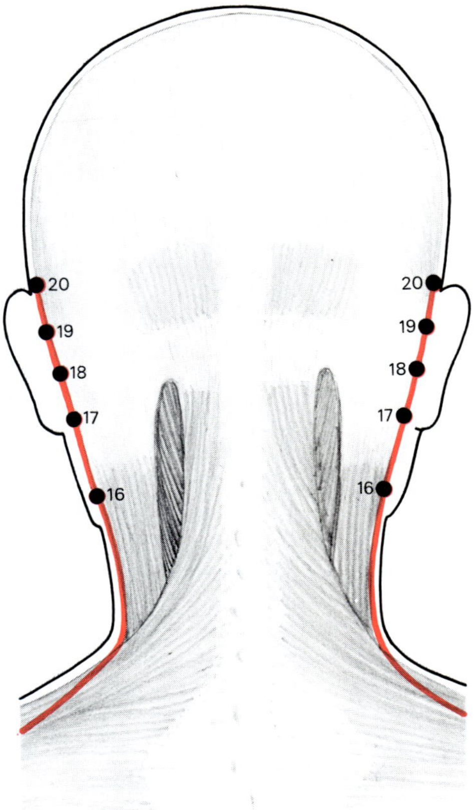
20
19
18
17
16
20
19
18
17
16

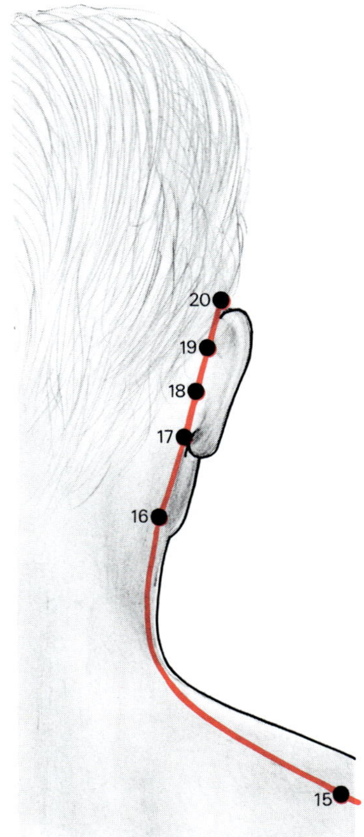
20
19
18
17
16
15

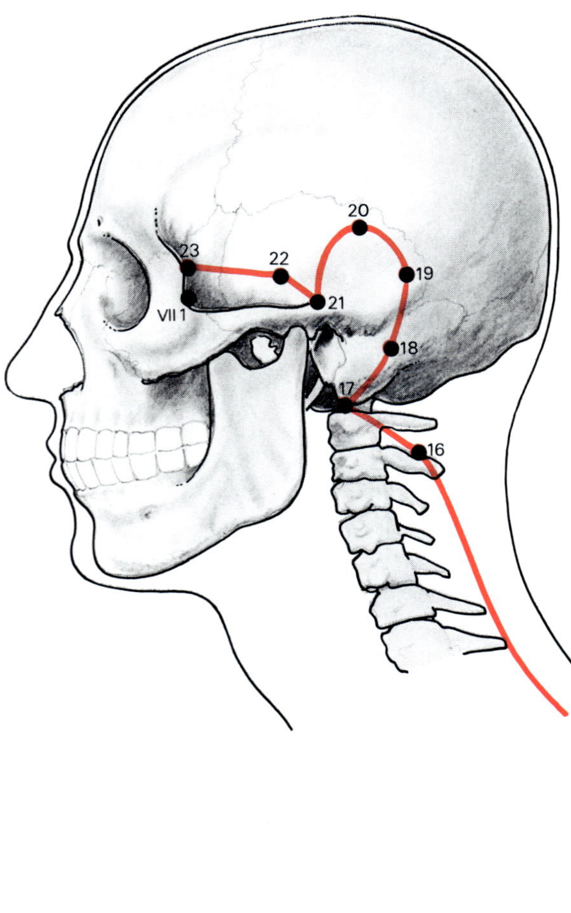
20
23
22
19
VII 1
21
18
17
16

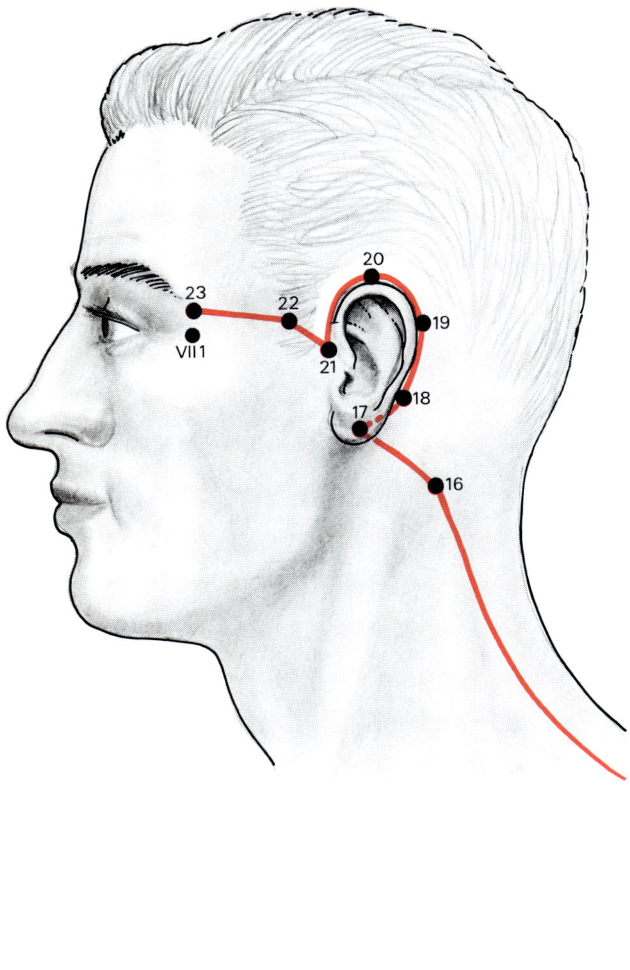
20
23
22
19
VII 1
21
18
17
16

VI **20** **Small Angle Of Ear** (Chuehsun)

⊥ X
△ 3–7

On the hair line, immediately superior to the level of the apex of the pinna.

VI **21** **Ear Gate** (Erhmen)

⊥ 3
△ 3–7

Anterior to the superior edge of the tragus of the ear, in the depression formed when the mouth is open.

VI **22** **Harmony Bone** (Holiao)

⊥ 3–7 Exit
△ 3–5

Anterior to the ear, on the hair line, on a level with the superior border of the root of the pinna.

VI **23** **Silk Bamboo Hollow** (Szuchukung)

⊥ 3
△ X

At the lateral end of the eyebrow, in the depression directly superior to VII 1.

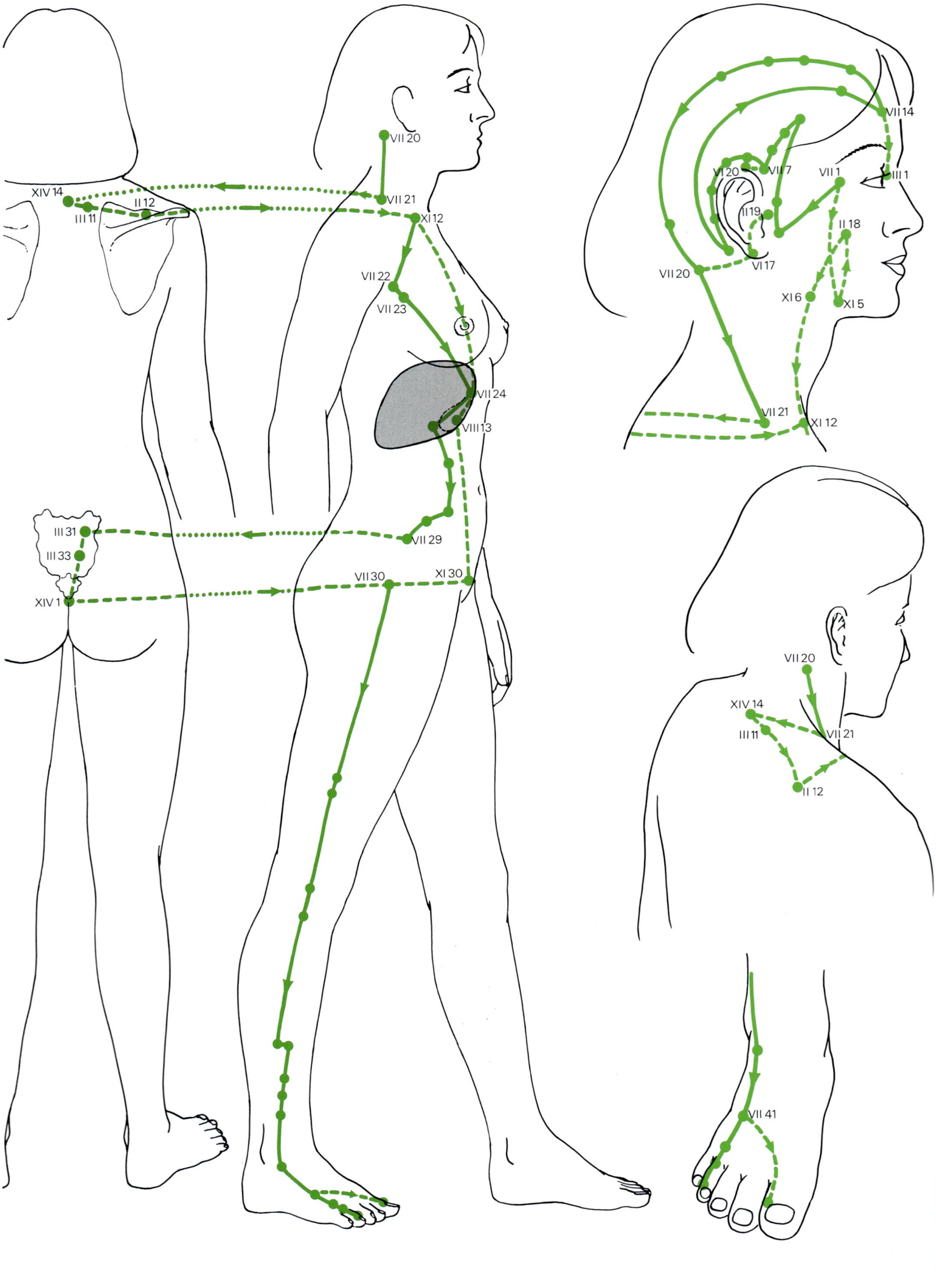
VII 20
VII 21
XIV 14
II 12
III 11
XI 12
VII 22
VII 23
VII 24
VIII 13
III 31
III 33
VII 29
VII 30
XI 30
XIV 1
VII 14
VI 20
VI 7
VII 1
III 1
II 19
II 18
VI 17
XI 6
XI 5
VII 41

The gall bladder superficial pathway begins at the level of the lateral canthus of the eye, at the entry point, VII 1. It runs inferiorly and laterally to a point anterior to the ear lobe, then ascends the temple to the fronto-parietal fissure. Here it curves down posterior to the ear, to the mastoid process. It returns forwards over the head to the superciliary arch of the forehead, VII 14. Again it turns posteriorly and travels over the head to the occipital region, down the back of the neck along the border of the trapezius to the shoulder, VII 21.

From VII 21 a deep branch goes posteriorly across the shoulder to the median line, inferior to the seventh cervical vertebra, XIV 14; then laterally and inferiorly to III 11, and finally descends laterally, via II 12, to the shoulder and the supraclavicular fossa, at XI 12. Here the meridian becomes superficial again.

There are four deep branches on the head: the first leaves VII 1, descends the cheek to the mandible, at XI 5, ascends to the lower border of the cheek bone, II 18, descends laterally to the angle of the jaw, at XI 6, and down the lateral side of the neck to the supraclavicular fossa, at XI 12. The second branch leaves VII 7 at the superior point of the ear and joins VI 20, which lies just posterior to VII 7. The third branch leaves VII 14 on the forehead and descends to the medial canthus of the eye, to III 1. The fourth branch leaves VII 20, goes anteriorly to VI 17 at the mastoid process, enters the ear and emerges in front of the ear, at II 19.

Both a superficial and a deep pathway descend the body from the supraclavicular fossa. The superficial pathway descends laterally to the fourth intercostal space, in the anterior axillary line at VII 22 then via VII 23 moves medially to the seventh intercostal space, in the line of the nipple, at VII 24; it then turns again laterally to reach the tip of the twelfth rib. It then travels to the anterior superior iliac spine and from there descends the hip laterally to VII 29.

Here the pathway becomes deep as it passes posteriorly and medially to descend the sacrum, via III 31 and III 33, to the tip of the coccyx, at XIV 1, and returns to join the superficial pathway at the depression posterior to the greater trochanter, at VII 30.

The deep pathway descends from the supraclavicular fossa to go through the thorax, passing the superficial pathway at VII 24, penetrates the diaphragm, connects to VIII 13, and then enters the liver and the gall bladder. From there it descends to the superior edge of the pubic bone, at XI 30, turns laterally, penetrating the pelvis, and joins the superficial pathway at the depression posterior to the greater trochanter, at VII 30. The meridian is now single and superficial as it descends the lateral border of the thigh to the lateral side of the knee. It runs down the lateral side of the calf, anterior to the fibula, passes anterior to the lateral malleolus, over the dorsal surface of the foot to run between the fourth and fifth metatarsal bones to end at its last point, the lateral nail point of the fourth toe.

A deep branch extends from the angle between the fourth and fifth metatarsal bones at the exit point, VII 41, travels to the cleft between the first and second metatarsal bones and on to the dorsal surface of the big toe. Here it connects with the liver meridian.

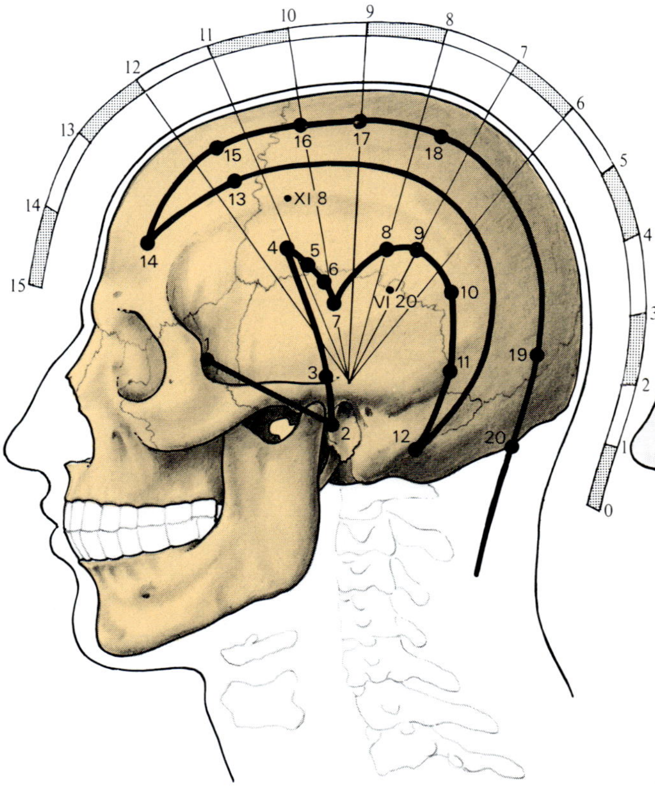

15
16
17
18
14
13
XI 8
4
5
6
7
8
9
VI 20
10
1
3
2
11
12
19
20

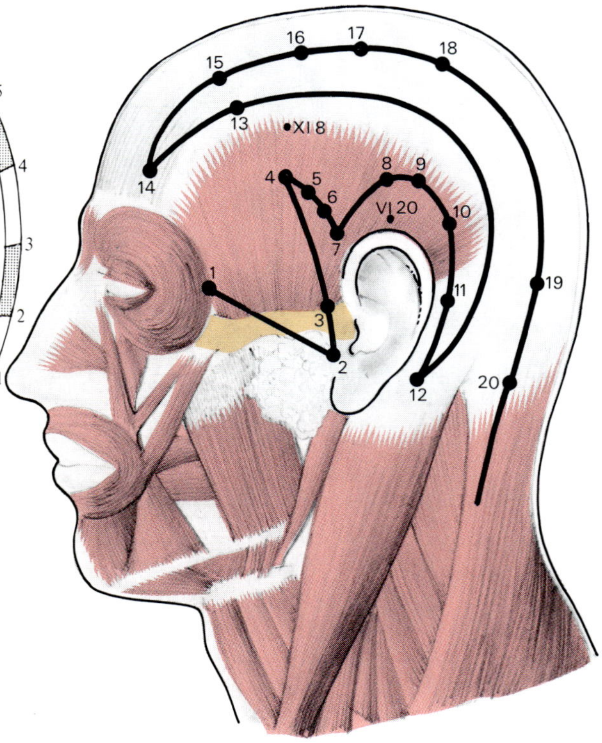

15
16
17
18
14
13
XI 8
4
5
6
7
8
9
VI 20
10
1
3
2
11
12
19
20

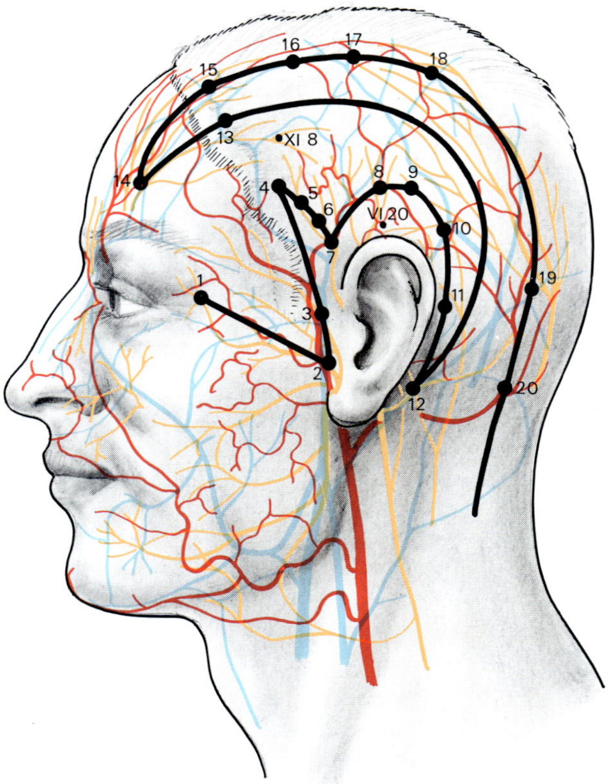

15
16
17
18
14
13
XI 8
4
5
6
7
8
9
VI 20
10
1
3
2
11
12
19
20

VII 1 In the depression just lateral to the orbital rim, at the level of the lateral canthus.

VII 2 On the posterior margin of the condyle of the mandible, anterior to the inferior border of the tragus. When the mouth is opened, a depression appears at this point.

VII 3 Anterior to the ear, immediately superior to the zygomatic arch, superior to VII 2.

VII 4 On the temple, $\frac{1}{2}$ ACI posterior to the natural hair line, 1 ACI inferior to XI 8.

VII 5 On the temple, $\frac{1}{2}$ ACI posterior to the natural hair line, one third of the distance from VII 4 to VII 7.

VII 6 On the temple, $\frac{1}{2}$ ACI posterior to the natural hair line, two thirds of the distance from VII 4 to VII 7.

VII 7 On the temple, $\frac{1}{2}$ ACI posterior to the natural hair line, at the level of the apex of the pinna, approximately 1 ACI anterior to and slightly inferior to VI 20.

VII 8 On the head, 1 ACI directly superior to VI 20.

VII 9 On the head, $\frac{1}{2}$ ACI posterior to VII 8 and 2 ACI superior to the natural hair line.

VII 10 On the head, posterior and slightly superior to the ear, 1 ACI posterior to the natural hair line, at the level of the superior edge of the root of the ear.

VII 11 On the head, posterior to the ear, mid-way between VII 10 and VII 12.

VII 12 On the head, within the angle formed by the posterior border of the mastoid process and the inferior edge of the occipital bone when the head is tilted forwards.

VII 13 On the head, $\frac{1}{2}$ ACI posterior to the natural hair line, on a vertical line superior to the lateral canthus.

VII 14 On the forehead, 1 ACI superior to the supra-orbital notch, which is found in the middle of the eyebrow.

VII 15 On the head, $\frac{1}{2}$ ACI posterior to the natural hair line, on a vertical line superior to the middle of the pupil when the eye is looking straight ahead.

VII 16 On the head, $1\frac{1}{2}$ ACI posterior to VII 15.

VII 17 On the head, 1 ACI posterior to VII 16.

VII 18 On the head, $1\frac{1}{2}$ ACI posterior to VII 17.

VII 19 On the head, lateral to the external occipital protruberance, $1\frac{1}{2}$ ACI superior to VII 20.

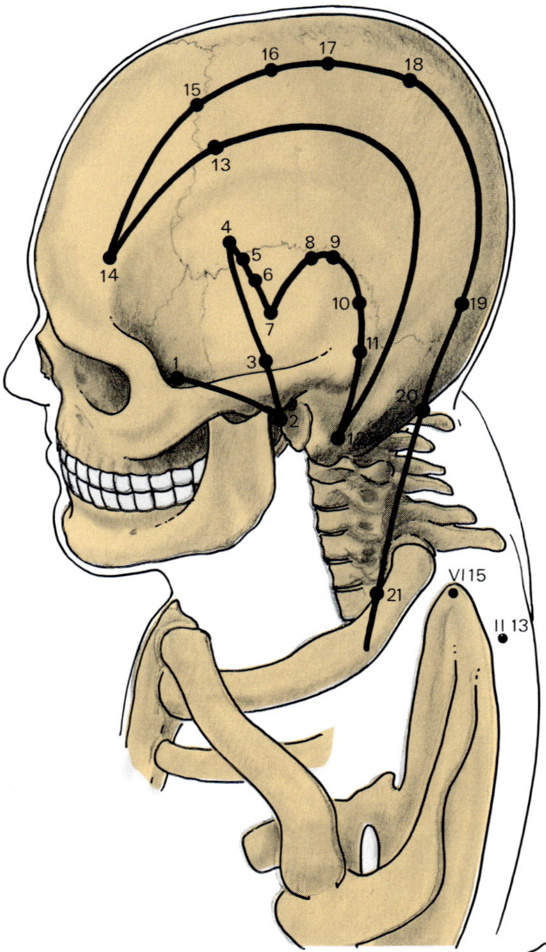
1
2
3
4
5
6
7
8
9
10
11
12
13
14
15
16
17
18
19
20
21
VI 15
II 13

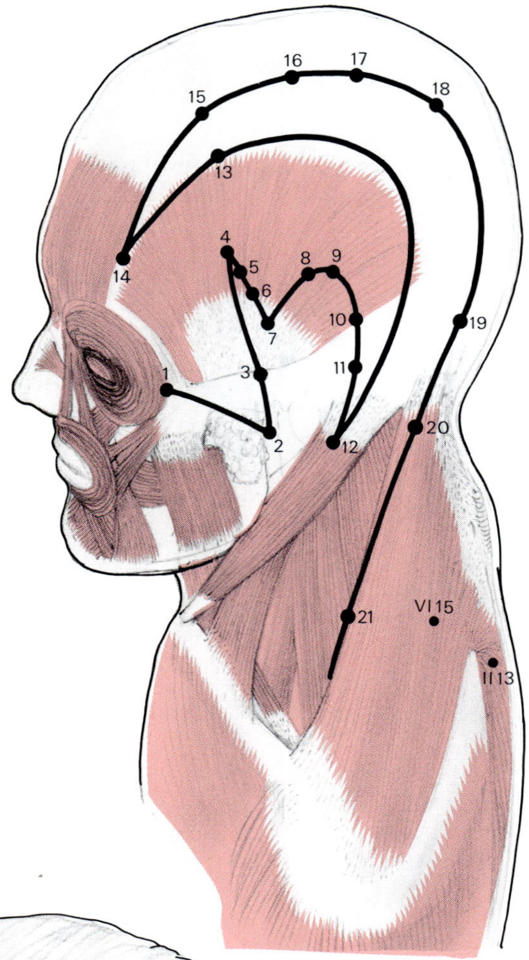
1
2
3
4
5
6
7
8
9
10
11
12
13
14
15
16
17
18
19
20
21
VI 15
II 13

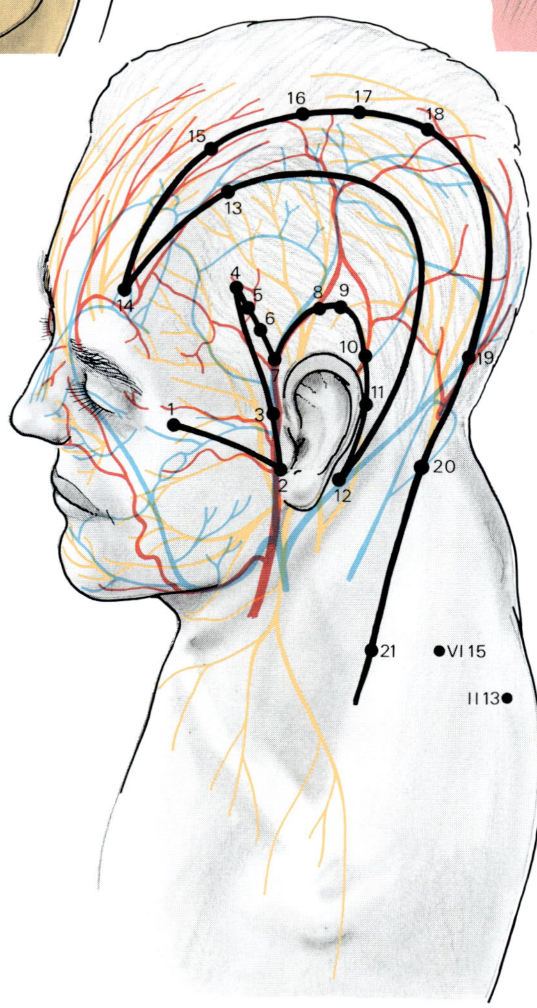
1
2
3
4
5
6
7
8
9
10
11
12
13
14
15
16
17
18
19
20
21
VI 15
II 13

VII 20 On the head, inferior to the occipital bone, in the centre of the depression between the external occipital protruberance and the mastoid process, superior to the natural hair line and lateral to the border of the trapezius.

VII 21 On the shoulder, mid-way between the spinous process of the seventh cervical vertebra and the lateral tip of the clavicle, upon the anterior border of the trapezius, in line with VI 15 and II 13.

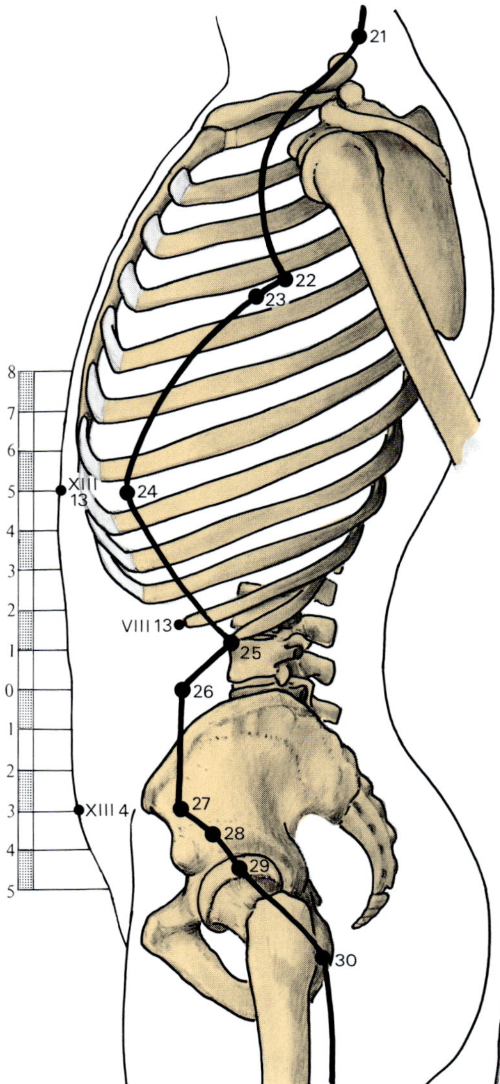
21
22
23
24
25
26
27
28
29
30
XIII 13
VIII 13
XIII 4
8
7
6
5
4
3
2
1
0
1
2
3
4
5

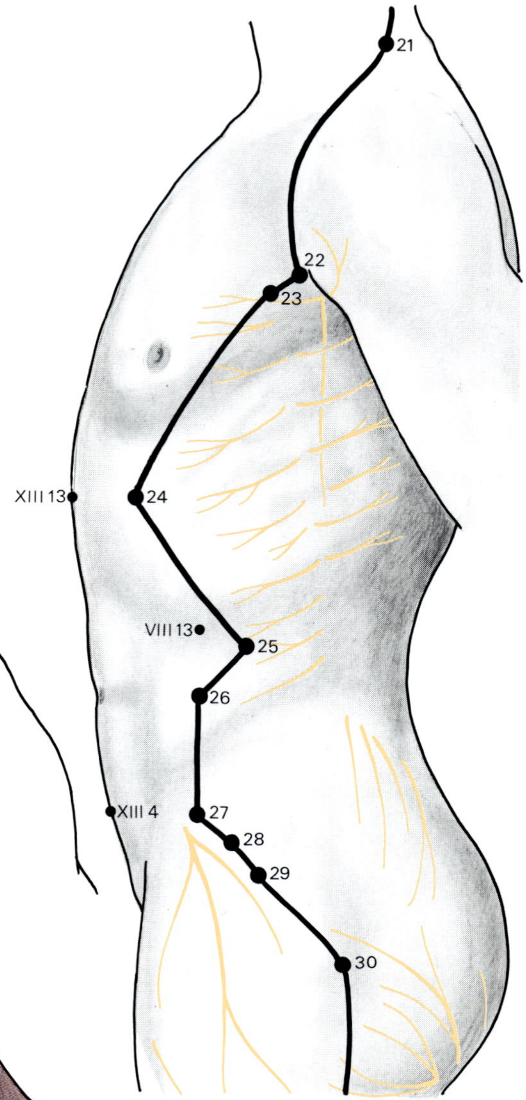
21
22
23
24
25
26
27
28
29
30
XIII 13
VIII 13
XIII 4

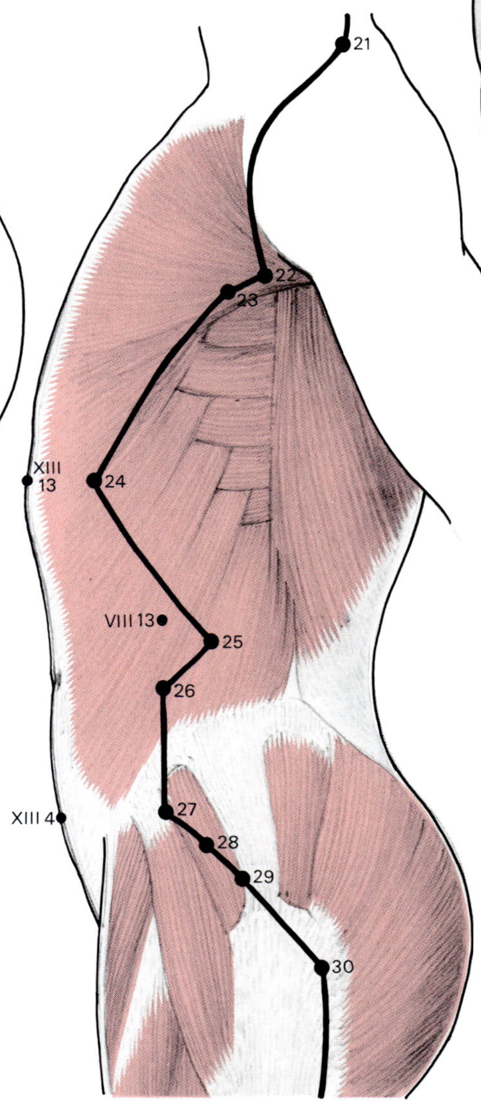
21
22
23
24
25
26
27
28
29
30
XIII 13
VIII 13
XIII 4

VII 21 On the shoulder, mid-way between the spinous process of the seventh cervical vertebra and the lateral tip of the clavicle, upon the anterior border of the trapezius, in line with VI 15 and II 13.

VII 22 In the fourth intercostal space, on the mid-axillary line.

VII 23 In the fourth intercostal space, 1 ACI medial to VII 22.

VII 24 In the seventh intercostal space, on the paramedian nipple line, approximately level with XIII 13.

VII 25 On the lateral surface of the abdomen, at the anterior tip of the twelfth rib.

VII 26 On the lateral surface of the abdomen, at the intersection of the vertical line passing through VIII 13 (or the anterior tip of the eleventh rib), and a horizontal line passing through the centre of the umbilicus.

VII 27 On the hip, inferior and slightly posterior to the anterior superior iliac spine, on a level with XIII 4.

VII 28 On the hip, mid-way between VII 27 and VII 29.

VII 29 On the hip, mid-way between the anterior superior iliac spine and the prominence of the greater trochanter.

VII 30 On the lateral surface of the hip, posterior to the prominence of the greater trochanter.

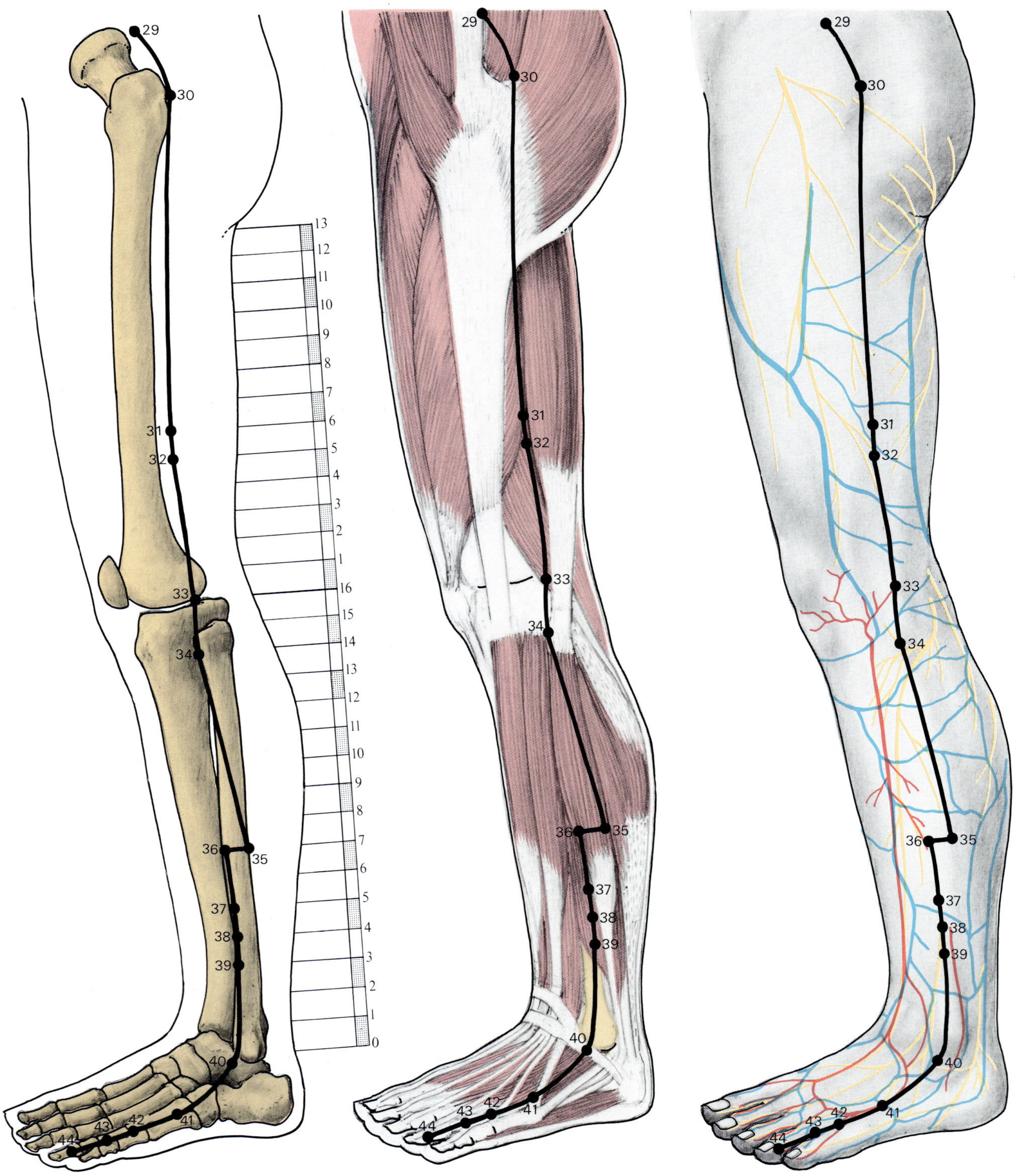
29
30
31
32
33
34
35
36
37
38
39
40
41
42
43
44
13
12
11
10
9
8
7
6
5
4
3
2
1
16
15
14
13
12
11
10
9
8
7
6
5
4
3
2
1
0

VII 29 On the hip, mid-way between the anterior superior iliac spine and the prominence of the greater trochanter.

VII 30 On the lateral surface of the hip, posterior to the prominence of the greater trochanter.

VII 31 On the lateral surface of the thigh, 6 ACI proximal to the flexure of the knee, between the vastus lateralis and the biceps femoris.

VII 32 On the lateral surface of the thigh, 5 ACI proximal to the flexure of the knee, between the vastus lateralis and the biceps femoris.

VII 33 On the lateral surface of the leg, between the lateral condyle of the femur and the lateral condyle of the tibia.

VII 34 On the lateral surface of the leg, 14 ACI proximal to the prominence of the lateral malleolus, anterior and just distal to the head of the fibula.

VII 35 On the lateral surface of the leg, 7 ACI proximal to the prominence of the lateral malleolus, posterior to the edge of the fibula, $\frac{1}{2}$ ACI posterior to VII 36.

VII 36 On the lateral surface of the leg, 7 ACI proximal to the prominence of the lateral malleolus. With the body supine and the knee semiflexed, the point lies anterior to the edge of the fibula.

VII 37 On the lateral surface of the leg, 5 ACi proximal to the prominence of the lateral malleolus. With the body supine and the knee semiflexed, the point lies anterior to the edge of the fibula.

VII 38 On the lateral surface of the leg, 4 ACI proximal to the prominence of the lateral malleolus. With the body supine and the knee semiflexed, the point lies anterior to the edge of the fibula.

VII 39 On the lateral surface of the leg, 3 ACI proximal to the prominence of the lateral malleolus. With the body supine and the knee semiflexed, the point lies anterior to the edge of the fibula.

VII 40 In the hollow anterior to the lateral malleolus, posterior to the tendon of the extensor digitorum longus.

VII 41 On the dorsal surface of the foot, in the angle between the fourth and fifth metatarsal bones.

VII 42 On the dorsal surface of the foot, between the fourth and fifth metatarsal bones, just proximal to the head of the fourth metatarsal bone.

VII 43 On the dorsal surface of the foot, between the fourth and fifth toes, just distal to the base of the proximal phalanx of the fourth toe.

VII 44 Lateral nail point of the fourth toe.

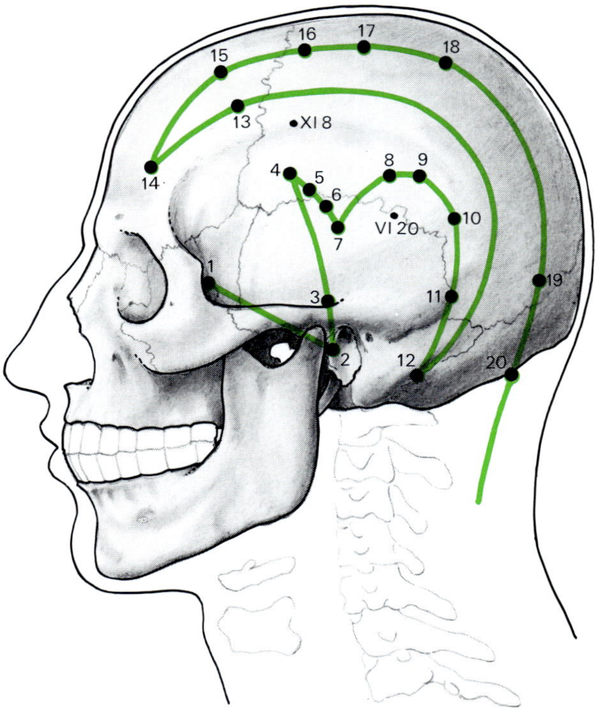
1
2
3
4
5
6
7
8
9
10
11
12
13
14
15
16
17
18
19
20
XI 8
VI 20

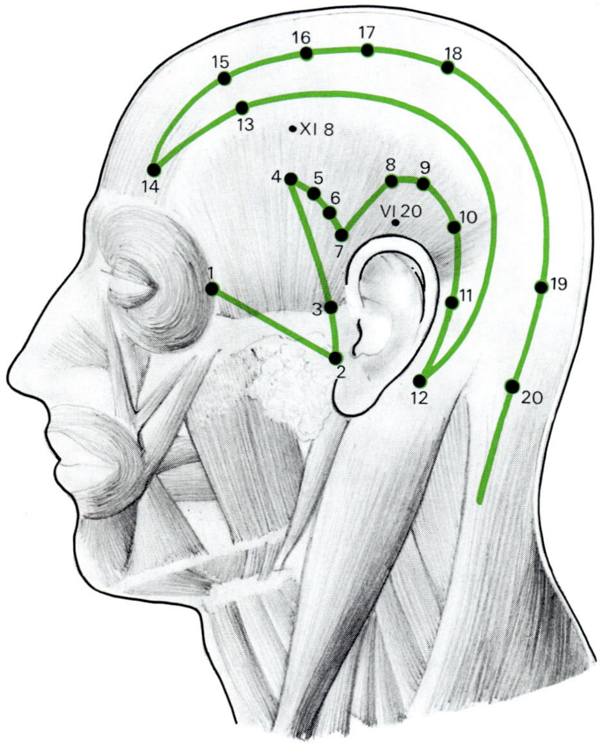
1
2
3
4
5
6
7
8
9
10
11
12
13
14
15
16
17
18
19
20
XI 8
VI 20

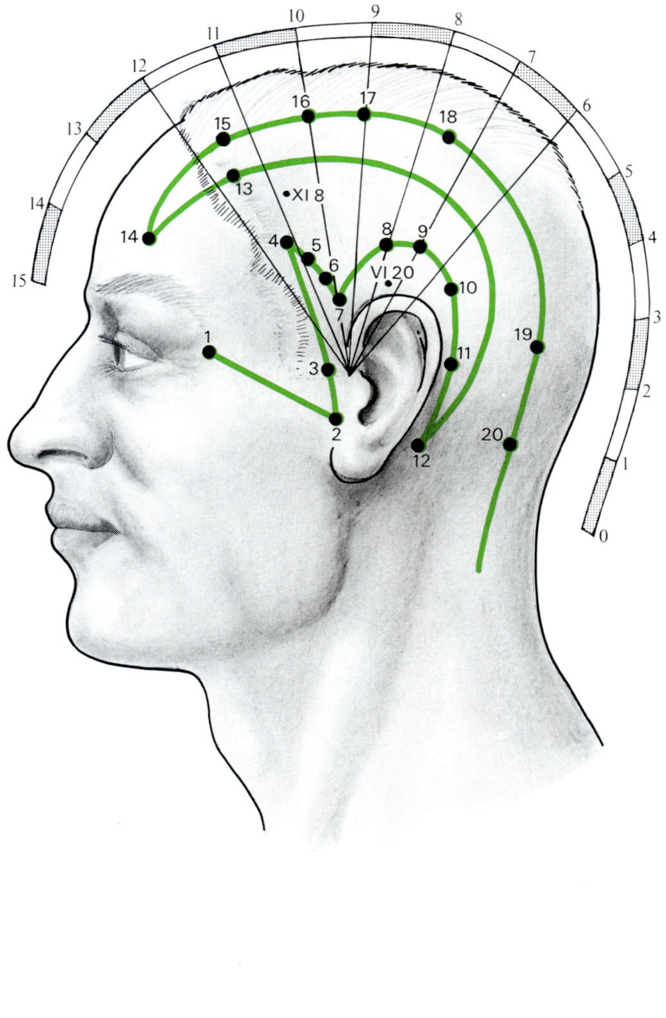
1
2
3
4
5
6
7
8
9
10
11
12
13
14
15
16
17
18
19
20
XI 8
VI 20
0
1
2
3
4
5
6
7
8
9
10
11
12
13
14
15

VII **1** **Orbit Bone** (Tungtzuliao)

⊥ 3 Entry
△ 5

In the depression just lateral to the orbital rim, at the level of the lateral canthus.

VII **2** **Hearing Assembly** (Tinghui)

⊥ 5
△ 5
XP1

On the posterior margin of the condyle of the mandible, anterior to the inferior border of the tragus. When the mouth is opened, a depression appears at this point.

VII **3** **Upper Pass** (Shangkuan)

⊥ X
△ 3–5

Anterior to the ear, immediately superior to the zygomatic arch, superior to VII 2.

VII **4** **Loathsome Jaws** (Hanyen)

⊥ 2
△ 3

On the temple, $\frac{1}{2}$ ACI posterior to the natural hair line, 1 ACI inferior to XI 8.

VII **5** **Suspended Skull** (Hsuanlu)

⊥ 3
△ 3

On the temple, $\frac{1}{2}$ ACI posterior to the natural hair line, one third of the distance from VII 4 to VII 7.

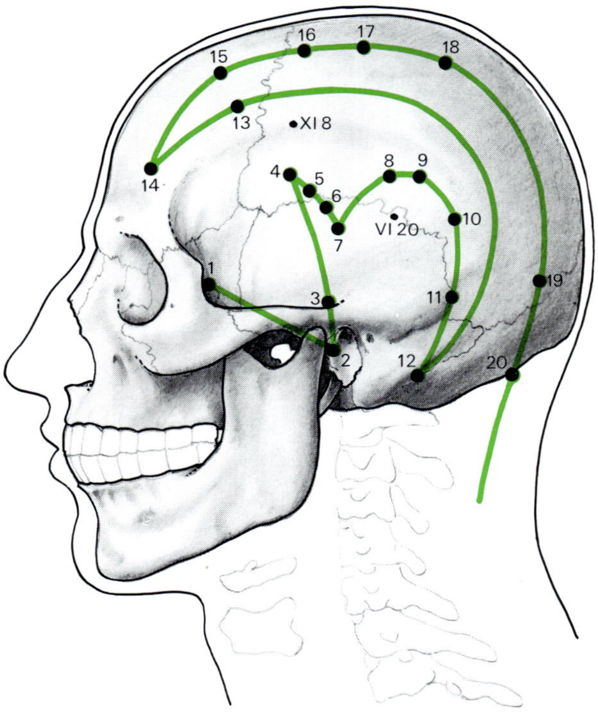
1
2
3
4
5
6
7
8
9
10
11
12
13
14
15
16
17
18
19
20
XI 8
VI 20

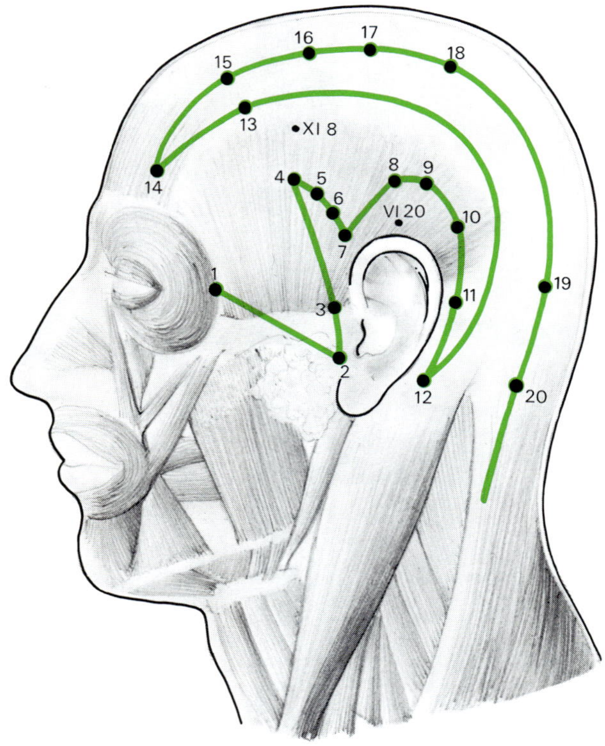
1
2
3
4
5
6
7
8
9
10
11
12
13
14
15
16
17
18
19
20
XI 8
VI 20

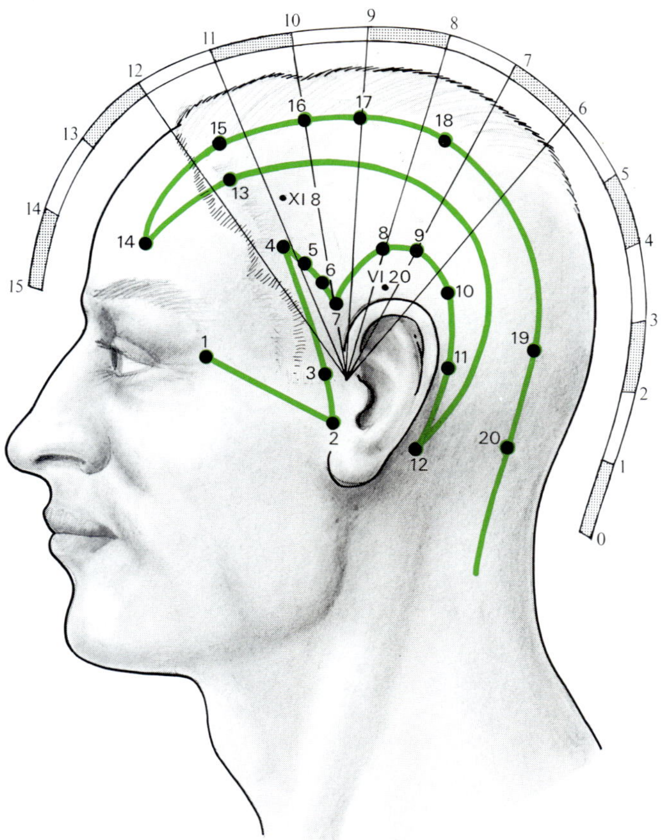
1
2
3
4
5
6
7
8
9
10
11
12
13
14
15
16
17
18
19
20
XI 8
VI 20
0
1
2
3
4
5
6
7
8
9
10
11
12
13
14
15

VII **6** **Suspended Regulator** (Hsuanli)

⊥ 2
△ 3

On the temple, $\frac{1}{2}$ ACI posterior to the natural hair line, two thirds of the distance from VII 4 to VII 7.

VII **7** **Crooked Hair On The Temples** (Chupin)

⊥ 3
△ 3–5

On the temple, $\frac{1}{2}$ ACI posterior to the natural hair line, at the level of the apex of the pinna, approximately 1 ACI anterior to and slightly inferior to VI 20.

VII **8** **Flowing Valley** (Shuaiku)

⊥ 3
△ 3–5

On the head, 1 ACI directly superior to VI 20.

VII **9** **Heaven Rushing** (Tienchung)

⊥ 3
△ 3–5
XP4

On the head, $\frac{1}{2}$ ACI posterior to VII 8 and 2 ACI superior to the natural hair line.

VII **10** **Floating White** (Fupai)

⊥ 3
△ 3–5

On the head, posterior and slightly superior to the ear, 1 ACI posterior to the natural hair line, at the level of the superior edge of the root of the ear.

VII **11** **Head Hole Yin** (Tou chiaoyin)

⊥ 3
△ 3–7

On the head, posterior to the ear, mid-way between VII 10 and VII 12.

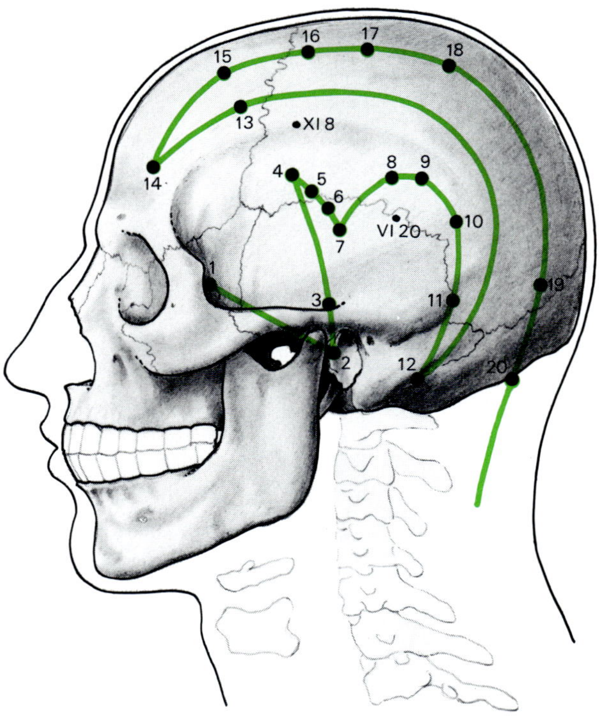
1
2
3
4
5
6
7
8
9
10
11
12
13
14
15
16
17
18
19
20
XI 8
VI 20

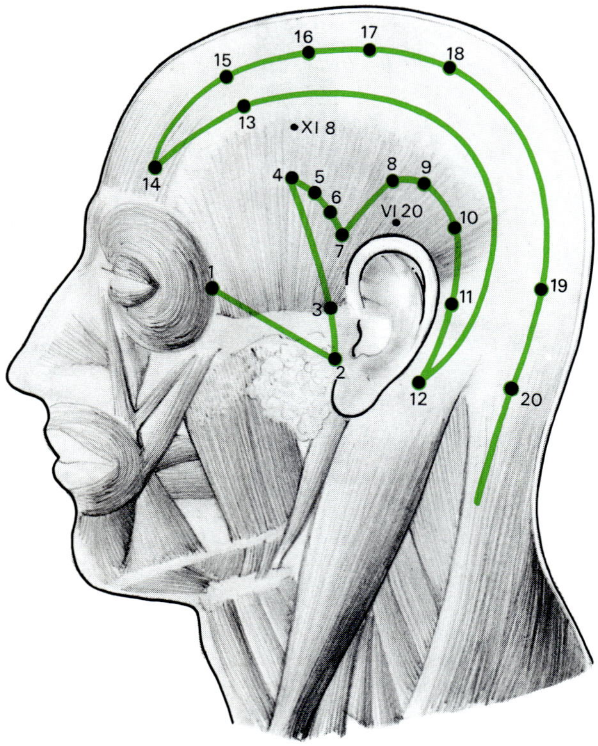
1
2
3
4
5
6
7
8
9
10
11
12
13
14
15
16
17
18
19
20
XI 8
VI 20

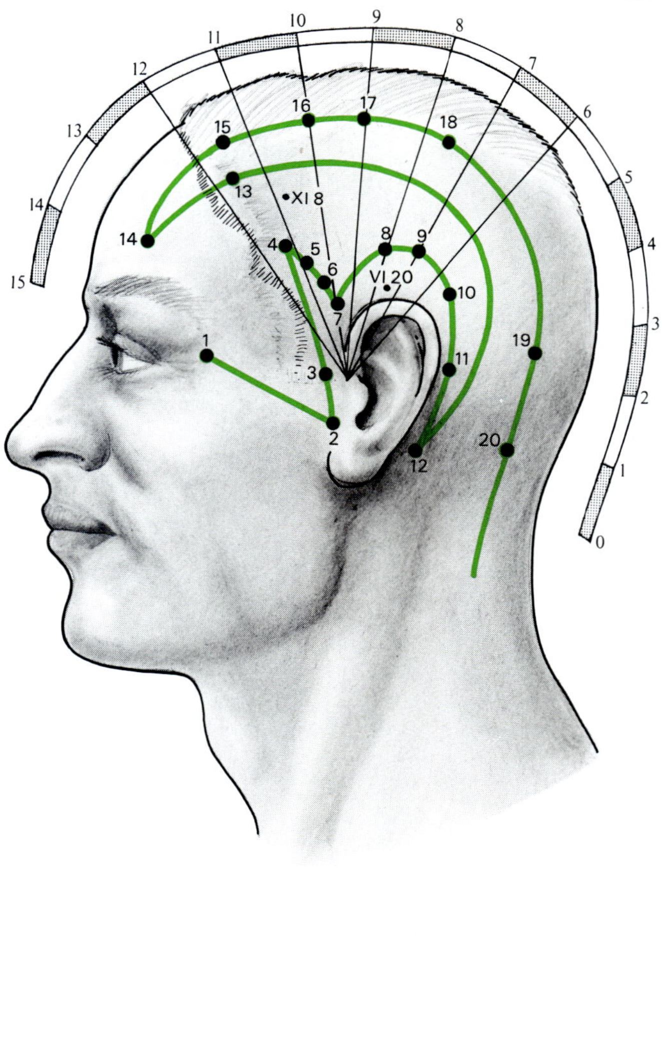
1
2
3
4
5
6
7
8
9
10
11
12
13
14
15
16
17
18
19
20
XI 8
VI 20
0
1
2
3
4
5
6
7
8
9
10
11
12
13
14
15

VII **12** **Final Bone** (Wanku)

⊥ 5
△ 3–7

On the head, within the angle formed by the posterior border of the mastoid process and the inferior edge of the occipital bone when the head is tilted forwards.

VII **13** **Root Spirit** (Penshen)

⊥ 3
△ 7

On the head, $\frac{1}{2}$ ACI posterior to the natural hair line, on a vertical line superior to the lateral canthus.

Point of Yang Wei Mo

VII **14** **Yang White** (Yangpai)

⊥ 2
△ 3

On the forehead, 1 ACI superior to the supra-orbital notch, which is found in the middle of the eyebrow.

Point of Yang Wei Mo

VII **15** **Head Above Tears** (Tou linchi)

⊥ 3
△ X

On the head, $\frac{1}{2}$ ACI posterior to the natural hair line, on a vertical line superior to the middle of the pupil when the eye is looking straight ahead.

VII **16** **Eye Window** (Muchuang)

⊥ 3
△ 5

On the head, $1\frac{1}{2}$ ACI posterior to VII 15.

Point of Yang Wei Mo

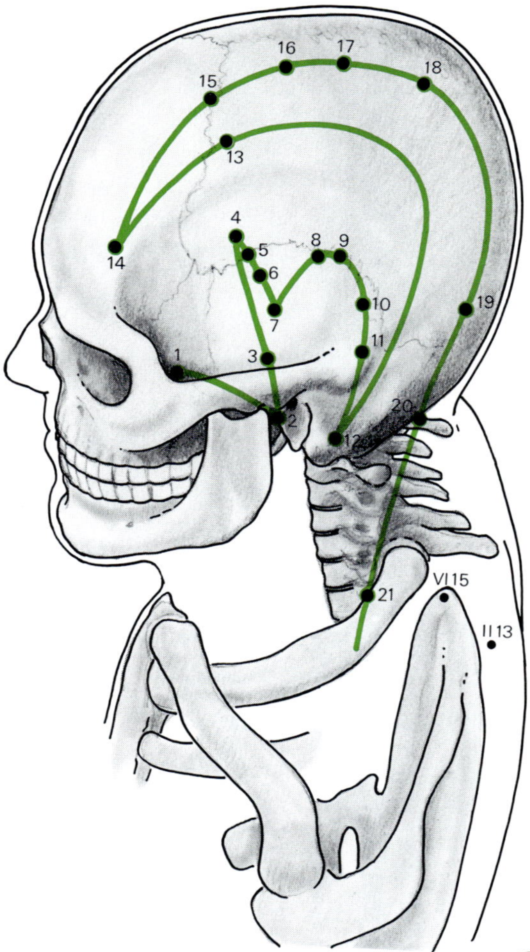
1
2
3
4
5
6
7
8
9
10
11
12
13
14
15
16
17
18
19
20
21
VI 15
II 13

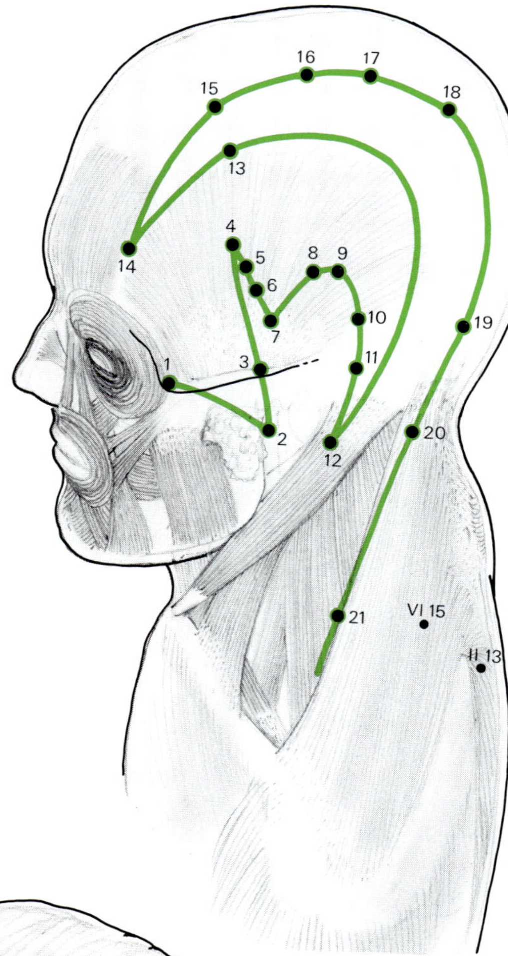
1
2
3
4
5
6
7
8
9
10
11
12
13
14
15
16
17
18
19
20
21
VI 15
II 13

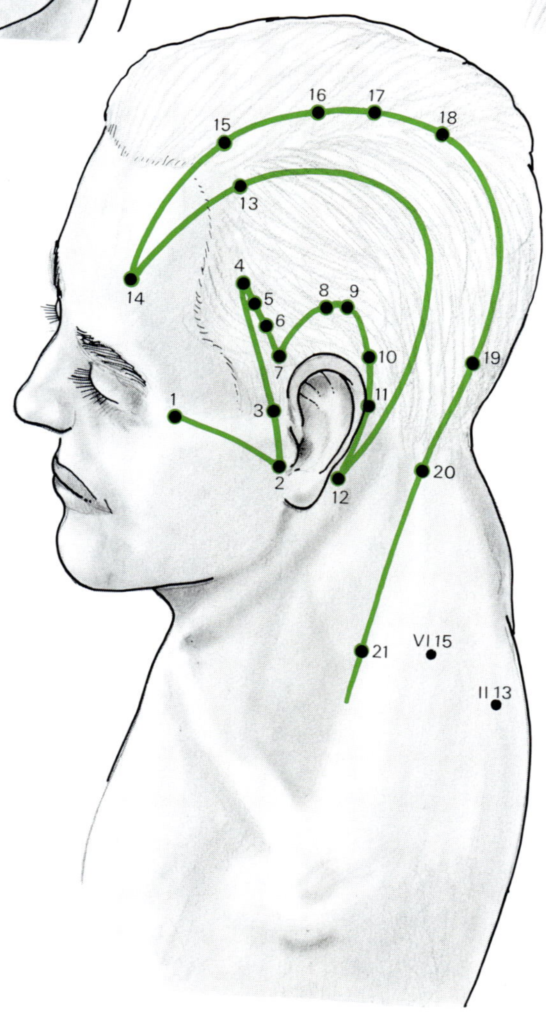
1
2
3
4
5
6
7
8
9
10
11
12
13
14
15
16
17
18
19
20
21
VI 15
II 13

VII **17** **Upright Living** (Chengying)

⊥ 3
△ 5

On the head, 1 ACI posterior to VII 16.

Point of Yang Wei Mo

VII **18** **Receiving Spirit** (Chengling)

⊥ X
△ 5

On the head, $1\frac{1}{2}$ ACI posterior to VII 17.

Point of Yang Wei Mo

VII **19** **Brain Hollow** (Naokung)

⊥ 3
△ 5

On the head, lateral to the external occipital protruberance, $1\frac{1}{2}$ ACI superior to VII 20.

Point of Yang Wei Mo

VII **20** **Wind Pond** (Fengchih)

⊥ 6
△ 7–10

Inferior to the occipital bone, in the centre of the depression between the external occipital protruberance and the mastoid process, superior to the natural hair line and lateral to the border of the trapezius.

Point of Yang Wei Mo
Point of Yang Qiao Mo
First Aid: poison

VII **21** **Shoulder Well** (Chienching)

⊥ 4–6
△ 7–15

Mid-way between the spinous process of the seventh cervical vertebra and the lateral tip of the clavicle, upon the anterior border of the trapezius, in line with VI 15 and II 13.

Point of Yang Wei Mo

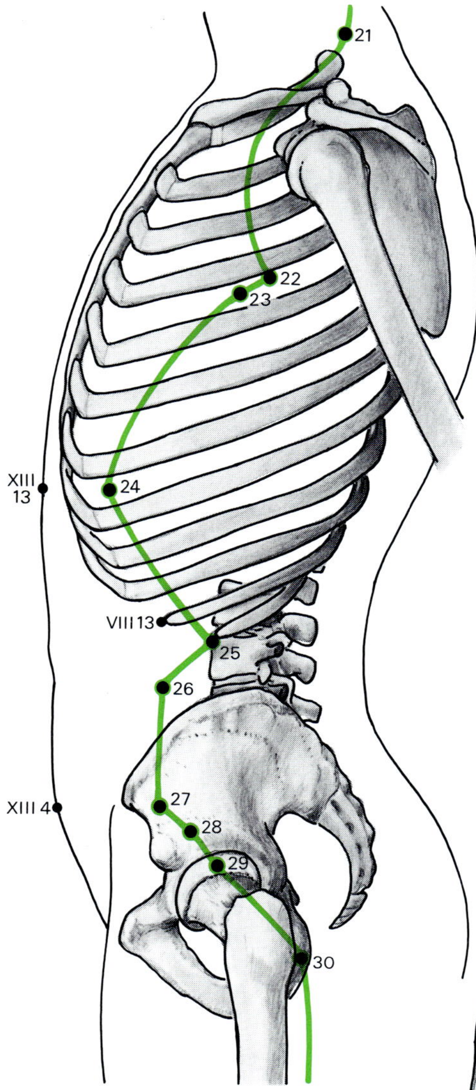
21
22
23
XIII
13
24
VIII 13
25
26
XIII 4
27
28
29
30

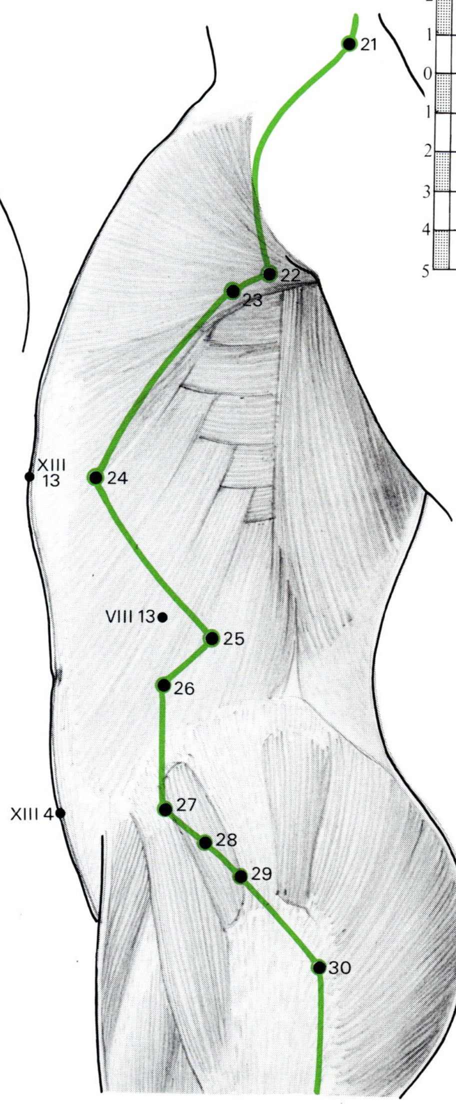
21
22
23
XIII
13
24
VIII 13
25
26
XIII 4
27
28
29
30

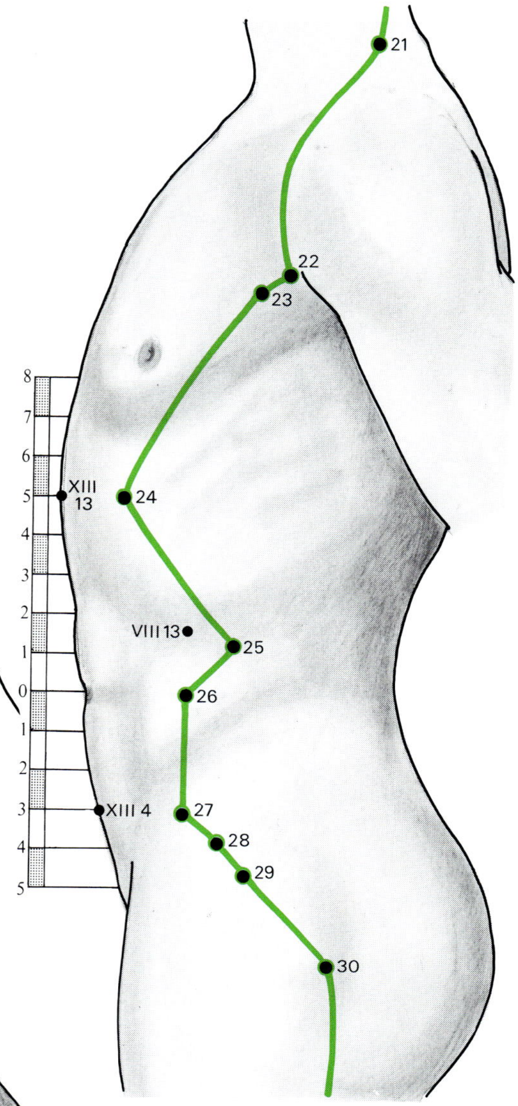
21
22
23
8
7
6
5
4
3
2
1
0
1
2
3
4
5
XIII
13
24
VIII 13
25
26
XIII 4
27
28
29
30

VII **22** **Armpit Abyss** (Yuanyeh)

⊥ 4
△ X

In the fourth intercostal space, on the mid-axillary line.

VII **23** **Neglected Muscles** (Chechin)

⊥ 5
△ 5

In the fourth intercostal space, 1 ACI medial to VII 22.

Alarm Point of VII

VII **24** **Sun And Moon** (Jihyueh)

⊥ 5
△ 5–7

In the seventh intercostal space, on the paramedian nipple line, approximately level with XIII 13.

Alarm Point of VII

VII **25** **Capital Gate** (Chingmen)

⊥ 7
△ 7–12

On the lateral surface of the abdomen, at the anterior tip of the twelfth rib.

Alarm Point of IV

VII **26** **Girdle Vessel** (Taimo)

⊥ 8
△ 5–15

On the lateral surface of the abdomen, at the intersection of the vertical line passing through VIII 13 (or the anterior tip of the eleventh rib), and a horizontal line passing through the centre of the umbilicus.

Point of Dai Mo

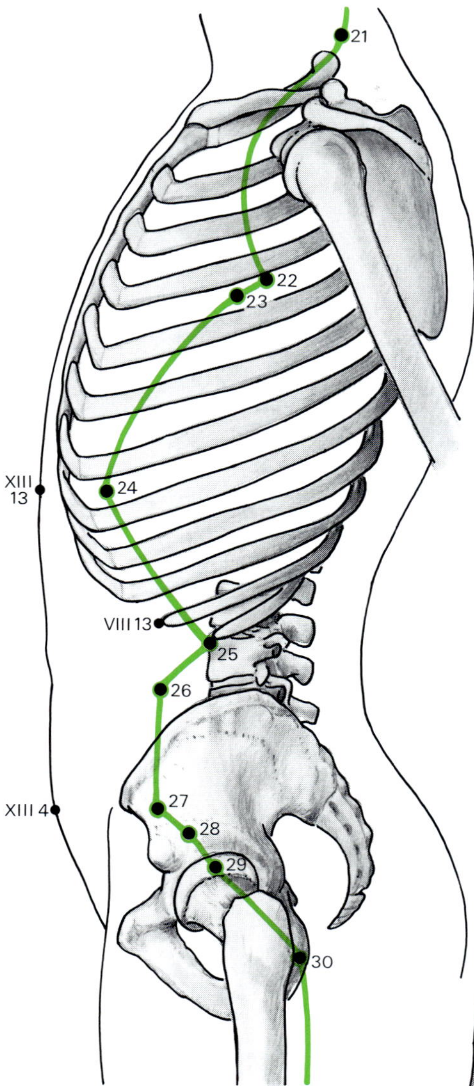
21
22
23
XIII 13
24
VIII 13
25
26
XIII 4
27
28
29
30

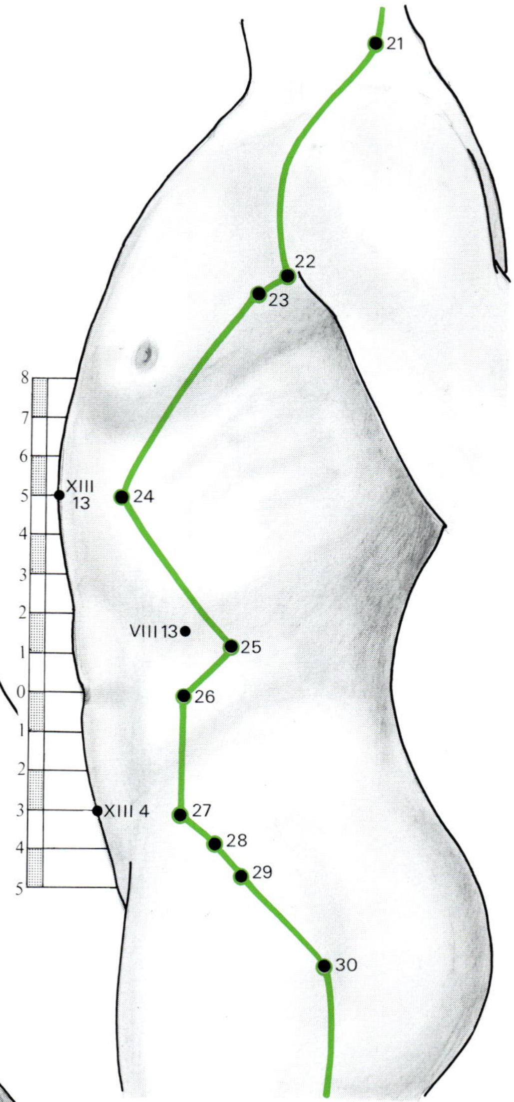
21
22
23
8
7
6
5
XIII 13
24
4
3
2
VIII 13
1
25
0
26
1
2
3
XIII 4
27
4
28
5
29
30

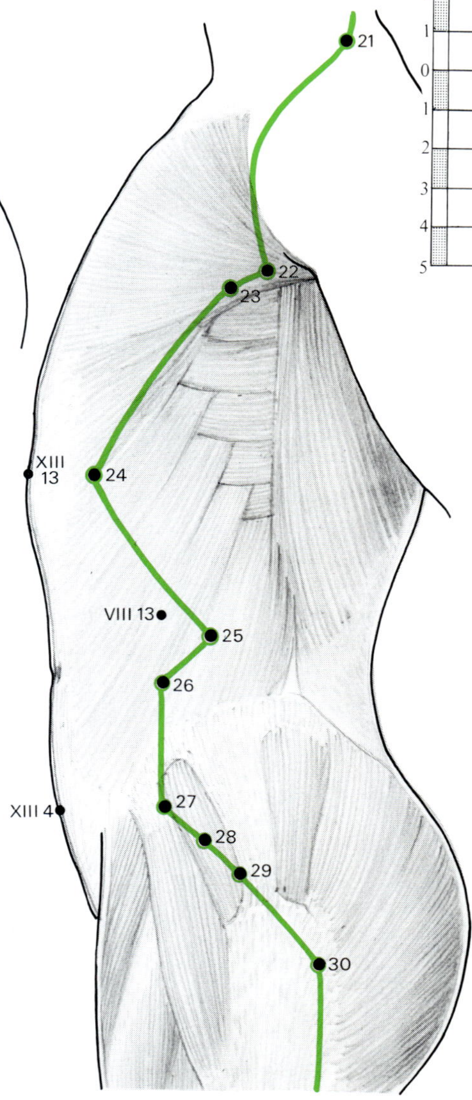
21
22
23
XIII 13
24
VIII 13
25
26
XIII 4
27
28
29
30

VII **27** **Five Pivots** (Wushu)

⊥ 7
△ 3–10

On the hip, inferior and slightly posterior to the anterior superior iliac spine, on a level with XIII 4.

Point of Dai Mo

VII **28** **Binding Path** (Weitao)

⊥ 8
△ 5–7

On the hip, mid-way between VII 27 and VII 29.

Point of Dai Mo

VII **29** **Dwelling In The Bone** (Chuliao)

⊥ 8
△ 5–7

On the hip, mid-way between the anterior superior iliac spine and the prominence of the greater trochanter.

Point of Yang Wei Mo
Point of Yang Qiao Mo

VII **30** **Jumping Circle** (Huantiao)

⊥ 10–15
△ 7–20

On the lateral surface of the hip, posterior to the prominence of the greater trochanter.

First Aid: fractures, sprains

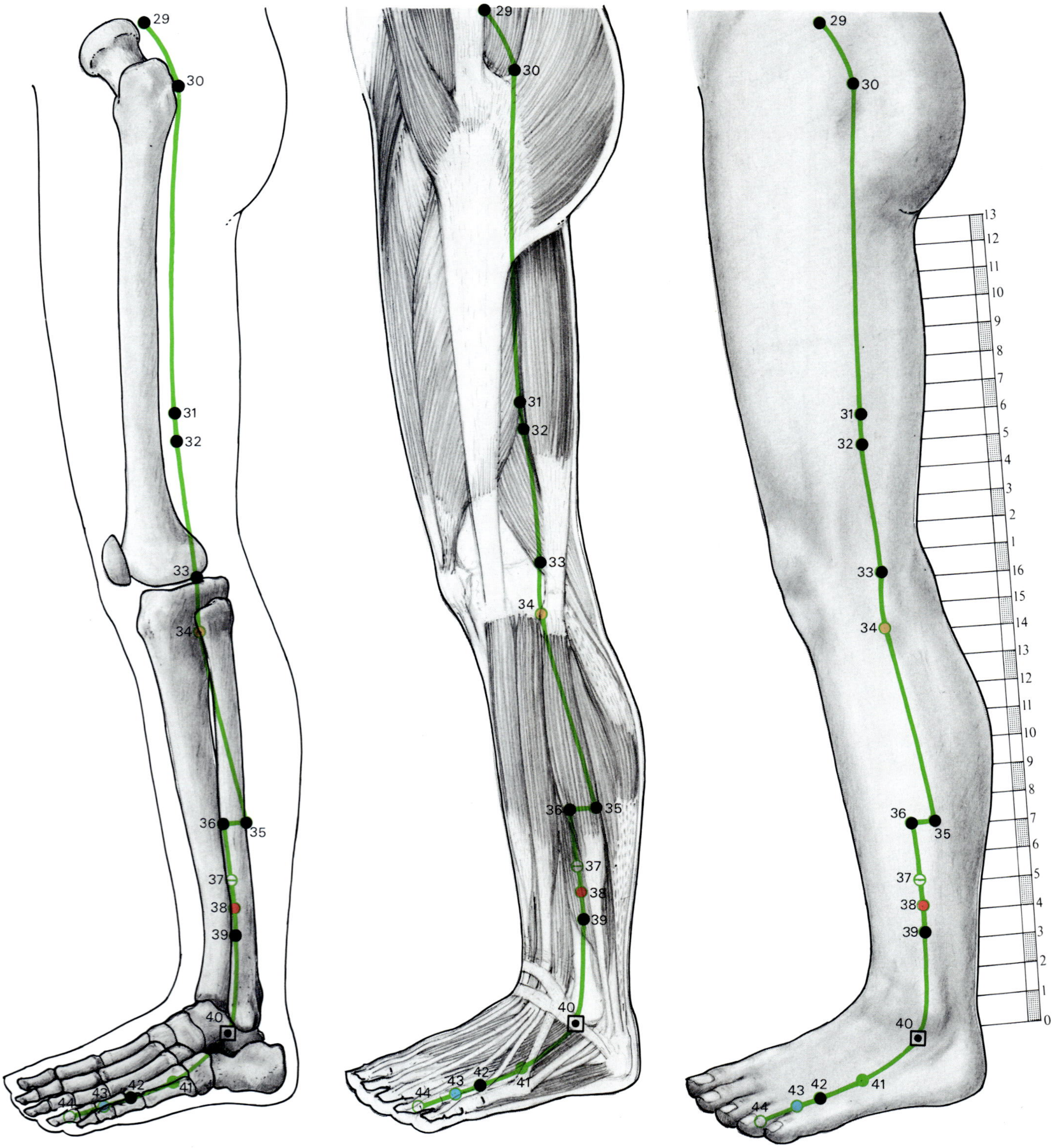
29
30
31
32
33
34
35
36
37
38
39
40
41
42
43
44
29
30
31
32
33
34
35
36
37
38
39
40
41
42
43
44
29
30
31
32
33
34
35
36
37
38
39
40
41
42
43
44
13
12
11
10
9
8
7
6
5
4
3
2
1
16
15
14
13
12
11
10
9
8
7
6
5
4
3
2
1
0

VII **31** **Wind Market** (Fengshih)

⊥ 5
△ 5

On the lateral surface of the thigh, 6 ACI proximal to the flexure of the knee, between the vastus lateralis and the biceps femoris.

VII **32** **Middle Ditch** (Chungtu)

⊥ 5
△ 5–7

On the lateral surface of the thigh, 5 ACI proximal to the flexure of the knee, between the vastus lateralis and the biceps femoris.

VII **33** **Knee Yang Border** (Tsu yangkuan)

⊥ 5
△ X

On the lateral surface of the leg, between the lateral condyle of the femur and the lateral condyle of the tibia.

VII **34** **Yang Mound Spring** (Yanglingchuan)

● ⊥ 6 Earth
△ 7–10
XP2

On the lateral surface of the leg. 14 ACI proximal to the prominence of the lateral malleolus, anterior and just distal to the head of the fibula.

Assembling Point of tendons
Point of Ho (Autumn)

VII **35** **Yang Crossing** (Yangchiao)

⊥ 6
△ 3–7

On the lateral surface of the leg, 7 ACI proximal to the prominence of the lateral malleolus, posterior to the edge of the fibula, $\frac{1}{2}$ ACI posterior to VII 36.

Point of Yang Wei Mo

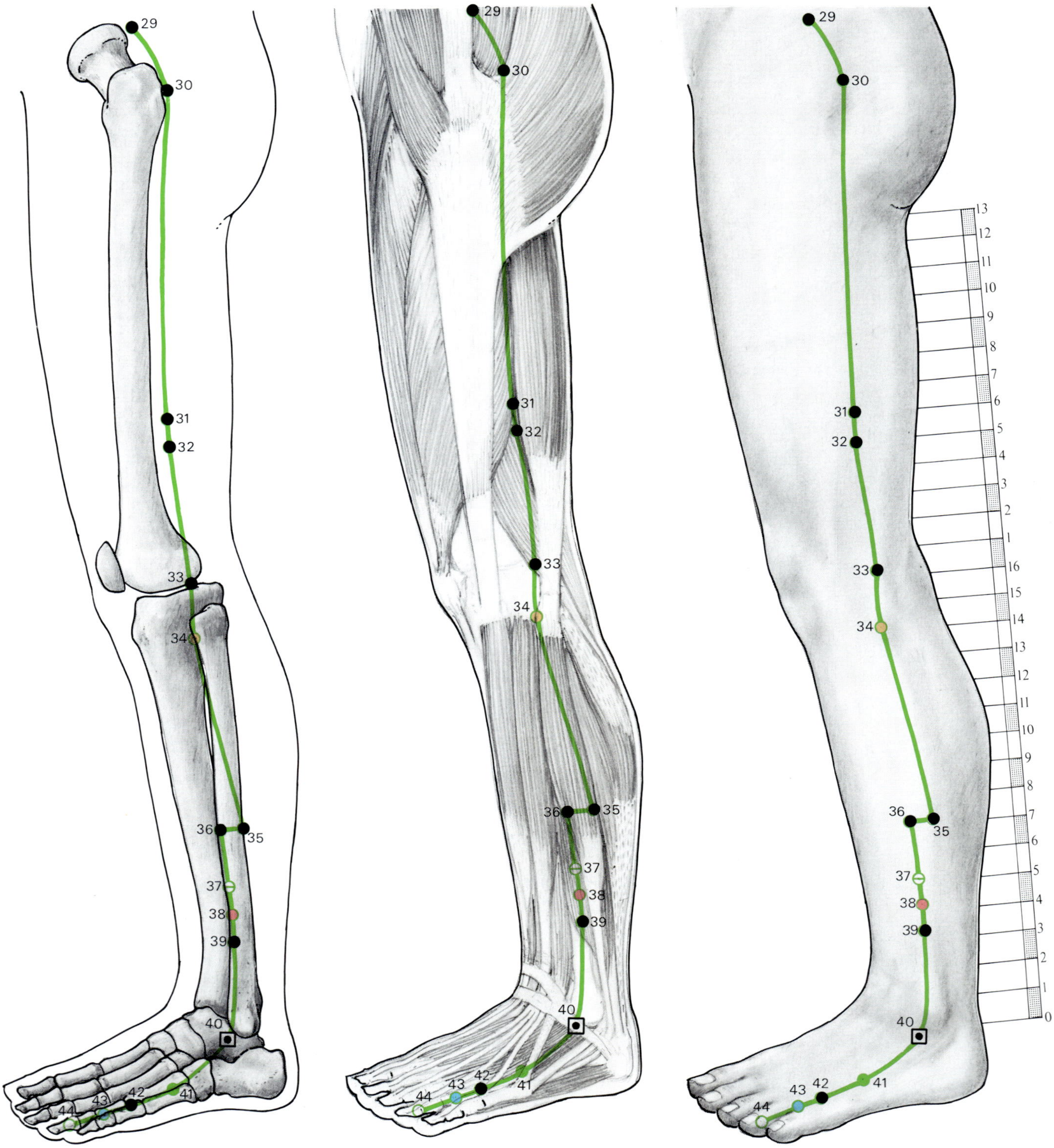
29
30
31
32
33
34
35
36
37
38
39
40
41
42
43
44
13
12
11
10
9
8
7
6
5
4
3
2
1
16
15
14
13
12
11
10
9
8
7
6
5
4
3
2
1
0

VII **36** **Outer Mound** (Waichiu)

⊥ 4
△ 3

On the lateral surface of the leg, 7 ACI proximal to the prominence of the lateral malleolus. With the body supine and the knee semiflexed, the point lies anterior to the edge of the fibula.

VII **37** **Bright And Clear** (Kuangming)

⊖ ⊥ 6 Junction
△ 7

On the lateral surface of the leg, 5 ACI proximal to the prominence of the lateral malleolus. With the body supine and the knee semiflexed, the point lies anterior to the edge of the fibula.

VII **38** **Yang Support** (Yangfu)

● ⊥ 6 Fire
△ 5–15 Sedation

On the lateral surface of the leg, 4 ACI proximal to the prominence of the lateral malleolus. With the body supine and the knee semiflexed, the point lies anterior to the edge of the fibula.

Point of Ching (late Summer)

VII **39** **Hanging Cup** (Hsuanchung)

⊥ 3
△ 5–15

On the lateral surface of the leg, 3 ACI proximal to the prominence of the lateral malleolus. With the body supine and the knee semiflexed, the point lies anterior to the edge of the fibula.

Assembling Point of marrow
Meeting Point of the three lower Yang meridians (III—VII—XI)

VII **40** **Wilderness Mound** (Chiuhsu)

□ ⊥ 5 Source
△ 3–7

In the hollow anterior to the lateral malleolus, posterior to the tendon of the extensor digitorum longus.

First Aid: food poisoning, poison

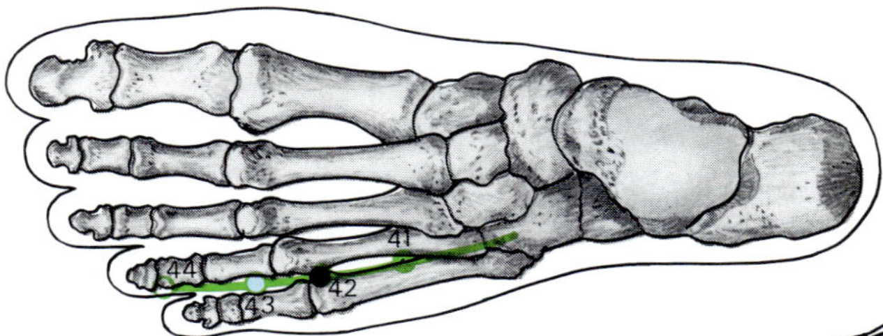
44
43
42
41

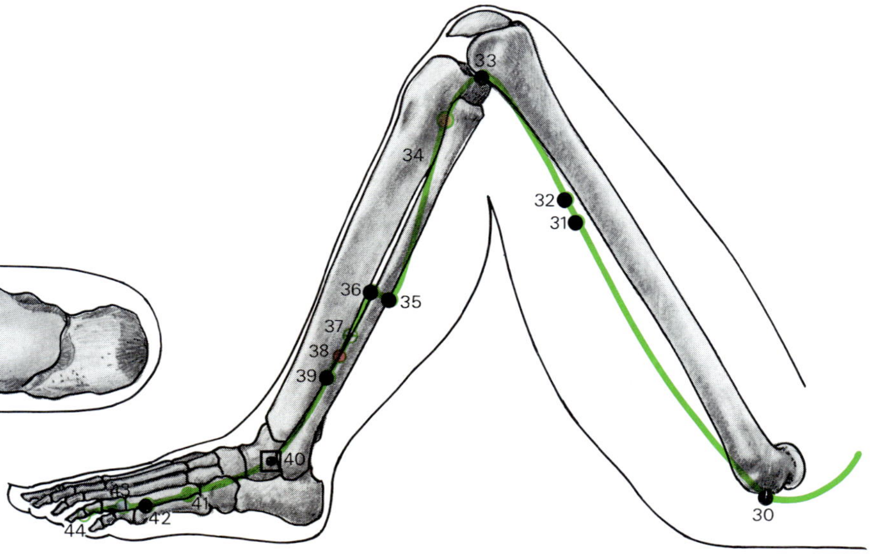
33
34
32
31
36
35
37
38
39
40
43
41
44
42
30

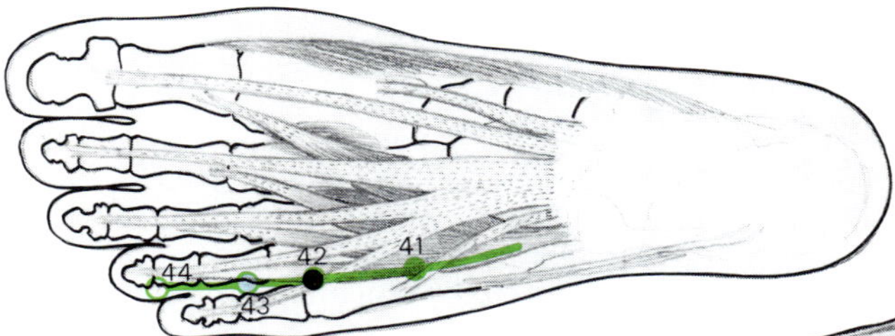
44
42
41
43

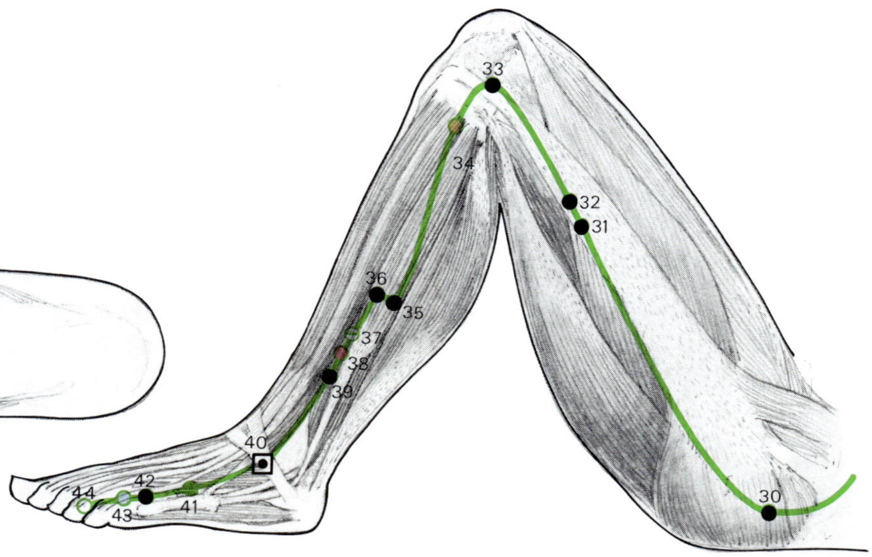
33
34
32
31
36
35
37
38
39
40
44
42
43
41
30

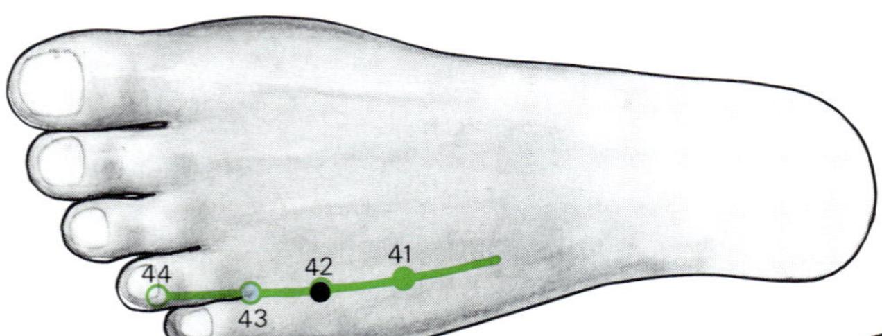
44
42
41
43

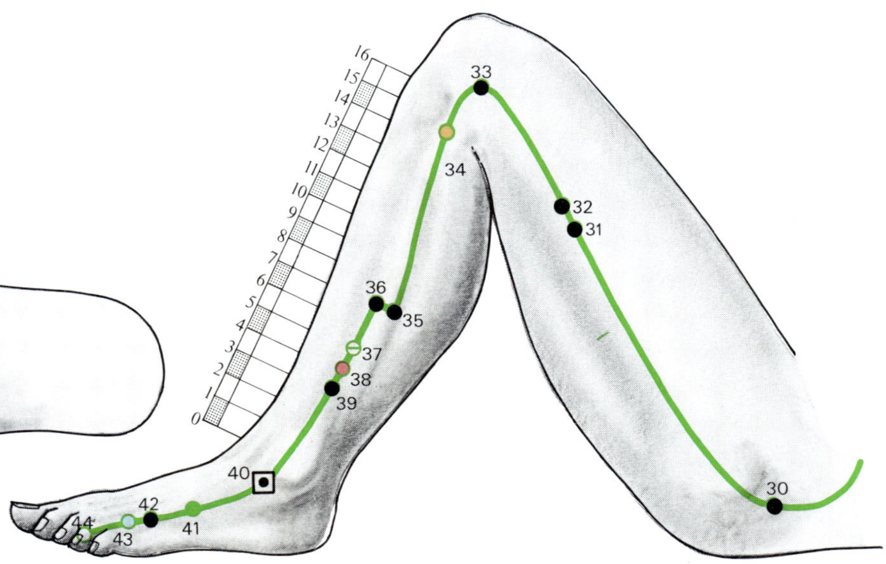
16
15
14
13
12
11
10
9
8
7
6
5
4
3
2
1
0
33
34
32
31
36
35
37
38
39
40
42
44
43
41
30

VII **41** **Foot Above Tears** (Tsu linchi)

⊥ 3 Wood
△ 5 Horary 11 p.m.–1 a.m.
Exit

On the dorsal surface of the foot, in the angle between the fourth and fifth metatarsal bones.

Point of Yu (Summer)
Master Point of Dai Mo
Coupled Point of Yang Wei Mo
First Aid: haemorrhage

VII **42** **Earth Five Meetings** (Tiwuhui)

⊥ 2
△ X

On the dorsal surface of the foot, between the fourth and fifth metatarsal bones, just proximal to the head of the fourth metatarsal bone.

VII **43** **Valiant Stream** (Hsiahsi)

⊥ 3 Water
△ 3–5 Tonification

On the dorsal surface of the foot, between the fourth and fifth toes, just distal to the base of the proximal phalanx of the fourth toe.

Point of Yung (Spring)

VII **44** **Foot Hole Yin** (Tsu chiaoyin)

⊥ 1 Metal
△ 3–5

Lateral nail point of the fourth toe.

Point of Cheng (Winter)

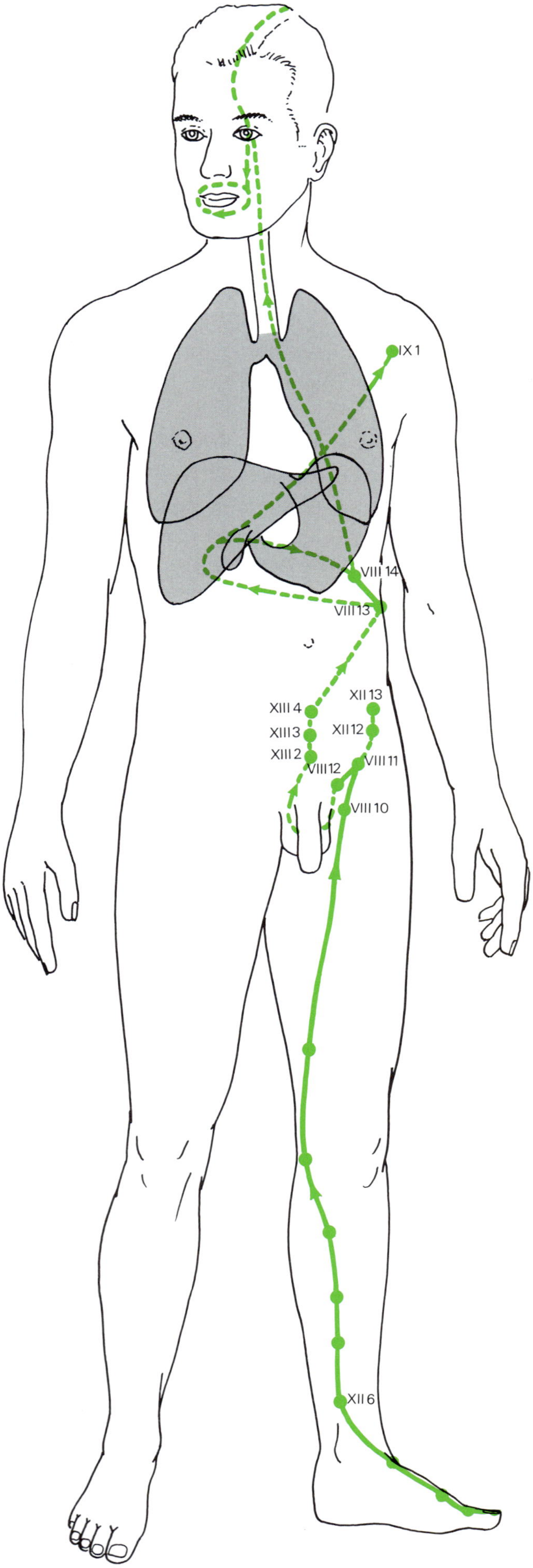
IX 1
VIII 14
VIII 13
XIII 4
XIII 3
XIII 2
XII 13
XII 12
VIII 12
VIII 11
VIII 10
XII 6

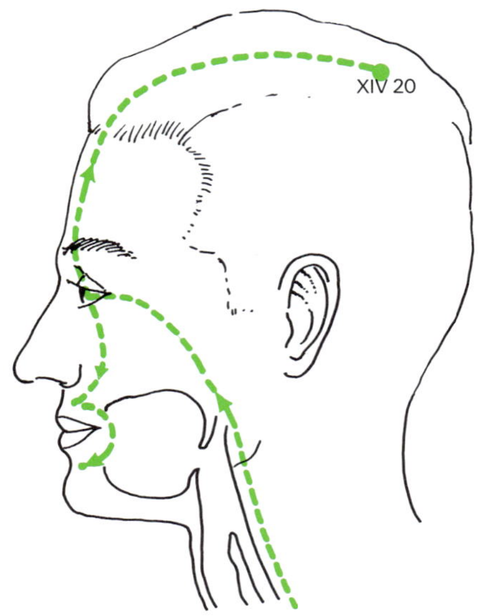
XIV 20

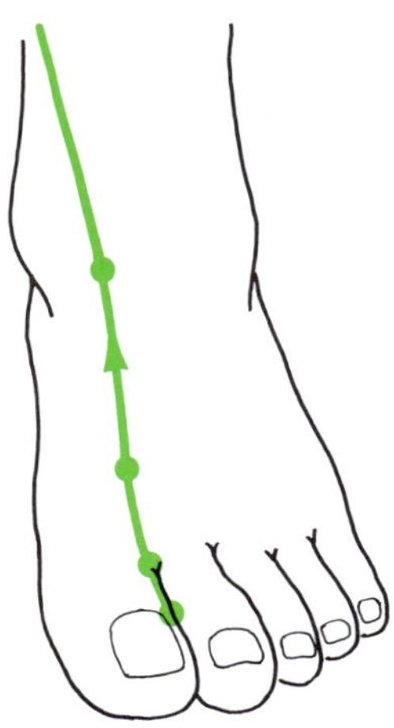

The liver meridian begins as the superficial pathway at the lateral nail point of the big toe, travels over the dorsal surface of the foot between the first and second metatarsal bones and passes anterior to the medial malleolus. It continues up the medial surface of the leg, posterior to the tibia, passing XII 6 at 4 ACI superior to the medial malleolus. It crosses medial to the patellar region to the medial side of the thigh, along the adductor longus through VIII 10, VIII 11 and VIII 12. A deep branch from VIII 11 ascends through XII 12 and XII 13. A further deep branch from VIII 12 runs medially to loop around the genitals and ascend the median line of the lower abdomen to XIII 2, XIII 3 and XIII 4, and then moves superiorly and laterally to the tip of the eleventh rib, at VIII 13. The final section of the superficial meridian then extends to a point on the inferior edge of the thoracic cage in line with the nipple, the exit point, VIII 14.

A deep branch runs from VIII 13 alongside the stomach to enter the liver and then connects with the gall bladder and returns to VIII 14. It then penetrates the diaphragm, radiates along the ribs and ascends posterior to the trachea and the larynx and pharynx to the nasal cavities and the nasal lacrimal canal. It connects with the eye and then rises up the forehead, crossing the frontal bone to the parietal bone at the top of the head, and terminates at XIV 20.

A branch leaves the deep pathway in the eye and travels down to the mandible and circles the mouth on the inside of the lips in the orbicularis oris. Another deep branch leaves the liver, penetrates the diaphragm and enters the lungs. Here it connects with the lung meridian, at IX 1.

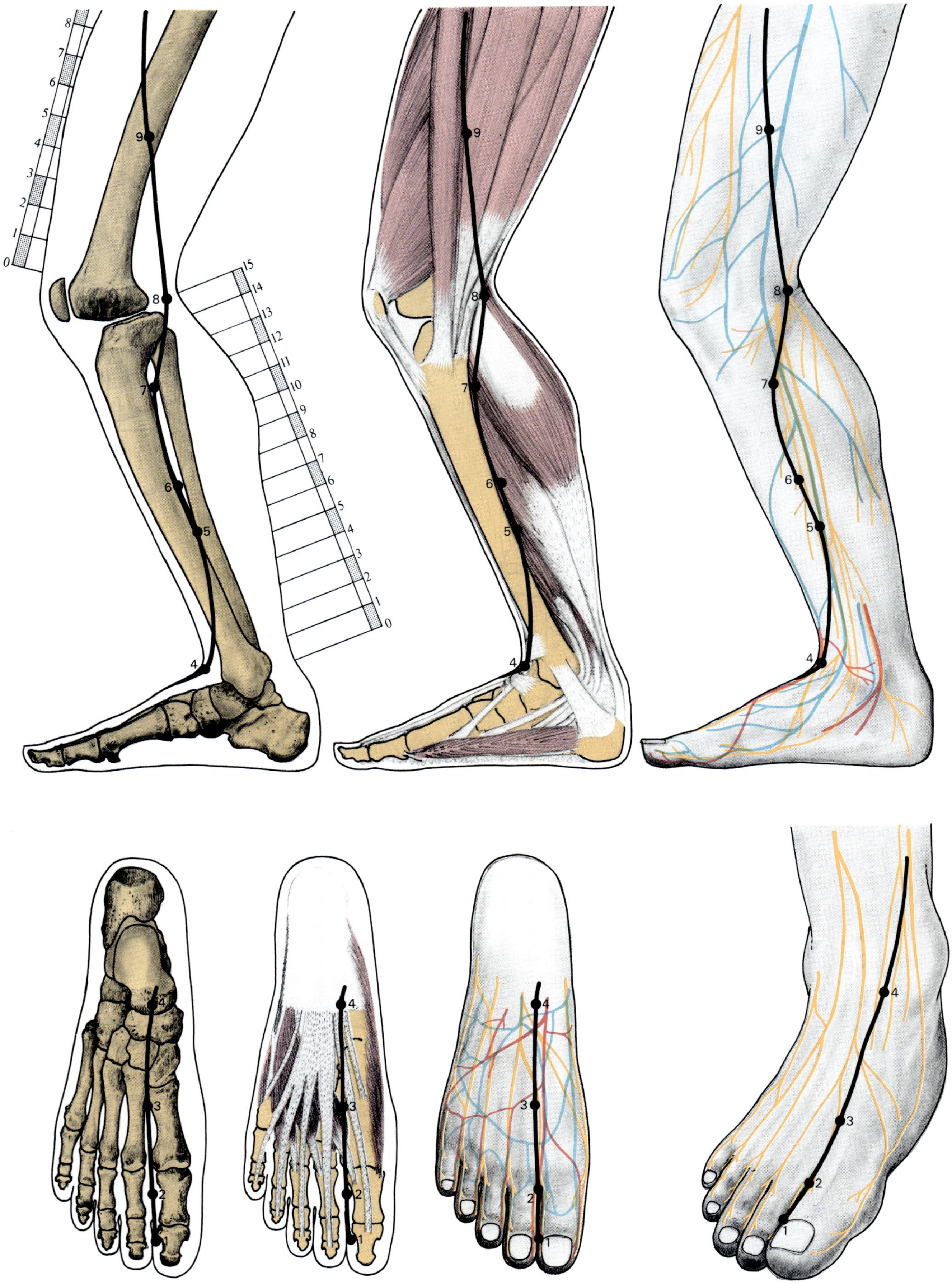
0
1
2
3
4
5
6
7
8
9
8
7
6
5
4
15
14
13
12
11
10
9
8
7
6
5
4
3
2
1
0
1
2
3
4

VIII 1 Lateral nail point of the big toe.

VIII 2 On the dorsal surface of the foot, between the big toe and the second toe, just distal to the base of the proximal phalanx of the big toe.

VIII 3 On the dorsal surface of the foot, in the angle between the first and second metatarsal bones.

VIII 4 At the anterior flexure of the ankle, between the tendons of the tibialis anterior and the extensor hallucis longus.

VIII 5 On the medial surface of the leg, 6 ACI proximal to the prominence of the medial malleolus, posterior to the edge of the tibia.

VIII 6 On the medial surface of the leg, 8 ACI proximal to the prominence of the medial malleolus, posterior to the edge of the tibia.

VIII 7 On the medial surface of the leg, 12 ACI proximal to the prominence of the medial malleolus, posterior to the edge of the tibia.

VIII 8 On the medial surface of the knee, posterior to the medial condyle of the tibia; close to the extremity of the crease formed when the knee is flexed.

VIII 9 On the medial surface of the thigh, 5 ACI proximal to the flexure of the knee, between the sartorius and the vastus medialis.

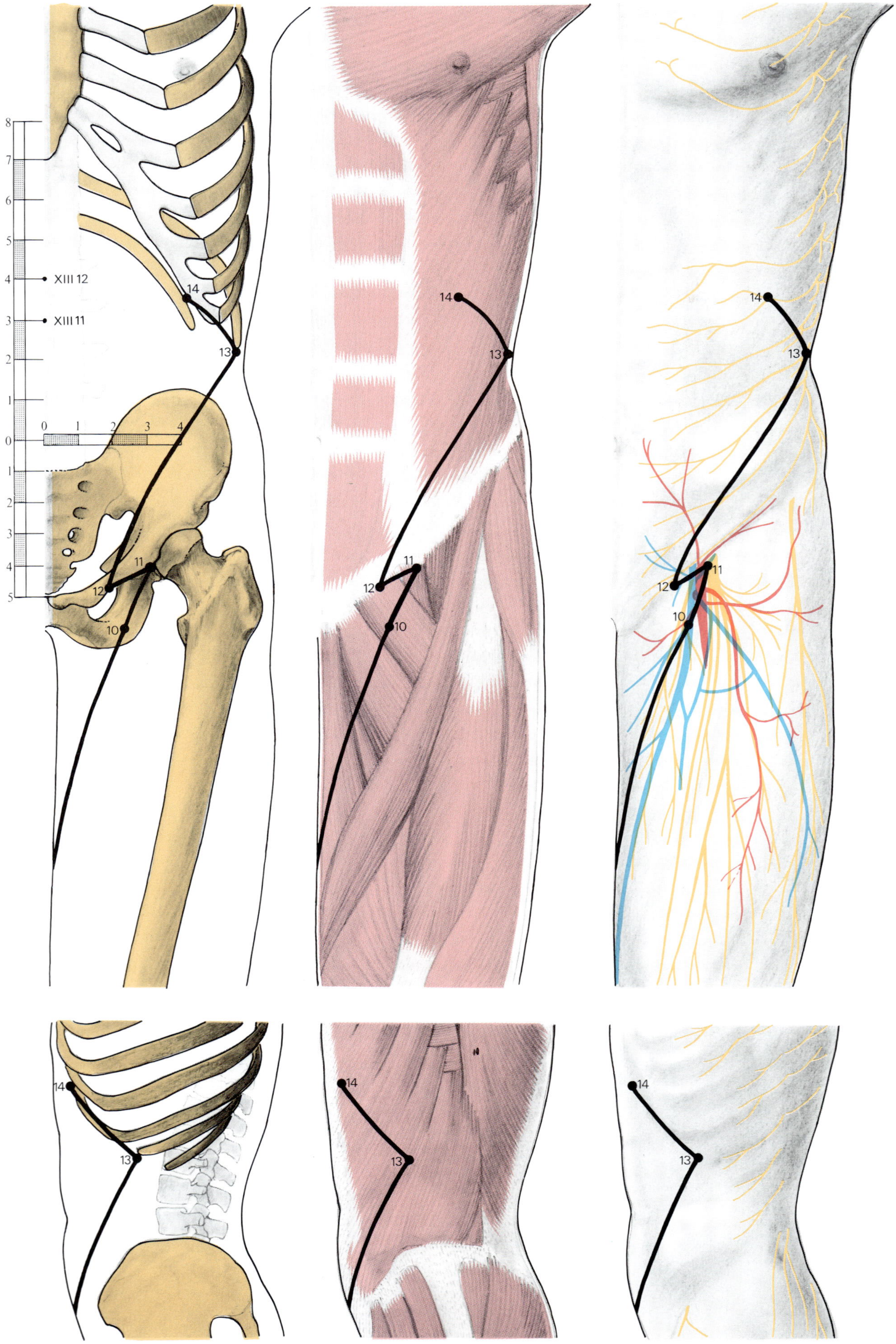
XIII 12
XIII 11
14
13
12
11
10

VIII **10** On the anterior surface of the thigh, lateral to the adductor longus, just medial to the femoral artery, 1 ACI distal to the flexure of the groin.

VIII **11** On the flexure of the groin, just lateral to the femoral artery.

VIII **12** On the flexure of the groin, 2 ACI lateral to the mid-line of the pubic symphysis.

VIII **13** At the anterior tip of the eleventh rib.

VIII **14** On the inferior edge of the thoracic cage, on the paramedian nipple line. The point lies at the level half-way between XIII 11 and XIII 12.

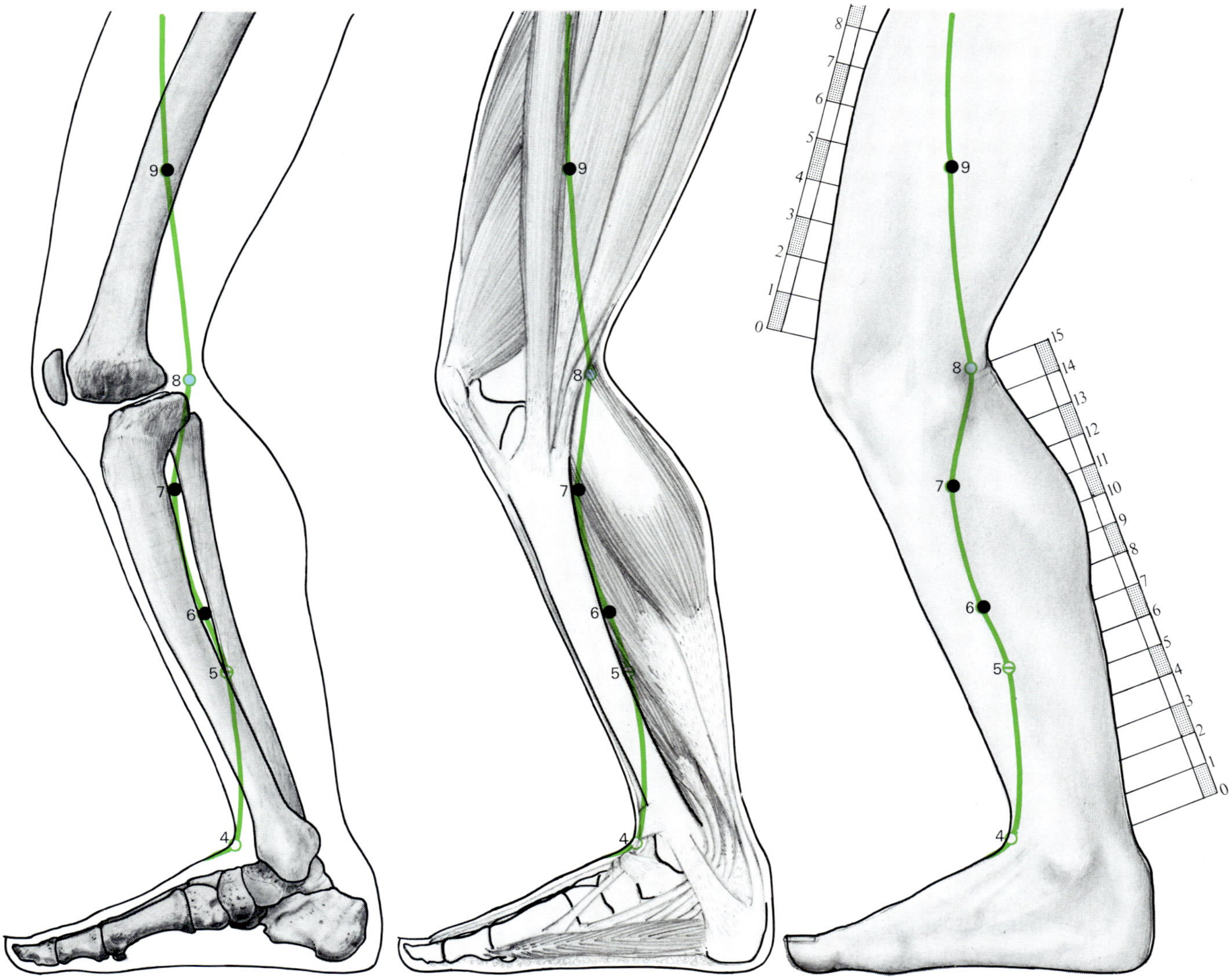

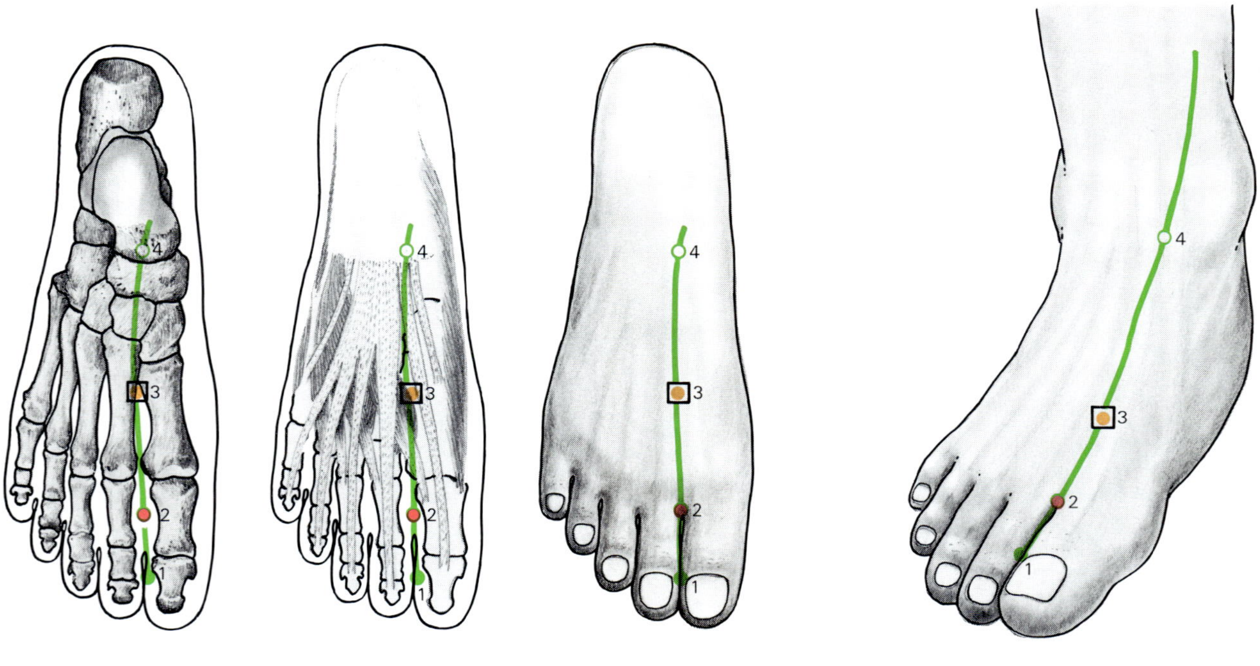

VIII **1** **Great Esteem** (Tatun)

● ⊥ 1 Wood
△ 5–7 Horary 1 a.m.–3 a.m.
Entry

Lateral nail point of the big toe.

Point of Cheng (Winter)

VIII **2** **Walk Between** (Hsingchien)

● ⊥ 3 Fire
△ 5–7 Sedation

On the dorsal surface of the foot, between the big toe and the second toe, just distal to the base of the proximal phalanx of the big toe.

Point of Yung (Spring)
First Aid: cramps, spasms, urine retention

VIII **3** **Supreme Rushing** (Taichung)

● ⊥ 3 Earth
□ △ 3–7 Source

On the dorsal surface of the foot, in the angle between the first and second metatarsal bones.

Point of Yu (Summer)
First Aid: asphyxia

VIII **4** **Middle Seal** (Chungfeng)

○ ⊥ 4 Metal
△ 3–5

At the anterior flexure of the ankle, between the tendons of the tibialis anterior and the extensor hallucis longus.

Point of Ching (late Summer)

VIII **5** **Insect Ditch** (Likou)

⊖ ⊥ 3 Junction
△ 3–7

On the medial surface of the leg, 6 ACI proximal to the prominence of the medial malleolus, posterior to the edge of the tibia.

A Centre of Energy

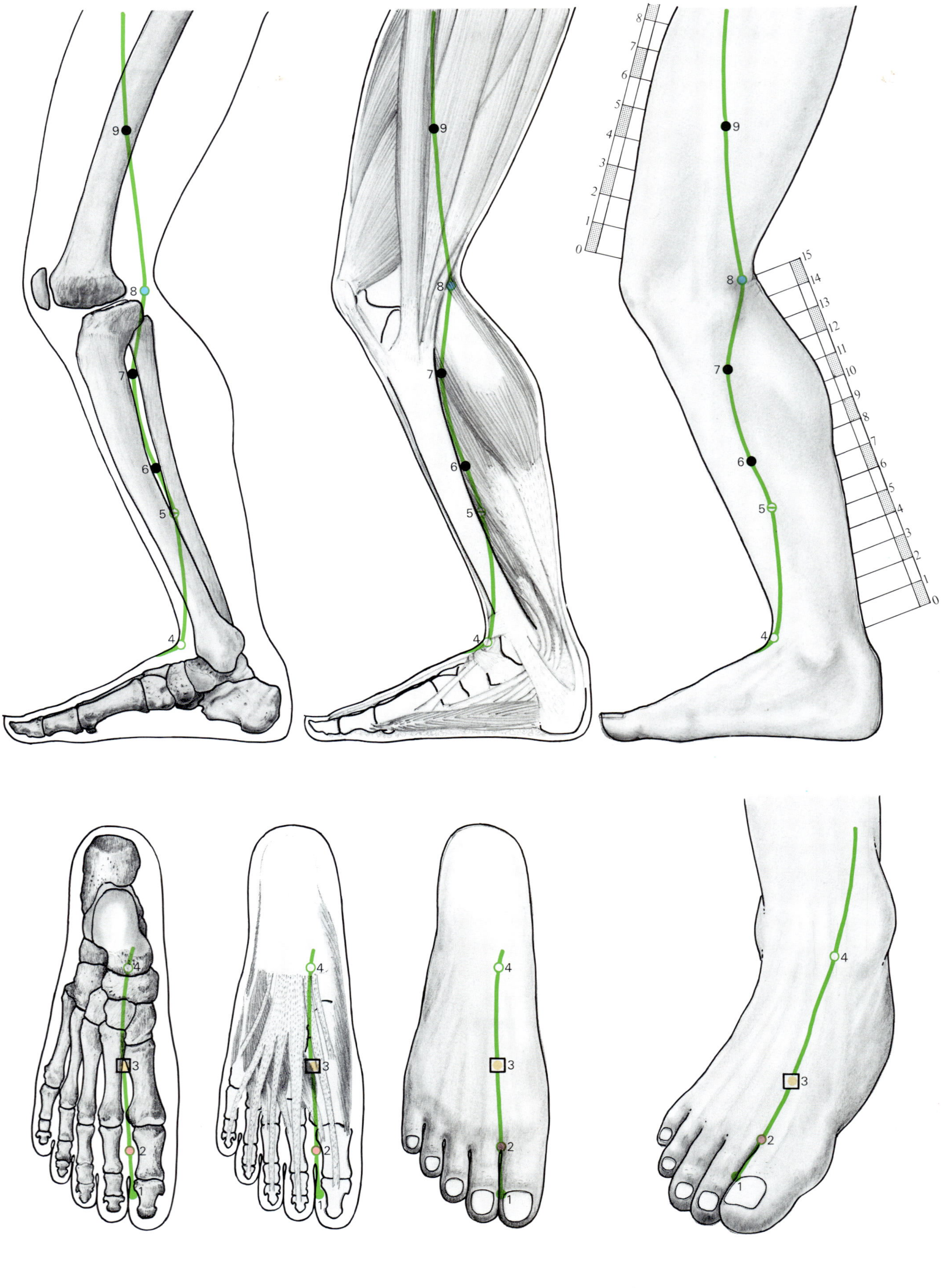
9
8
7
6
5
4
4
3
2
1

VIII **6** **Middle Capital** (Chungtu)

⊥ 3
△ 3

On the medial surface of the leg, 8 ACI proximal to the prominence of the medial malleolus, posterior to the edge of the tibia.

A Centre of Energy
First Aid: cramps, spasms, urine retention

VIII **7** **Knee Border** (Hsikuan)

⊥ 4
△ 5

On the medial surface of the leg, 12 ACI proximal to the prominence of the medial malleolus, posterior to the edge of the tibia.

VIII **8** **Crooked Spring** (Chuchuan)

● ⊥ 6 Water
△ 3–5 Tonification

On the medial surface of the knee, posterior to the medial condyle of the tibia; close to the extremity of the crease formed when the knee is flexed.

Point of Ho (Autumn)

VIII **9** **Yin Wrapping** (Yinpao)

⊥ 5
△ 3

On the medial surface of the thigh, 5 ACI proximal to the flexure of the knee, between the sartorius and the vastus medialis.

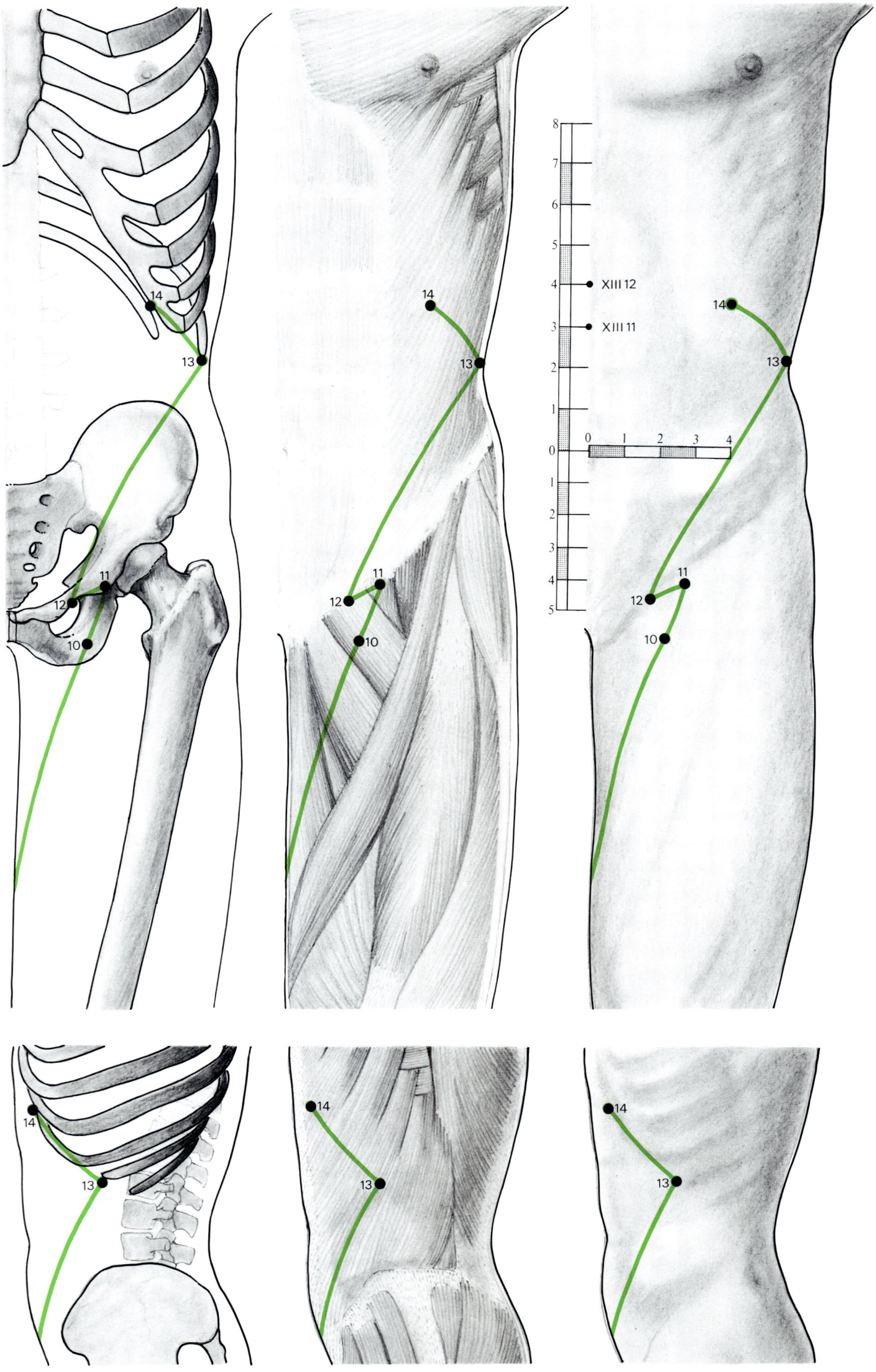
14
13
11
12
10
XIII 12
XIII 11
14
13
14
13
14
13

VIII **10** **Five Miles** (Tsu wuli)

⊥ 5
△ 5

On the anterior surface of the thigh, lateral to the adductor longus, just medial to the femoral artery, 1 ACI distal to the flexure of the groin.

VIII **11** **Yin Angle** (Yinlien)

⊥ 3
△ 3

On the flexure of the groin, just lateral to the femoral artery.

VIII **12** **Hasty Pulse** (Chimo)

⊥ X
△ 3

On the flexure of the groin, 2 ACI lateral to the mid-line of the pubic symphysis.

VIII **13** **Chapter Gate** (Changmen)

⊥ 6–8
△ 7–20

At the anterior tip of the eleventh rib.

Point of Dai Mo
Alarm Point of XII
Assembling Point of solid organs
Meeting Point of the five Yin organs

VIII **14** **Gate Of Hope** (Chimen)

⊥ 4 Exit
△ 5–7

On the inferior edge of the thoracic cage, on the paramedian nipple line. The point lies at the level half-way between XIII 11 and XIII 12.

Point of Yin Wei Mo
Alarm Point of VIII

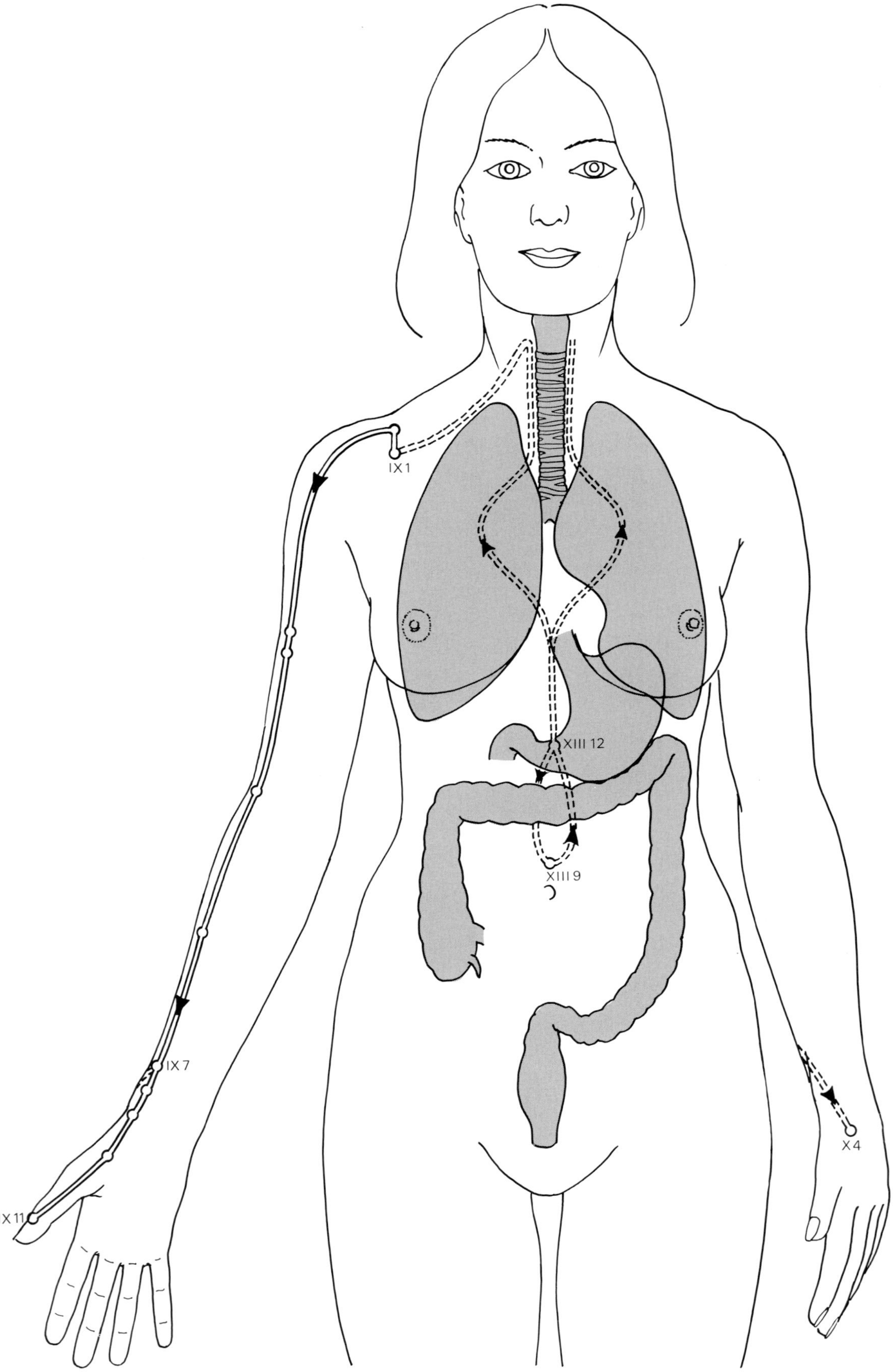
IX 1
XIII 12
XIII 9
IX 7
X 4
IX 11

The lung meridian begins at a deep level in the region of the stomach, at XIII 12. It descends to loop around the transverse colon, at XIII 9, then travels up the median line, passes the stomach and penetrates the diaphragm. Here it branches into each lobe of the lung. The meridian rejoins the median line above the lungs and ascends in two bilateral branches, on either side of the trachea, to the level of the larynx. Each branch then descends laterally to the inferior border of the clavicle and emerges to become the superficial pathway at a point lateral to the second rib, the entry point, IX 1.

The superficial meridian arches over the anterior surface of the shoulder and travels down the lateral side of the biceps to the flexure of the elbow. It then runs over the anterior radial side of the forearm to the region of the pulse, over the wrist on to the thenar eminence, along the anterolateral edge of the thumb to its last point, the lateral nail point, IX 11.

Proximal to the styloid process of the radius, a deep branch leaves the exit point, IX 7, and travels to the dorsal surface of the hand. It passes between the first and second metacarpal bones where it connects to the colon meridian, at X 4.

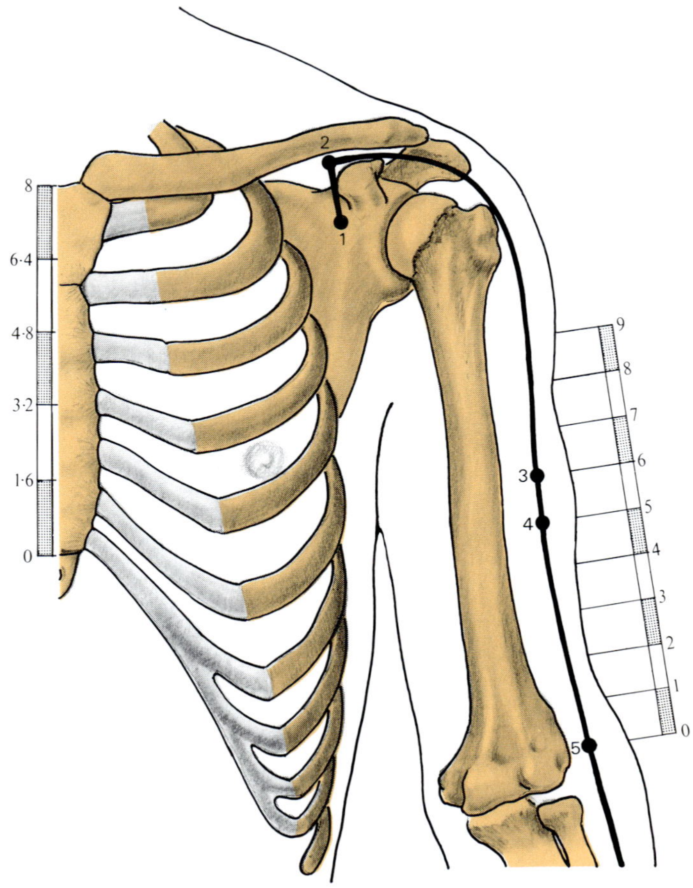
2
1
8
6·4
4·8
3·2
1·6
0
9
8
7
6
5
4
3
2
1
0
3
4
5

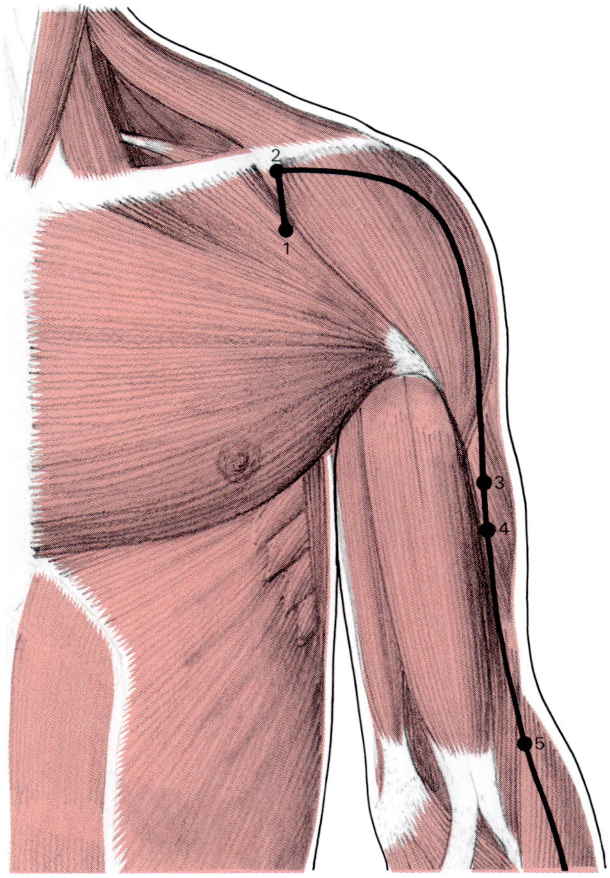
2
1
3
4
5

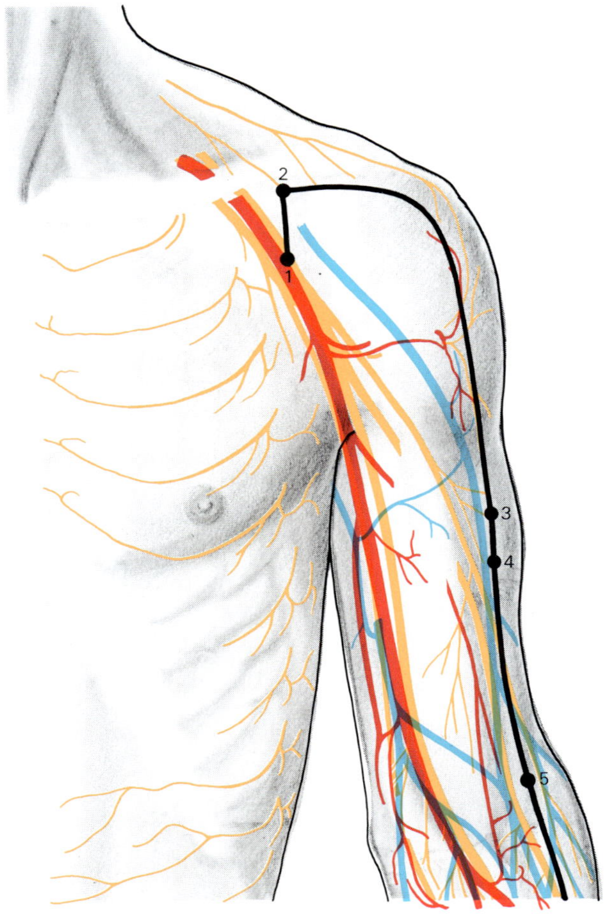
2
1
3
4
5

IX 1 On the chest, on a level with the space between the first and second ribs, 1.6 ACI inferior to IX 2.

IX 2 On the chest, in the depression which is found inferior to the clavicle and medial to the apex of the coracoid process.

IX 3 On the anterolateral surface of the arm, on the lateral border of the biceps, 6 ACI proximal to the flexure of the elbow. To find, the arm must be extended and rotated laterally at the shoulder joint, and the forearm fully supinated (i.e. in the anatomical position).

IX 4 On the anterolateral surface of the arm, on the lateral border of the biceps, 5 ACI proximal to the flexure of the elbow with the arm extended.

IX 5 On the elbow crease, approximately 1 ACI lateral to the tendon of the biceps.

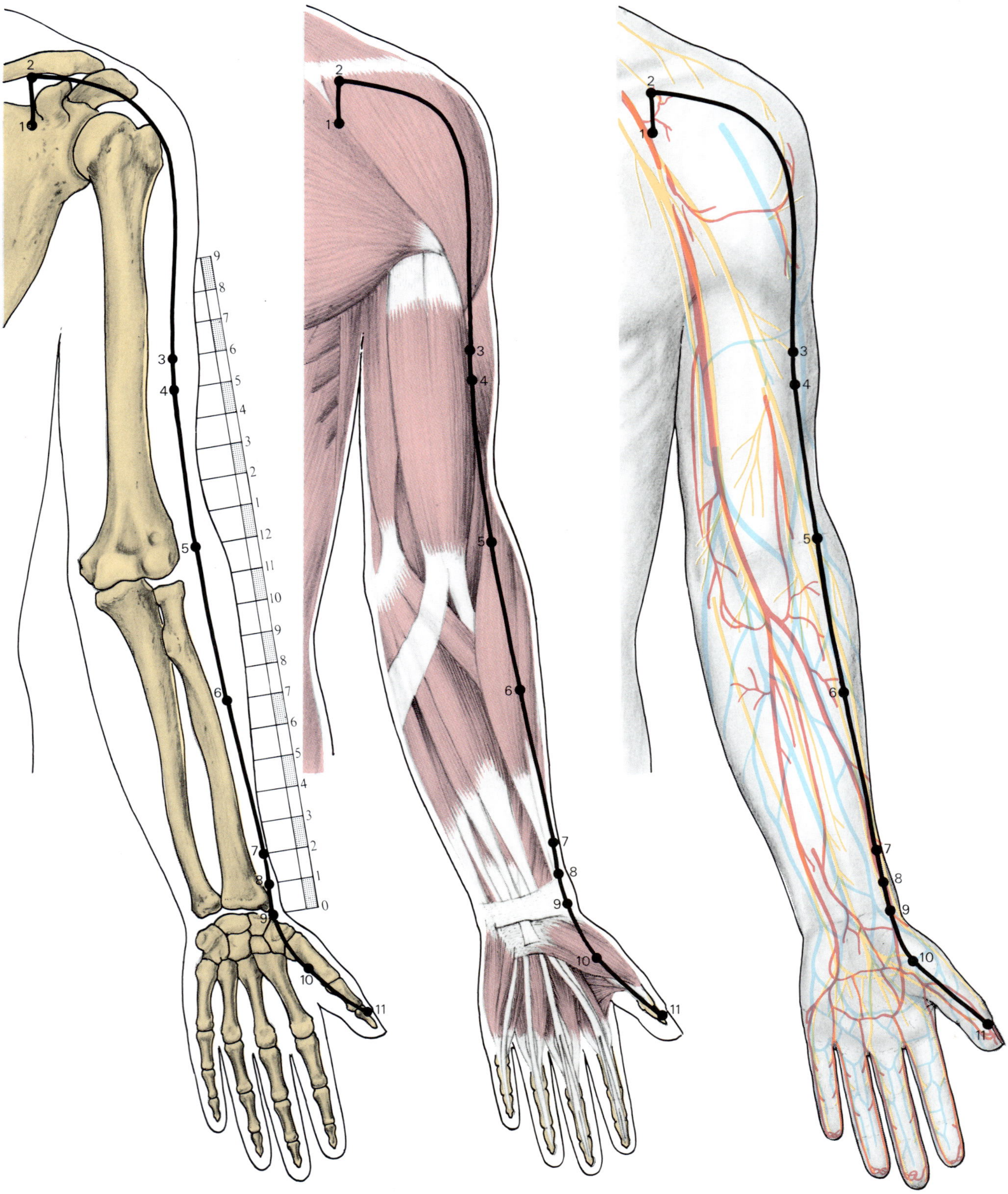
1 2 3 4 5 6 7 8 9 10 11
1 2 3 4 5 6 7 8 9 10 11
1 2 3 4 5 6 7 8 9 10 11

IX	6	On the anterior surface of the forearm, 7 ACI proximal to IX 9, lateral to the flexor carpi radialis.
IX	7	On the anterior surface of the forearm, 2 ACI proximal to IX 9, just lateral to the radial artery.
IX	8	On the anterior surface of the forearm, 1 ACI proximal to IX 9, upon the radial artery.
IX	9	On the crease of the flexure of the wrist, between the radius and the scaphoid bone, upon the radial artery.
IX	10	On the palmar surface of the hand, mid-way along the ulnar side of the first metacarpal bone.
IX	11	Radial nail point of the thumb.

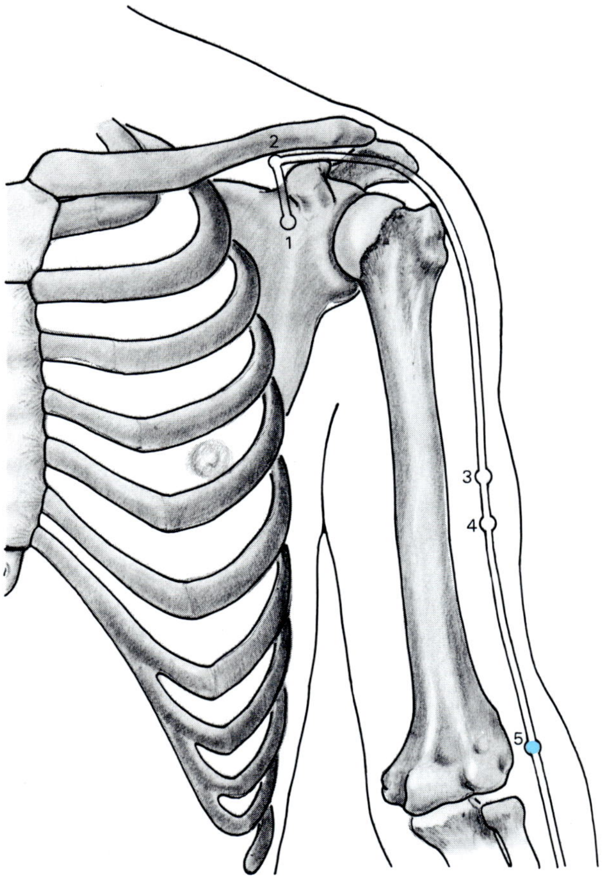

2
1
3
4
5

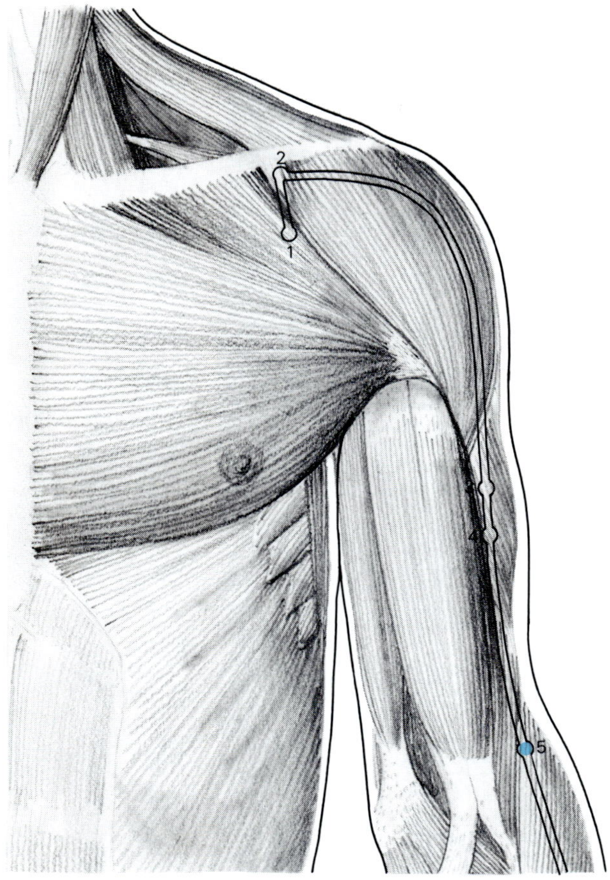

2
1
4
5

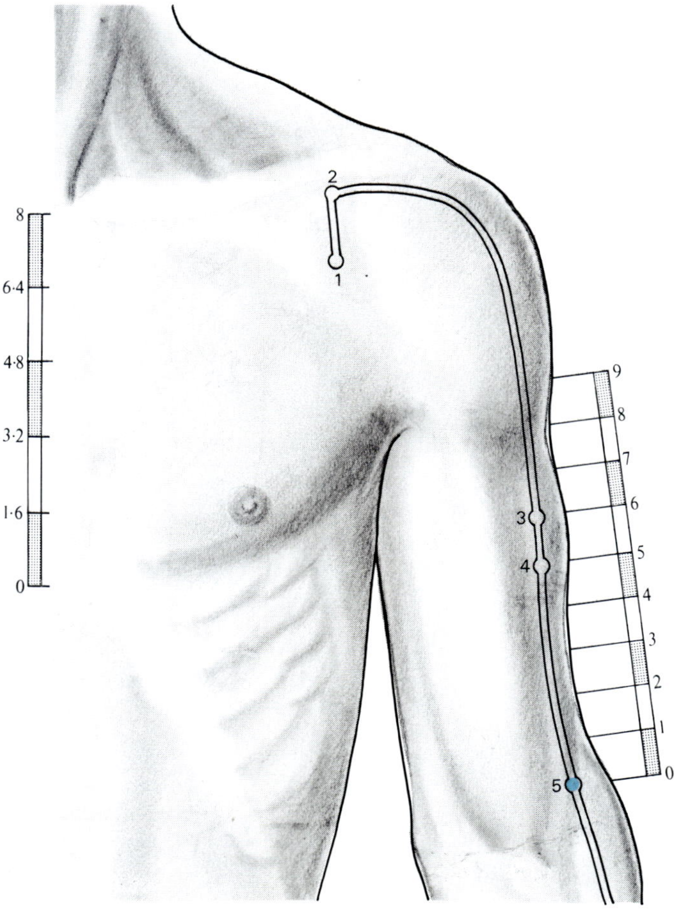

2
1
3
4
5
8
6·4
4·8
3·2
1·6
0
9
8
7
6
5
4
3
2
1
0

IX **1** **Middle Palace** (Chungfu)

⊥ 3–5 Entry
△ 5–10

On the chest, on a level with the space between the first and second ribs, 1.6 ACI inferior to IX 2.

Alarm Point of IX
First Aid: drowning

IX **2** **Cloud Gate** (Yunmen)

⊥ 3–5
△ 5–10

On the chest, in the depression which is found inferior to the clavicle and medial to the apex of the coracoid process.

IX **3** **Heavenly Palace** (Tienfu)

⊥ 4–6
△ X

On the anterolateral surface of the arm, on the lateral border of the biceps, 6 ACI proximal to the flexure of the elbow. To find, the arm must be extended and rotated laterally at the shoulder joint, and the forearm fully supinated (i.e. in the anatomical position).

Window of the Sky
First Aid: poison

IX **4** **Valiant White** (Hsiapai)

⊥ 3–5
△ 5

On the anterolateral surface of the arm, on the lateral border of the biceps, 5 ACI proximal to the flexure of the elbow with the arm extended.

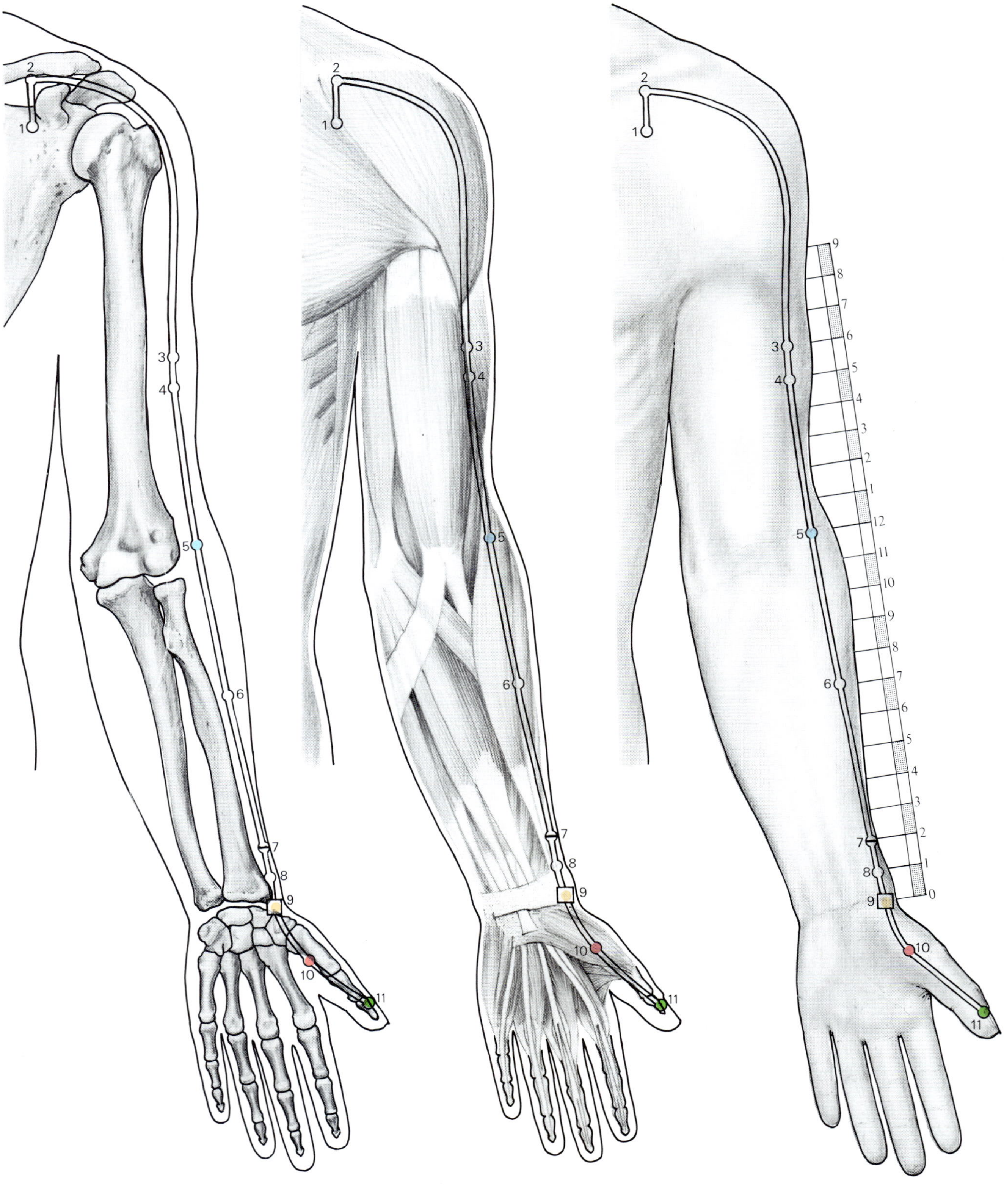
1
2
3
4
5
6
7
8
9
10
11
1
2
3
4
5
6
7
8
9
10
11
1
2
3
4
5
6
7
8
9
10
11
9
8
7
6
5
4
3
2
1
12
11
10
9
8
7
6
5
4
3
2
1
0

	IX	**5**	**Outside Marsh** (Chihtse)
●	⊥	3–5	Water
	△	3–5	Sedation

On the elbow crease, approximately 1 ACI lateral to the tendon of the biceps.

Point of Ho (Autumn)

	IX	**6**	**Greatest Hole** (Kungtsui)
	⊥	5	
	△	5	

On the anterior surface of the forearm, 7 ACI proximal to IX 9, lateral to the flexor carpi radialis.

	IX	**7**	**Narrow Defile** (Liehchueh)
⊖	⊥	2–3	Junction
	△	3–5	Exit
		XP6	

On the anterior surface of the forearm, 2 ACI proximal to IX 9, just lateral to the radial artery.

Master Point of Ren Mo
Coupled Point of Yin Qiao Mo

	IX	**8**	**Meridian Gutter** (Chingchu)
○	⊥	2–3	Metal
	△	X	Horary 3 a.m.–5 a.m.

On the anterior surface of the forearm, 1 ACI proximal to IX 9, upon the radial artery.

Point of Ching (late Summer)
First Aid: electric shock

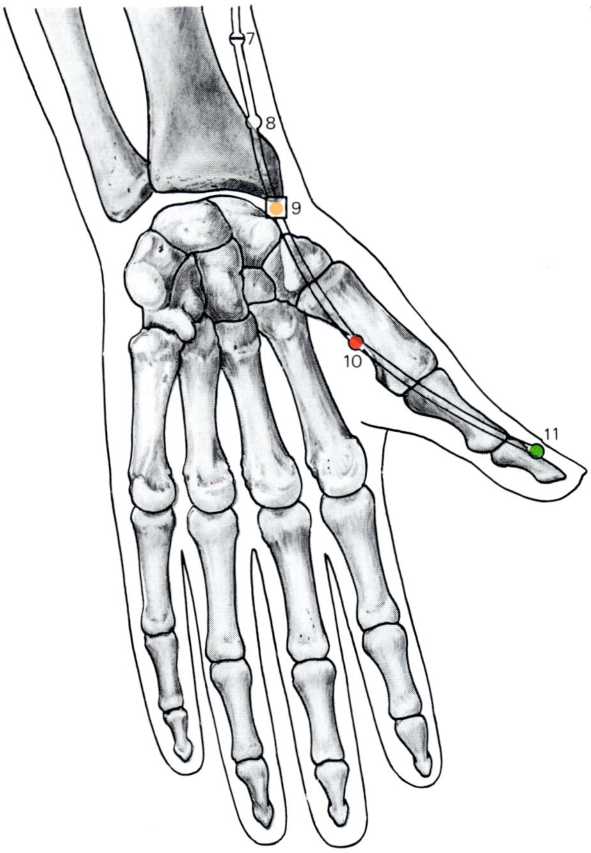
7
8
9
10
11

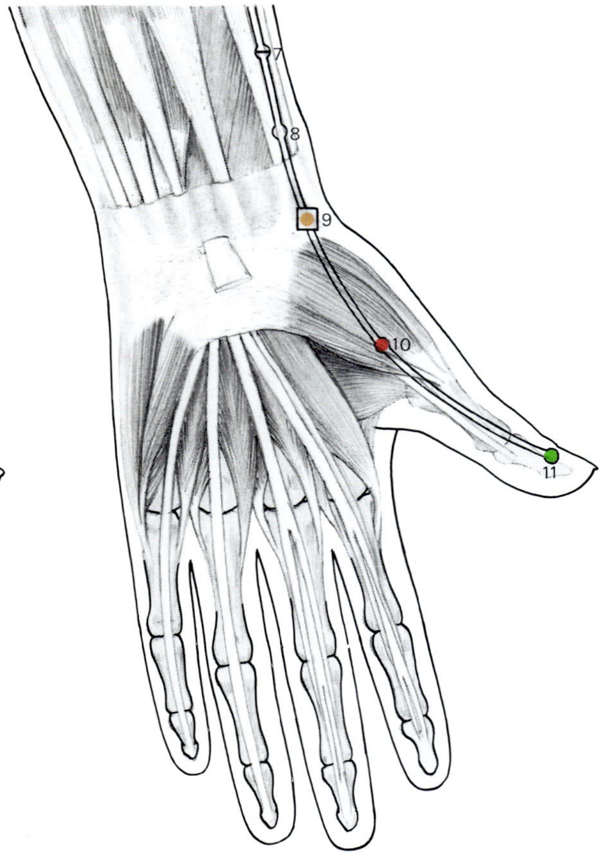
7
8
9
10
11

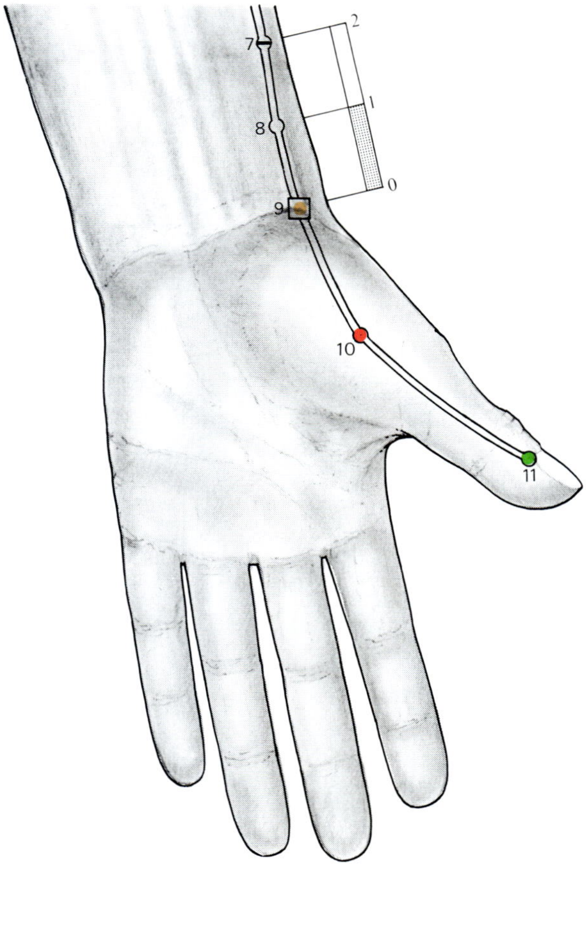
2
7
1
8
0
9
10
11

IX **9** **Very Great Abyss** (Taiyuan)

● ⊥ 2 Earth
△ 3 Tonification
□ Source

On the crease of the flexure of the wrist, between the radius and the scaphoid bone, upon the radial artery.

Point of Yu (Summer)
Assembling Point of meridians
Reunion of arteries and veins
First Aid: asphyxia, collapse, concussion, food poisoning, insensibility, poison, shock

IX **10** **Fish Region** (Yuchi)

● ⊥ 3–5 Fire
△ X

On the palmar surface of the hand, mid-way along the ulnar side of the first metacarpal bone.

Point of Yung (Spring)

IX **11** **Little Merchant** (Shaoshang)

● ⊥ 1 Wood
△ X
XP7

Radial nail point of the thumb.

Point of Cheng (Winter)
First Aid: convulsions, insensibility, sunstroke

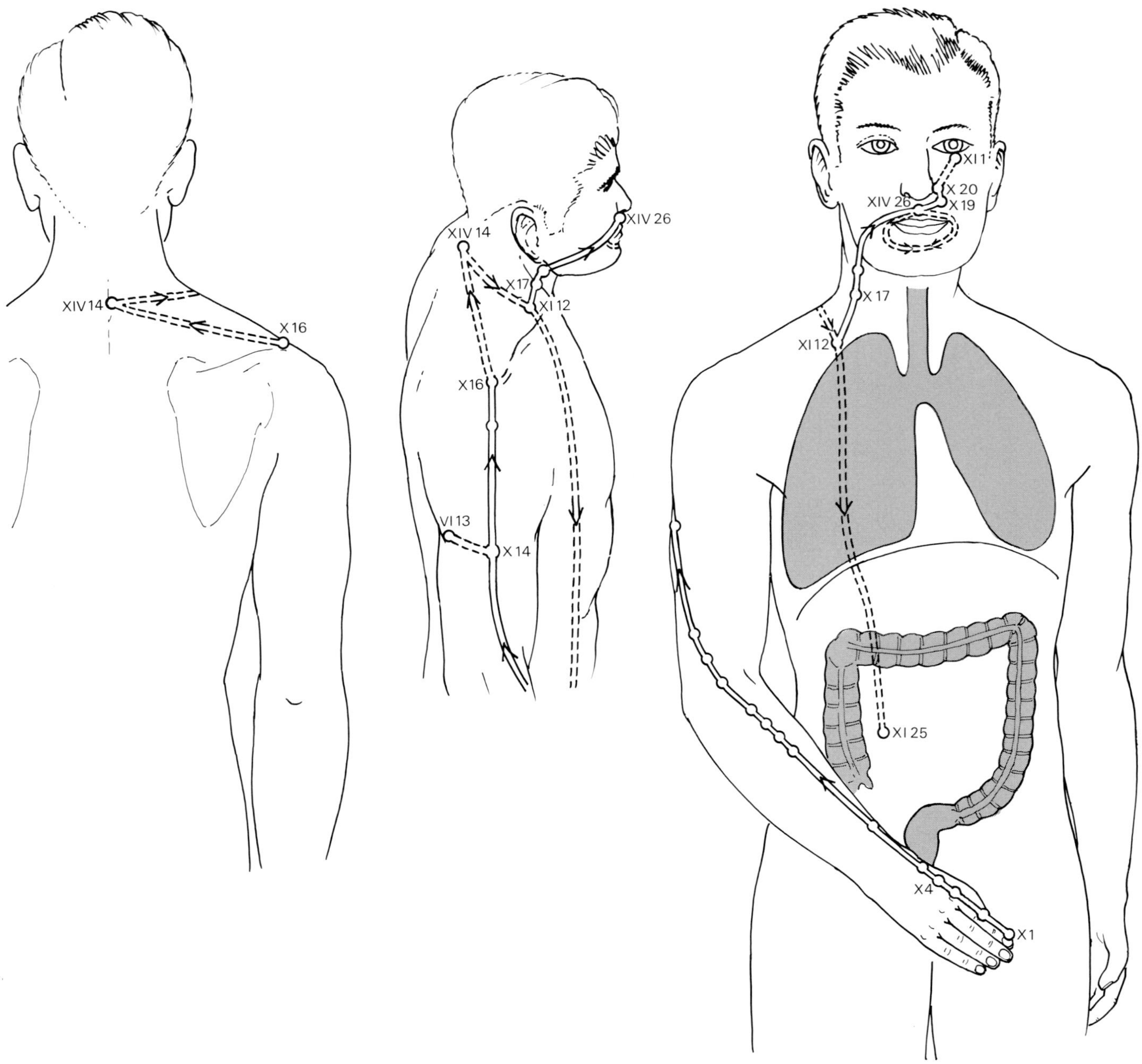
XIV14
X16
XIV 14
X17
XI 12
XIV 26
X16
VI 13
X 14
XI 1
X 20
XIV 26
X 19
X 17
XI 12
XI 25
X4
X1

The colon meridian begins as the superficial pathway at the radial nail point of the index finger, X 1. The meridian travels along the dorsal surface of the index finger on the lateral side, passes through the angle of the first and second metacarpal bones, at the entry point, X 4, through the anatomical snuffbox, up the radial margin of the forearm to the lateral border of the elbow, lateral to the epicondyle of the humerus. It then ascends the lateral border of the biceps to the insertion of the deltoid. From this point, X 14, a short deep branch extends posteriorly to VI 13.

The main meridian continues to the shoulder passing through the cleft between the acromion and the clavicle, to X 16. From X 16 a deep section of the meridian travels across the trapezius to the median line at the base of the seventh cervical vertebra, at XIV 14. It returns anteriorly over the shoulder to the supraclavicular fossa, at XI 12. Here the meridian divides.

A deep branch continues down through the chest, enters the lungs, penetrates the diaphragm and travels through the abdomen to connect with the large intestines, at XI 25. The other superficial branch continues medially to the base of the neck, at X 17, travels up a portion of the sternocleidomastoid to the posterior region of the mandible. From there it runs to the upper jaw and the upper lip. At the philtrum, at XIV 26, it crosses over to the opposite side of the face to X 19 and ends at the inferior edge of the alum of the nose, at the exit point, X 20. From here it connects to the stomach meridian, at XI 1.

A deep branch leaves the meridian in the upper jaw and travels through the gum of the lower jaw, encircling the mouth.

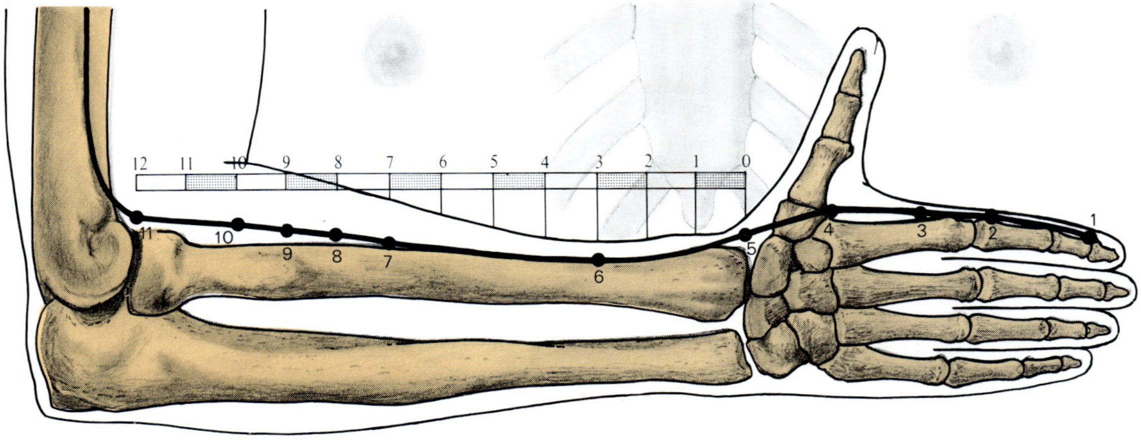
12
11
10
9
8
7
6
5
4
3
2
1
0
11
10
9
8
7
6
5
4
3
2
1

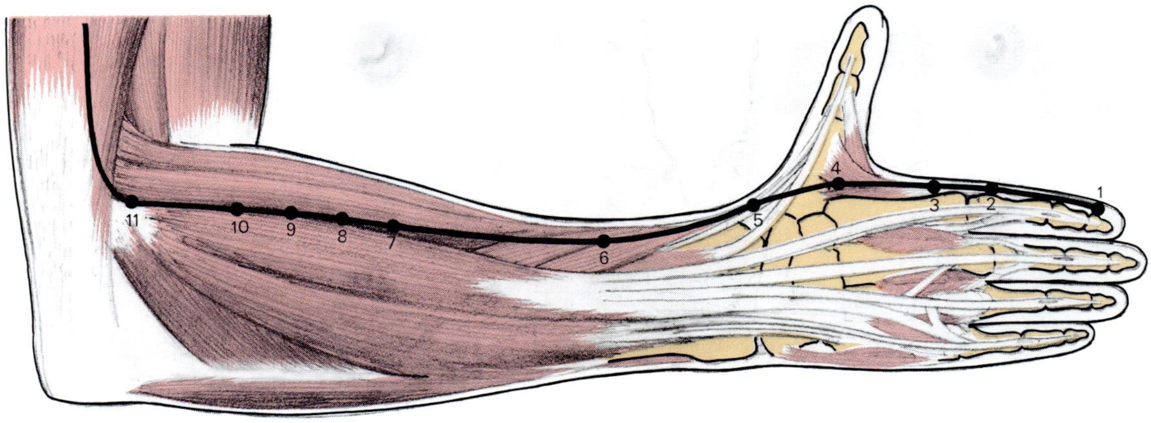
11
10
9
8
7
6
5
4
3
2
1

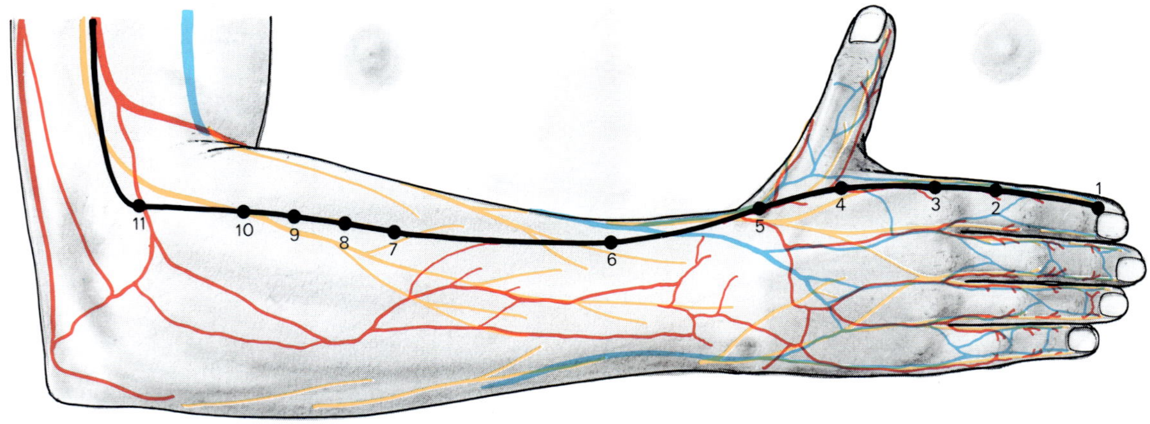
11
10
9
8
7
6
5
4
3
2
1

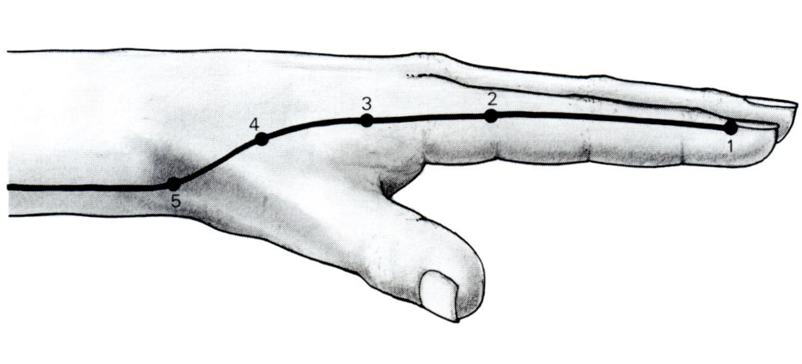
5
4
3
2
1

X 1 Radial nail point of the index finger.

X 2 On the posterolateral surface of the index finger, just distal to the base of the proximal phalanx.

X 3 On the dorsal surface of the hand, immediately proximal and radial to the head of the second metacarpal bone.

X 4 On the dorsal surface of the hand, in the angle between the proximal ends of the first and second metacarpal bones.

X 5 On the radial edge of the wrist, between the styloid process of the radius and the base of the scaphoid bone, between the extensor pollicis longus and the extensor pollicis brevis, in the anatomical snuffbox.

X 6 On the posterior radial surface of the forearm, 3 ACI proximal to the flexure of the wrist, along the radius. With the anterior surface of the forearm across the chest, the point lies ulnar to the radial edge of the radius.

X 7 On the posterior radial surface of the forearm, 7 ACI proximal to the flexure of the wrist. With the anterior surface of the forearm across the chest, the point lies on the radial border of the extensor digitorum.

X 8 On the posterior radial surface of the forearm, 8 ACI proximal to the flexure of the wrist. With the anterior surface of the forearm across the chest, the point lies on the radial border of the extensor digitorum.

X 9 On the posterior radial surface of the forearm, 9 ACI proximal to the flexure of the wrist. With the anterior surface of the forearm across the chest, the point lies on the radial border of the extensor digitorum.

X 10 On the posterior radial surface of the forearm, 10 ACI proximal to the flexure of the wrist. With the anterior surface of the forearm across the chest, the point lies on the radial border of the extensor digitorum.

X 11 On the posterior radial surface of the forearm. With the anterior surface of the forearm across the chest, the point lies between the lateral end of the elbow crease and the lateral epicondyle of the humerus.

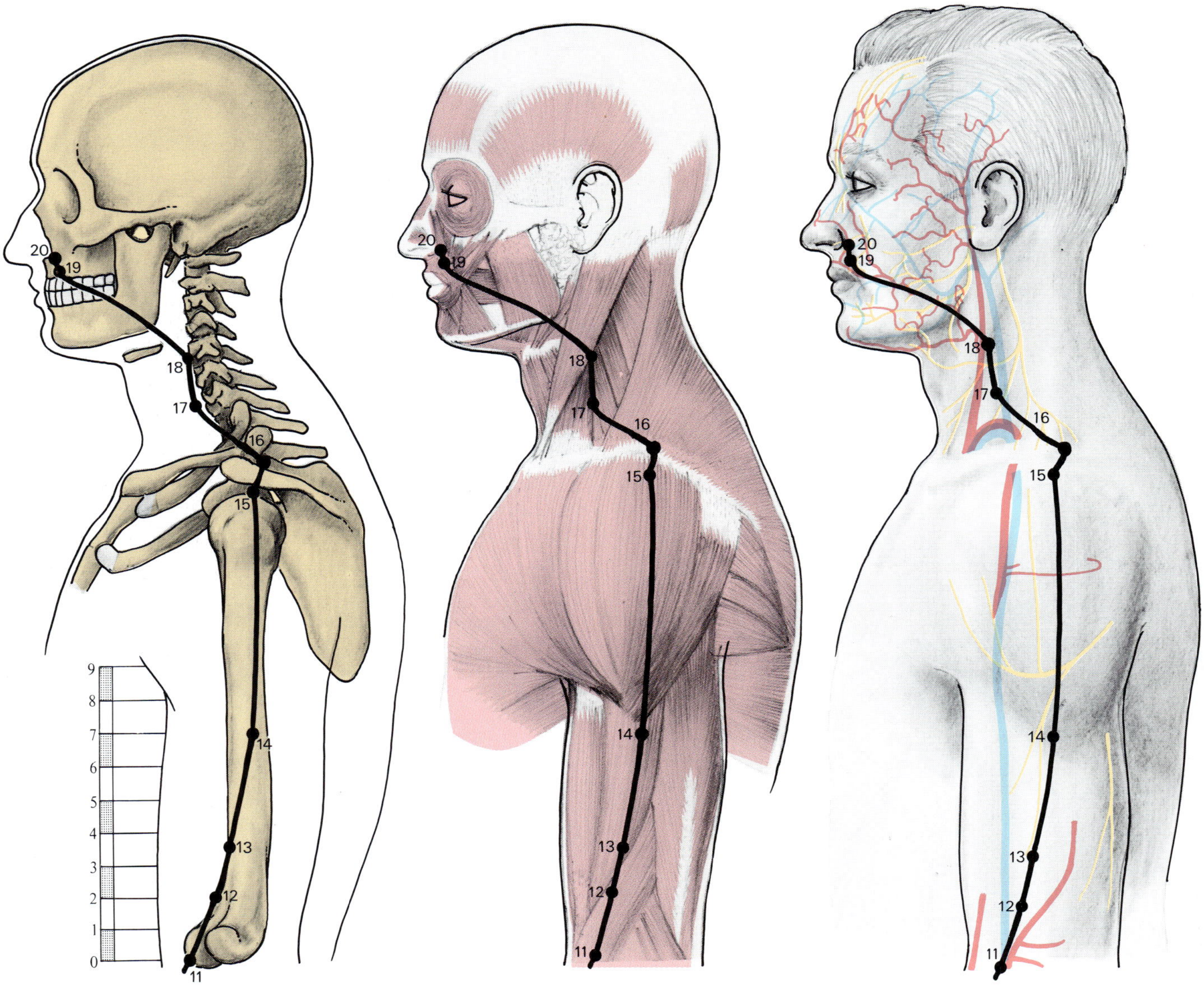

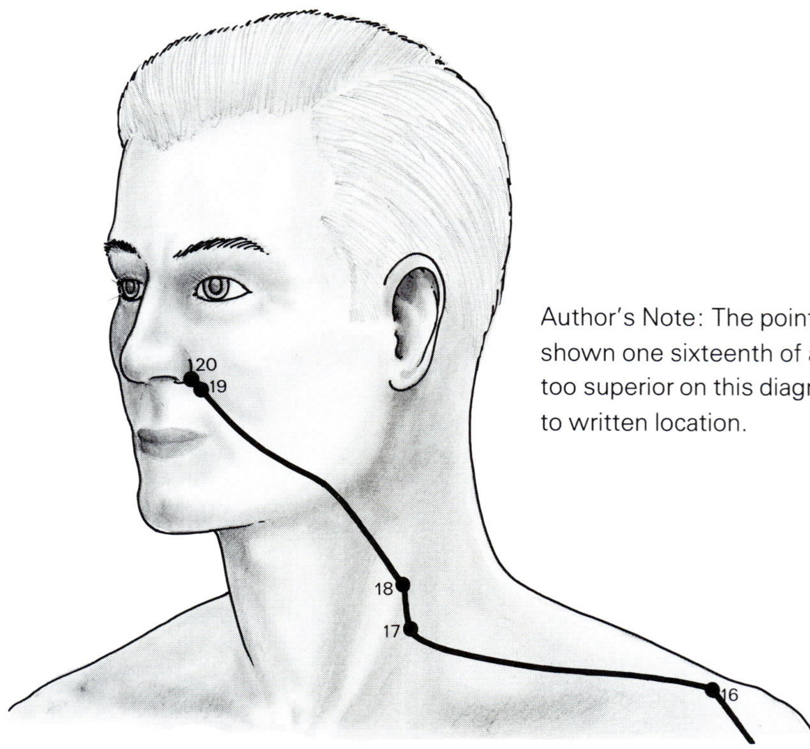

Author's Note: The point X19 is shown one sixteenth of an inch too superior on this diagram. Refer to written location.

X	12	On the lateral surface of the arm, 2 ACI proximal to the lateral epicondyle of the humerus.
X	13	On the lateral surface of the arm, $3\frac{1}{2}$ ACI proximal to the lateral epicondyle of the humerus.
X	14	On the anterolateral surface of the arm, 7 ACI proximal to the flexure of the elbow, on the distal border of the 'V' of the insertion of the deltoid.
X	15	On the lateral surface of the shoulder, distal to the acromioclavicular joint, in the concavity between the acromion and the greater tubercle of the humerus, formed when the arm is abducted.
X	16	In the depression between the acromial end of the clavicle and the spine of the scapula.
X	17	On the posterior border of the sternocleidomastoid, approximately 1 ACI inferior to X 18.
X	18	Between the two heads of the sternocleidomastoid, lateral to, and on a level with, the middle of the laryngeal prominence, and XI 9.
X	19	Half-way between the inferior border of the nose and the edge of the upper lip, $\frac{1}{2}$ ACI medial to the nasolabial fold.
X	20	On the face, at the inferior edge of the alum, 1 fen lateral to the alum.

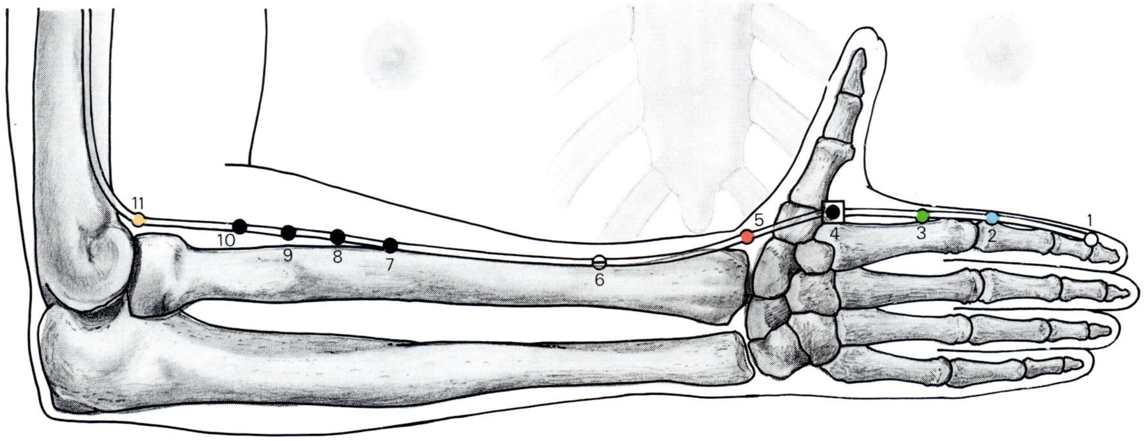
11
10
9
8
7
6
5
4
3
2
1

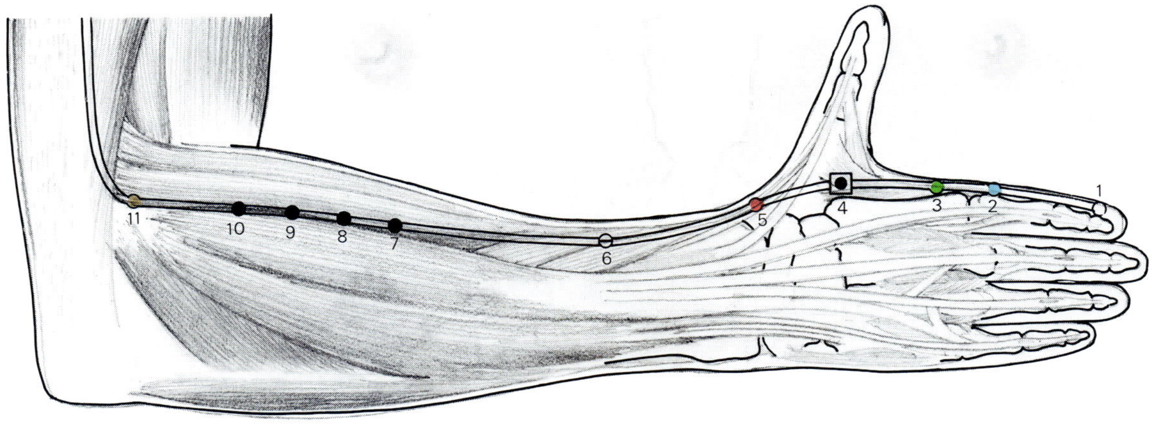
11
10
9
8
7
6
5
4
3
2
1

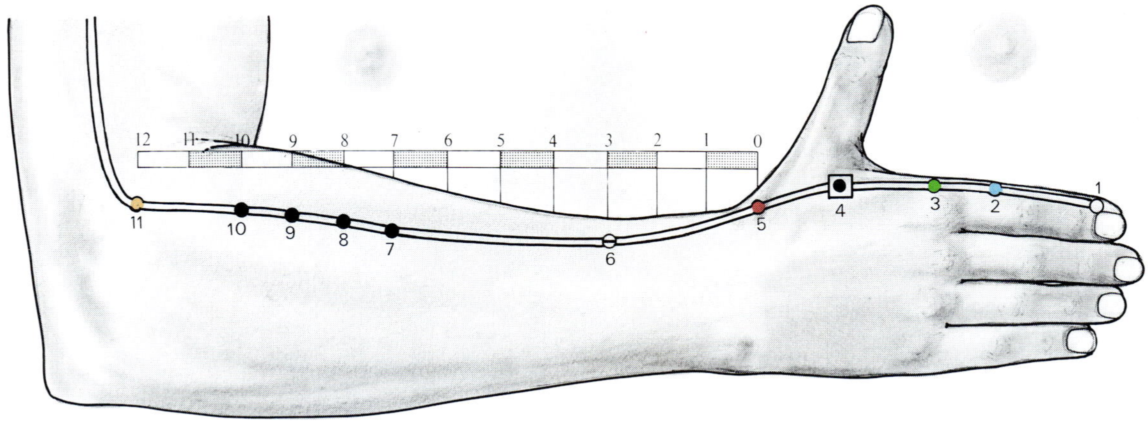
12 11 10 9 8 7 6 5 4 3 2 1 0
11
10
9
8
7
6
5
4
3
2
1

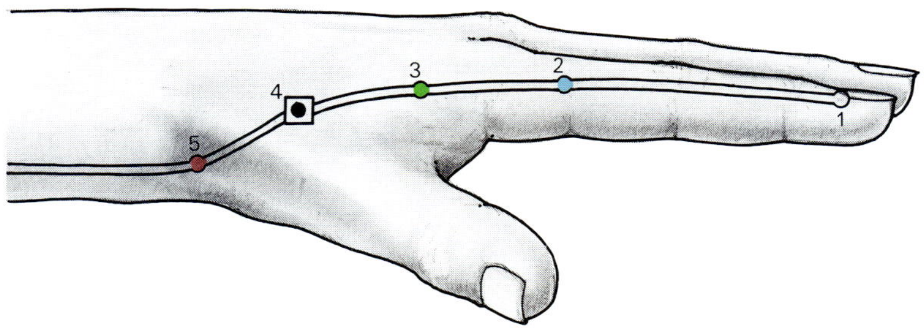
5
4
3
2
1

X **1** **Merchant Yang** (Shangyang)

○ ⊥ 1 Metal
△ 3 Horary 5 a.m.–7 a.m.

Radial nail point of the index finger.

Point of Cheng (Winter)
First Aid: toothache

X **2** **Second Interval** (Erhchien)

● ⊥ 3 Water
△ 3 Sedation
XP9

On the posterolateral surface of the index finger, just distal to the base of the proximal phalanx.

Point of Yung (Spring)

X **3** **Third Interval** (Sanchien)

● ⊥ 3 Wood
△ 3

On the dorsal surface of the hand, immediately proximal and radial to the head of the second metacarpal bone.

Point of Yu (Summer)

X **4** **Joining Of The Valleys** (Hoku)

□ ⊥ 5 Source
△ 5–7 Entry
XP1

On the dorsal surface of the hand, in the angle between the proximal ends of the first and second metacarpal bones.

Point for acupuncture blackout
Centre Reunion General Point of Yang
Greater Assembling Point of the face and mouth
A Centre of Energy
First Aid: dull pains, earache, fainting, food poisoning, poison, toothache

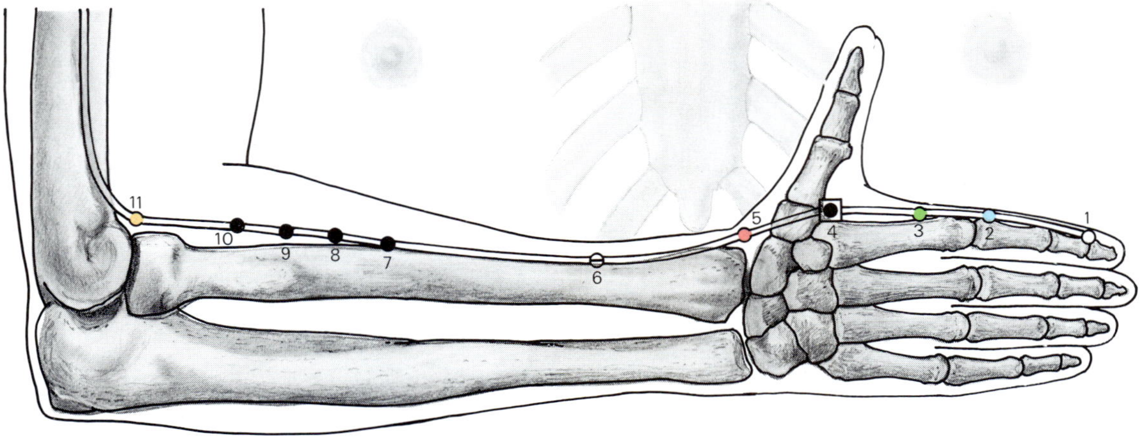
11
10
9
8
7
6
5
4
3
2
1

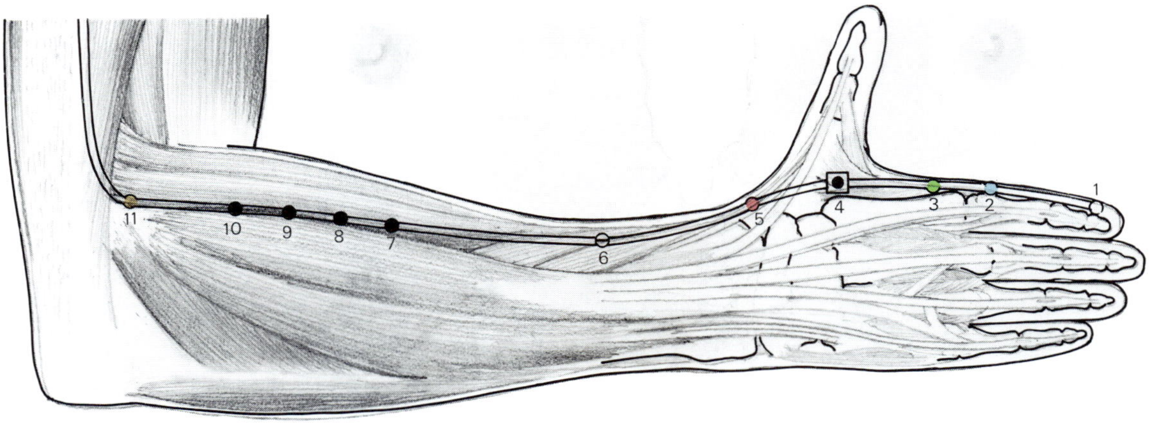
11
10
9
8
7
6
5
4
3
2
1

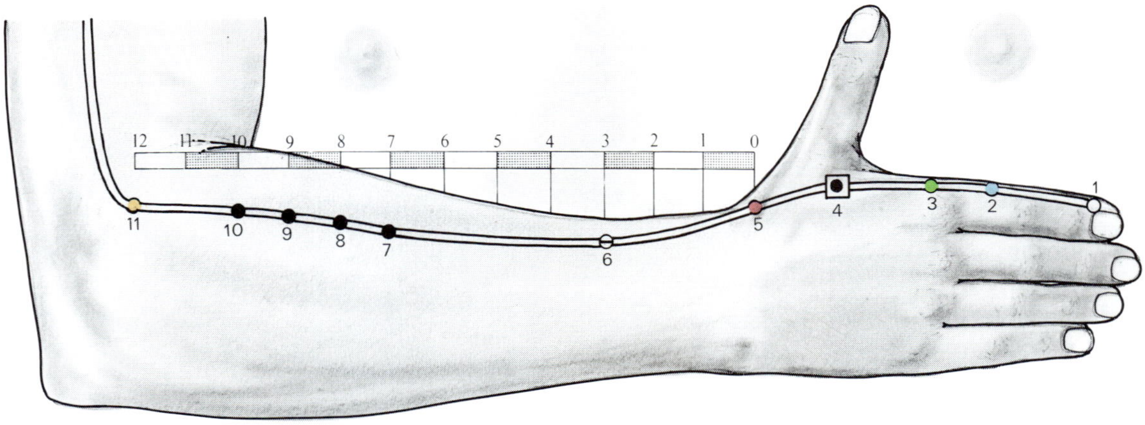
12 11 10 9 8 7 6 5 4 3 2 1 0
11
10
9
8
7
6
5
4
3
2
1

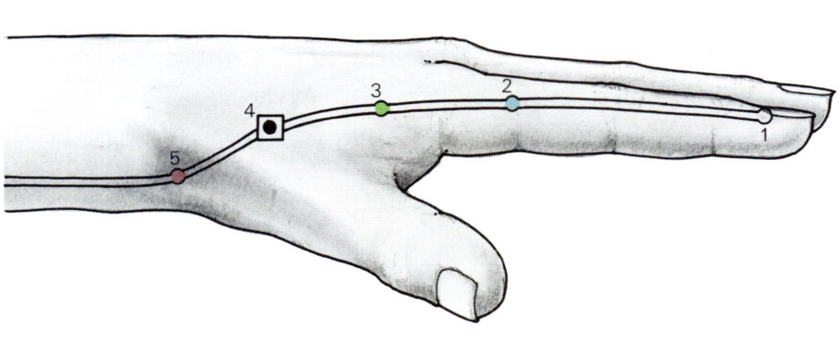
5
4
3
2
1

X **5** **Yang Stream** (Yanghsi)

⊥ 3 Fire
△ 5

On the radial edge of the wrist, between the styloid process of the radius and the base of the scaphoid bone, between the extensor pollicis longus and the extensor pollicis brevis, in the anatomical snuffbox.

Point of Ching (late Summer)

X **6** **Side Passage** (Pienli)

⊖ ⊥ 3 Junction
△ 5–7

On the posterior radial surface of the forearm, 3 ACI proximal to the flexure of the wrist, along the radius. With the anterior surface of the forearm across the chest, the point lies ulnar to the radial edge of the radius.

X **7** **Warm Current** (Wenliu)

⊥ 3
△ 5–30

On the posterior radial surface of the forearm, 7 ACI proximal to the flexure of the wrist. With the anterior surface of the forearm across the chest, the point lies on the radial border of the extensor digitorum.

X **8** **Lower Side** (Hsialien)

⊥ 4
△ 6

On the posterior radial surface of the forearm, 8 ACI proximal to the flexure of the wrist. With the anterior surface of the forearm across the chest, the point lies on the radial border of the extensor digitorum.

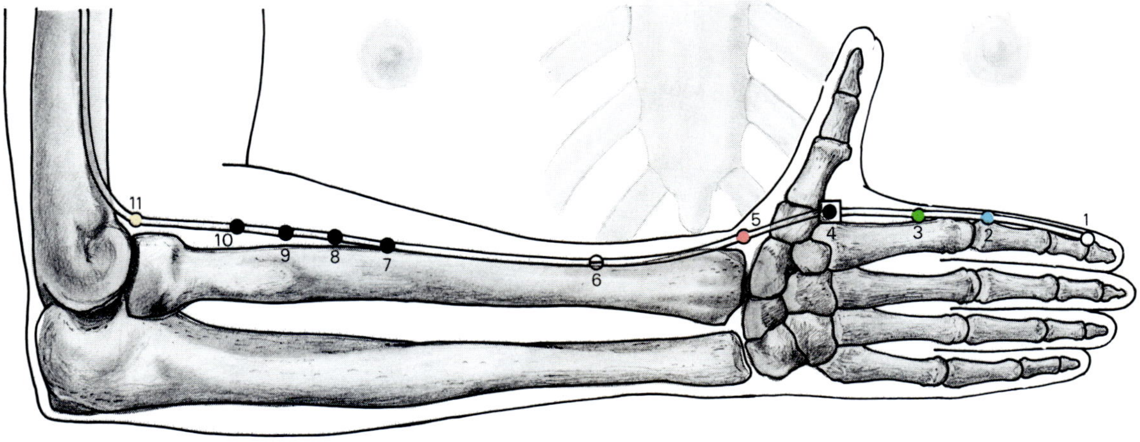
11
10
9
8
7
6
5
4
3
2
1

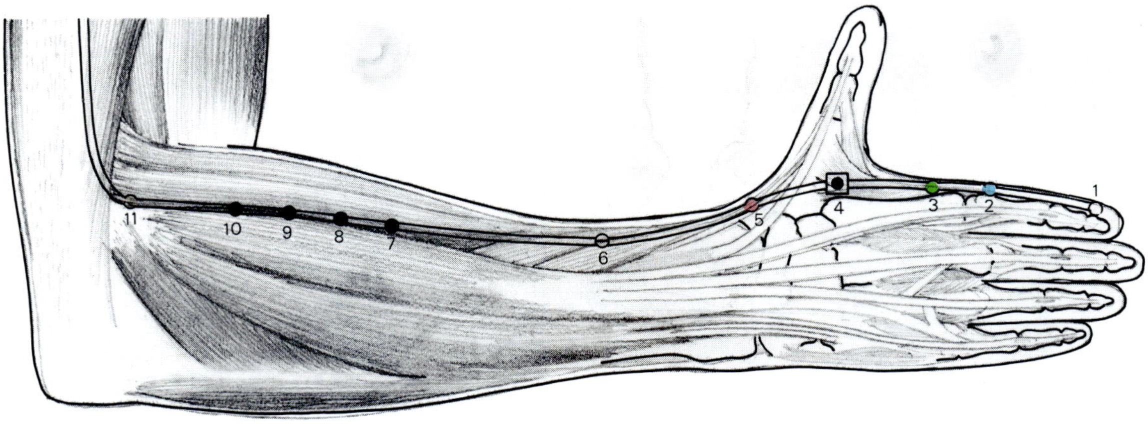
11
10
9
8
7
6
5
4
3
2
1

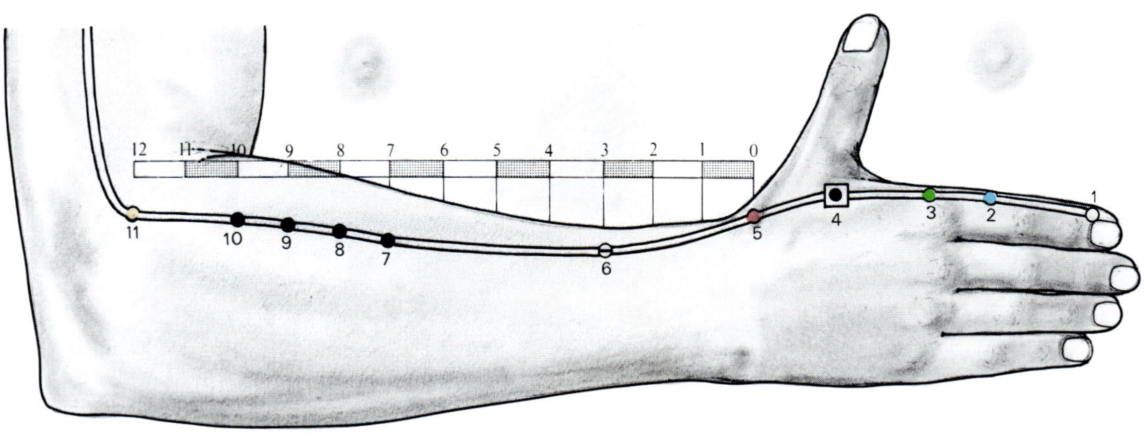
12 11 10 9 8 7 6 5 4 3 2 1 0
11
10
9
8
7
6
5
4
3
2
1

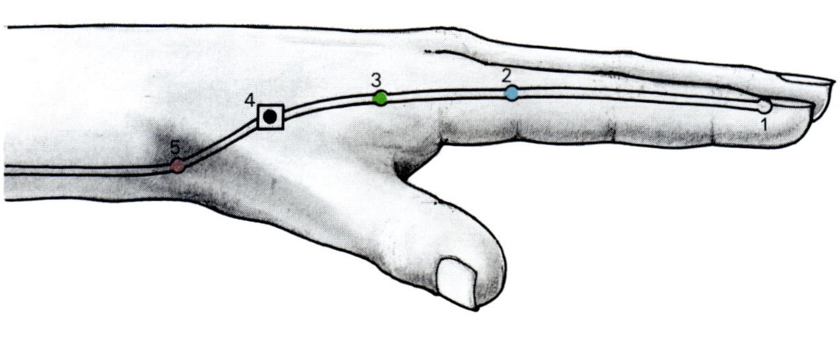
5
4
3
2
1

X **9** **Upper Angle** (Shanglien)

⊥ 4
△ 5–10

On the posterior radial surface of the forearm, 9 ACI proximal to the flexure of the wrist. With the anterior surface of the forearm across the chest, the point lies on the radial border of the extensor digitorum.

X **10** **Arm Three Miles** (Shou sanli)

⊥ 5
△ 5–10
XP9

On the posterior radial surface of the forearm, 10 ACI proximal to the flexure of the wrist. With the anterior surface of the forearm across the chest, the point lies on the radial border of the extensor digitorum.

X **11** **Crooked Pond** (Chuchih)

⊥ 5–8 Earth
△ 5–10 Tonification

On the posterior radial surface of the forearm. With the anterior surface of the forearm across the chest, the point lies between the lateral end of the elbow crease and the lateral epicondyle of the humerus.

Point of Ho (Autumn)

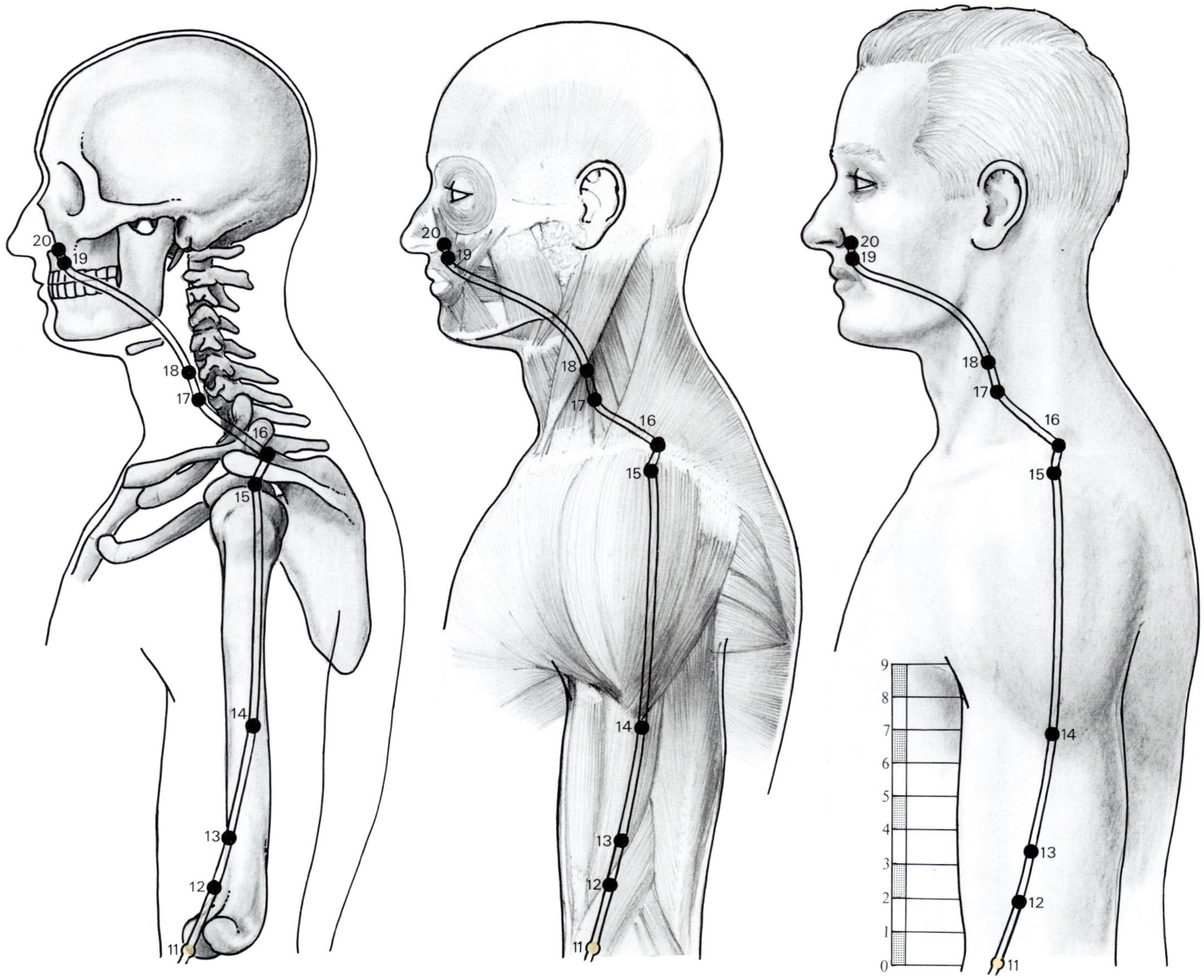

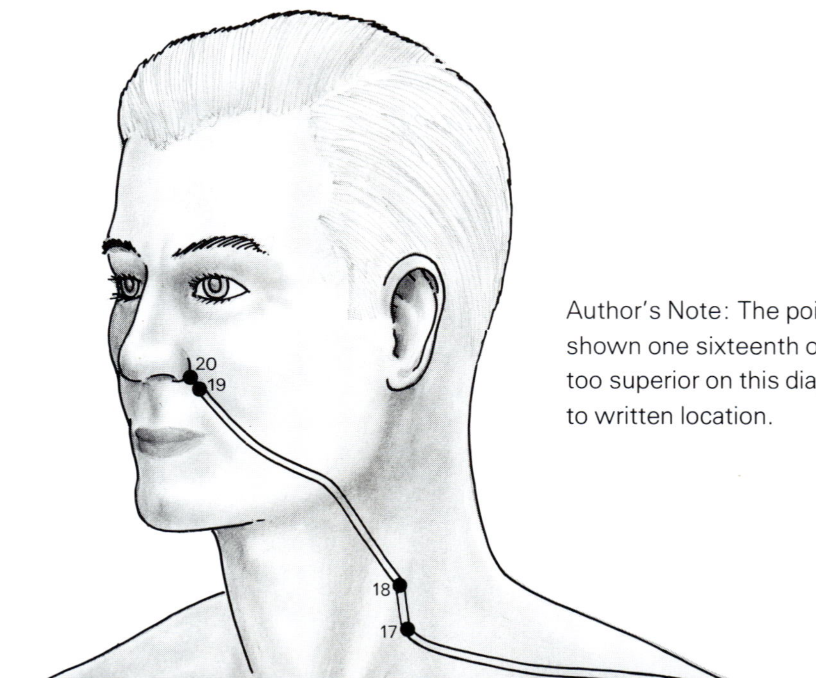

Author's Note: The point X19 is shown one sixteenth of an inch too superior on this diagram. Refer to written location.

X **12** **Elbow Bone** (Chouliao)

⊥ 3
△ 3

On the lateral surface of the arm, 2 ACI proximal to the lateral epicondyle of the humerus.

X **13** **Arm Five Miles** (Shou wuli)

⊥ X
△ 7

On the lateral surface of the arm, $3\frac{1}{2}$ ACI proximal to the lateral epicondyle of the humerus.

X **14** **Outer Bone Of The Arm** (Pinao)

⊥ 3
△ 3–7

On the anterolateral surface of the arm, 7 ACI proximal to the flexure of the elbow, on the distal border of the 'V' of the insertion of the deltoid.

X **15** **Shoulder Joint** (Chienyu)

⊥ 6
△ 7

On the lateral surface of the shoulder, distal to the acromioclavicular joint, in the concavity between the acromion and the greater tubercle of the humerus, formed when the arm is abducted.

Point of Yang Qiao Mo
First Aid: apoplexy, concussion, electric shock, exhaustion, haemorrhage, head injury, insensibility, shock

X **16** **Great Bone** (Chuku)

⊥ 6
△ 3–7

In the depression between the acromial end of the clavicle and the spine of the scapula.

Point of Yang Qiao Mo

X **17** **Heavenly Vessel** (Tienting)

⊥ 3
△ 3–7

On the posterior border of the sternocleidomastoid, approximately 1 ACI inferior to X 18.

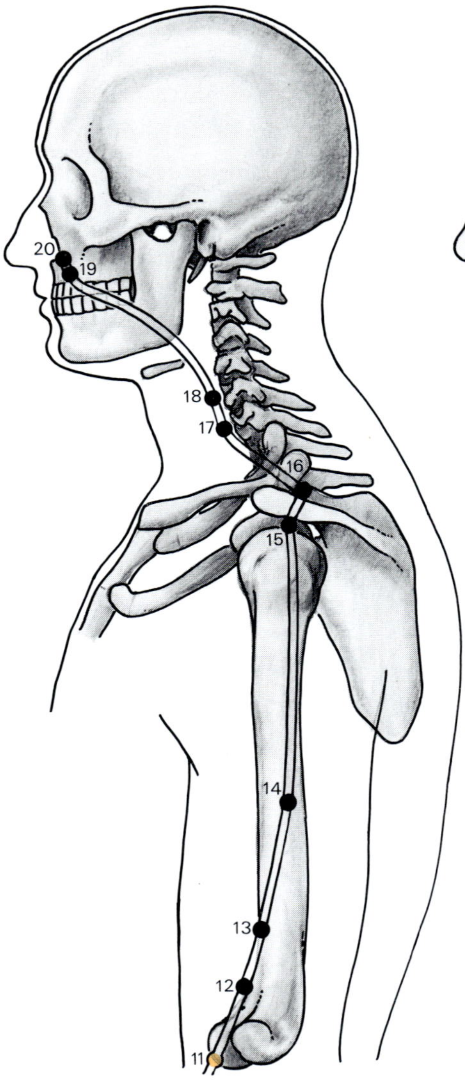

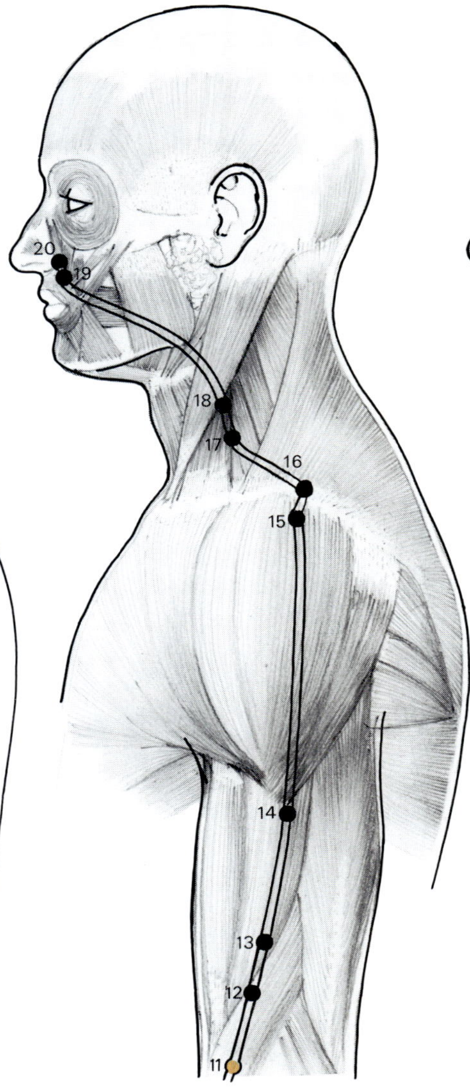

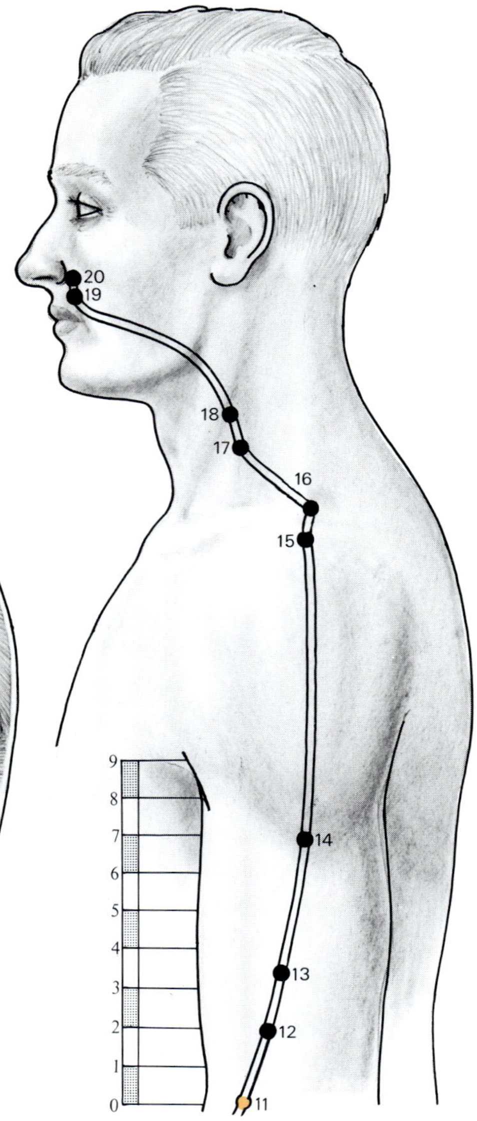

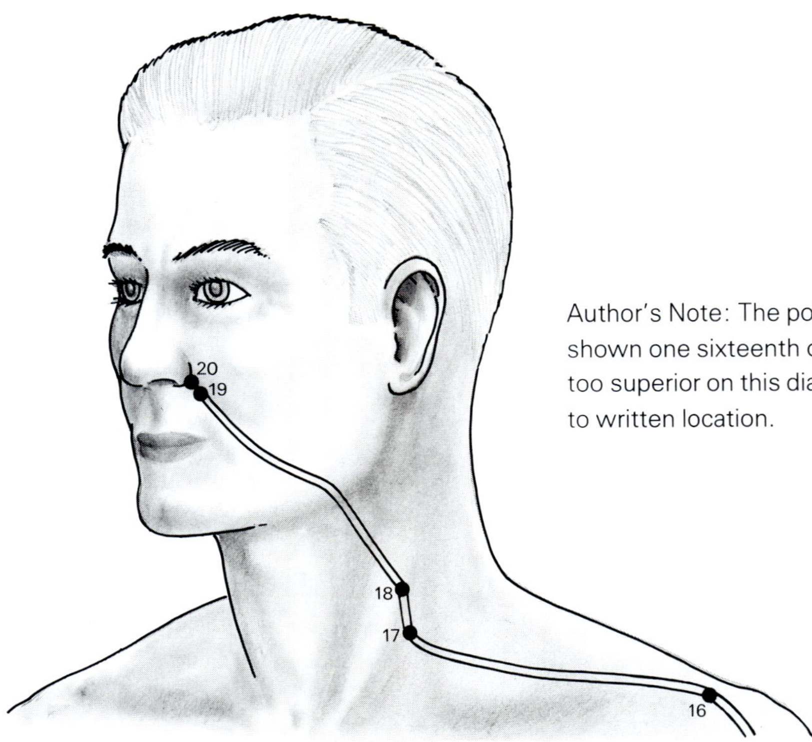

Author's Note: The point X19 is shown one sixteenth of an inch too superior on this diagram. Refer to written location.

X **18** **Support And Rush Out** (Futu)

⊥ 4
△ 3

Between the two heads of the sternocleidomastoid, lateral to, and on a level with, the middle of the laryngeal prominence, and XI 9.

Window of the Sky

X **19** **Grain Bone** (Holiao)

⊥ 1–3
△ X

Half-way between the inferior border of the nose and the edge of the upper lip, $\frac{1}{2}$ ACI medial to the nasolabial fold.

X **20** **Welcome Fragrance** (Yinghsiang)

⊥ 1–3 Exit
△ X

On the face, at the inferior edge of the alum, 1 fen lateral to the alum.

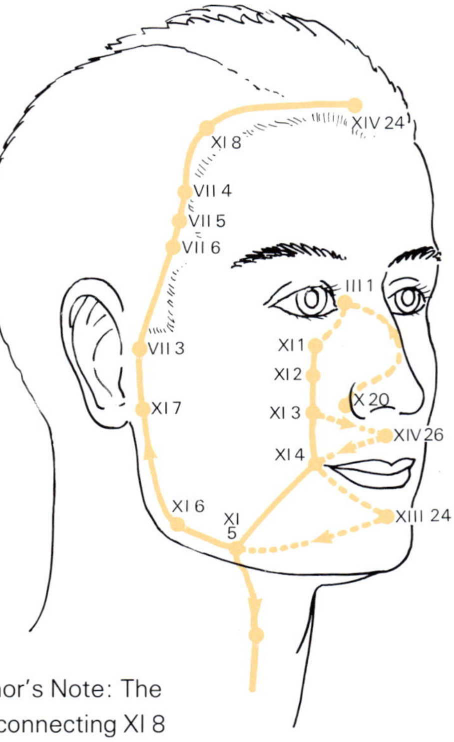

Author's Note: The line connecting XI 8 and XIV 24 should be a broken line rather than a solid one.

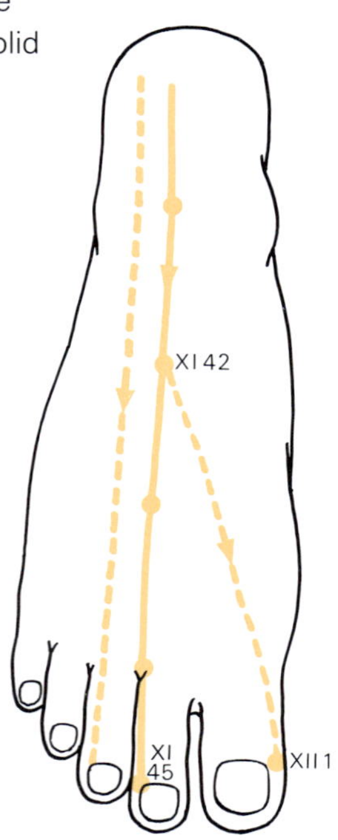

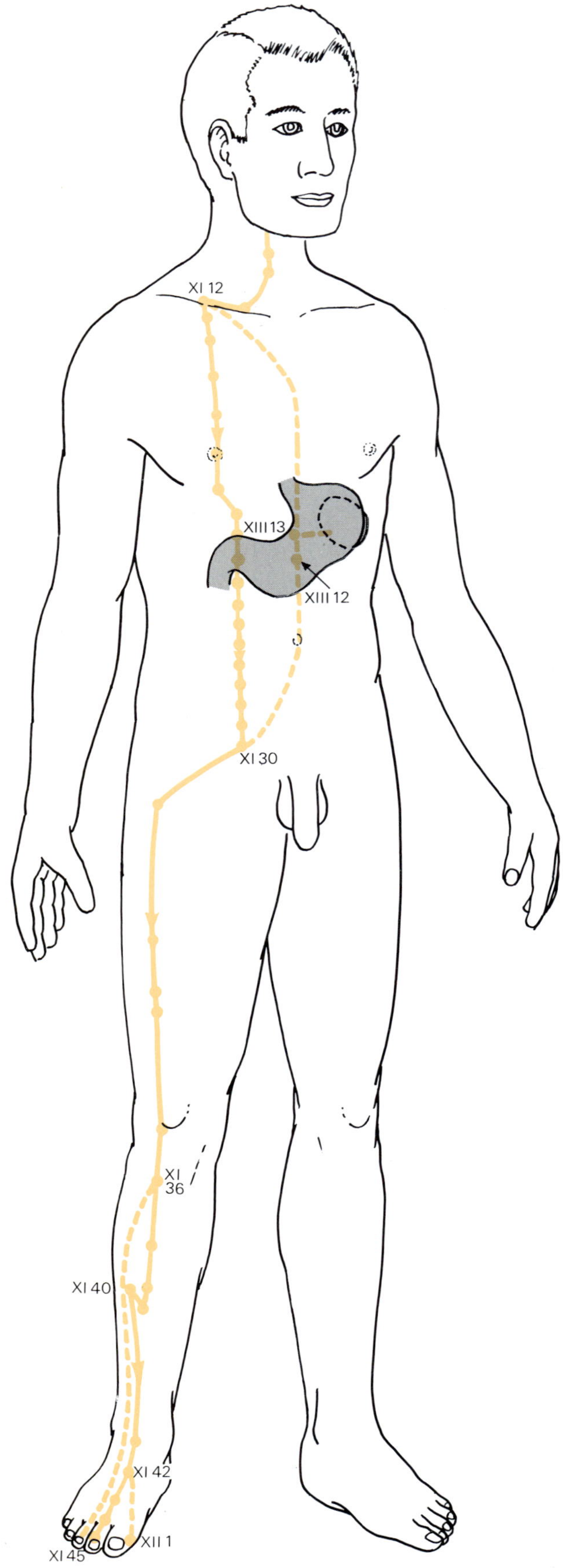

The stomach meridian begins at a deep level in the region of the nasal alum at X 20. It rises up the side of the nose to the mid-line of the bridge of the nose, then turns to the medial corner of the eye, at III 1. It travels laterally to the centre of the inferior border of the orbit, where the meridian becomes superficial, at XI 1. The superficial meridian descends the cheek in line with the pupil of the eye, through XI 2, XI 3 and XI 4. From XI 3 a deep pathway crosses to the philtrum on the upper lip at XIV 26 and contours the mouth through XI 4. It continues to the centre of the lower lip at XIII 24 and then on to rejoin the superficial meridian. The meridian then passes laterally to XI 5 at the masseter at the angle of the lower jaw, ascends through XI 6 anterior to the ear, to XI 7, and from there to the hair line on the temple, and up over the frontal bone, passing points VII 3, 6, 5 and 4, and then through XI 8 to the mid-point of the hair line above the forehead, at XIV 24.

The first branch leaves the meridian from the mandible and continues the superficial pathway down the side of the trachea to the medial end of the clavicle. It then runs laterally to the supraclavicular fossa, at XI 12, where it divides into a superficial and a deep pathway. The superficial pathway descends the chest in the line of the nipple. In the fifth intercostal space it deviates medially to continue down the abdomen in the paramedian line to the inguinal ligament, at XI 30. The deep pathway leaves XI 12 and travels medially and inferiorly through the chest, penetrates the diaphragm and enters the stomach in the median line, at XIII 13. A branch leaves from here to connect with the spleen.

The deep pathway continues down the median line to XIII 12 and then travels inferiorly and laterally to meet the superficial meridian at XI 30. The pathway is now single and superficial as it descends the anterior surface of the leg along the lateral edge of the rectus femoris, through the lateral border of the patella and down the lateral edge of the tibia. At 9 ACI inferior to the patella the meridian detours superiorly and laterally to XI 40 and thence to the centre of the ankle joint. It travels along the mid-line of the dorsal surface of the foot, between the second and third metatarsal bones to end at the lateral nail point of the second toe at the last point, XI 45.

A deep branch leaves the superficial meridian from the point 3 ACI below the patella, XI 36, travels lateral to the superficial pathway and ends at the lateral nail point of the middle toe. A second branch leaves the superficial meridian from the middle of the dorsal surface of the foot, at the exit point, XI 42, and runs to the medial nail point of the big toe, where it connects with the spleen meridian, at XII 1.

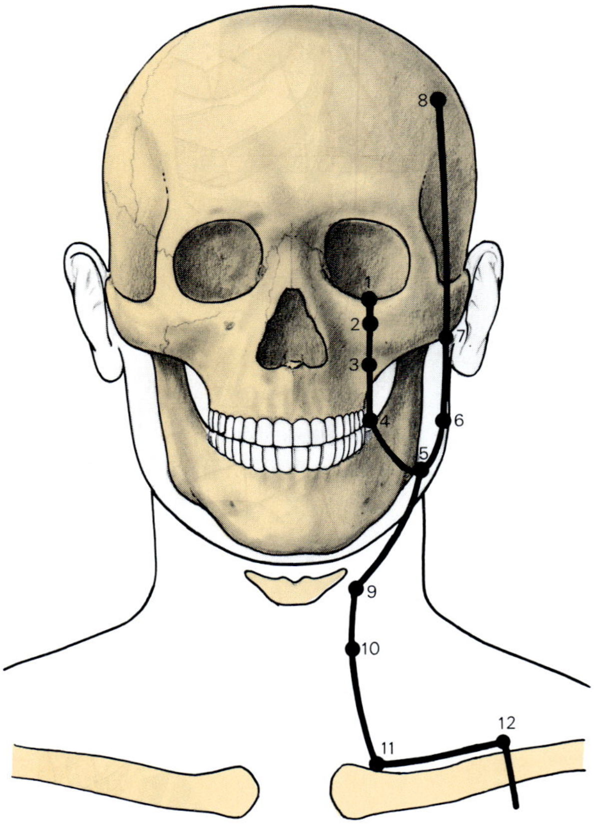
1
2
3
4
5
6
7
8
9
10
11
12

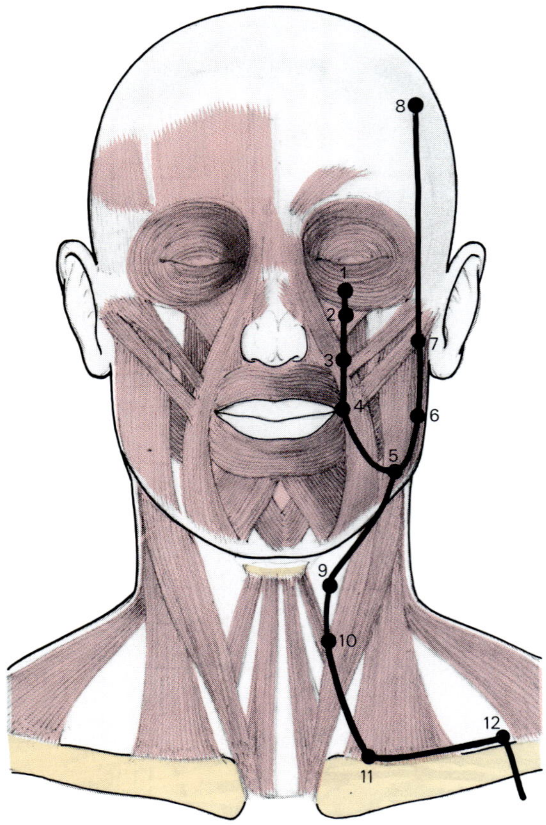
1
2
3
4
5
6
7
8
9
10
11
12

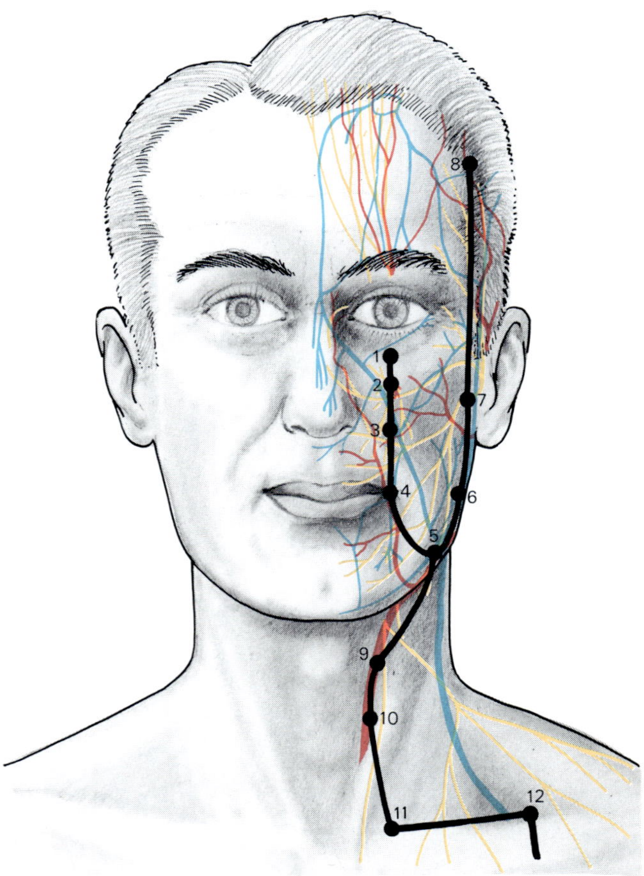
1
2
3
4
5
6
7
8
9
10
11
12

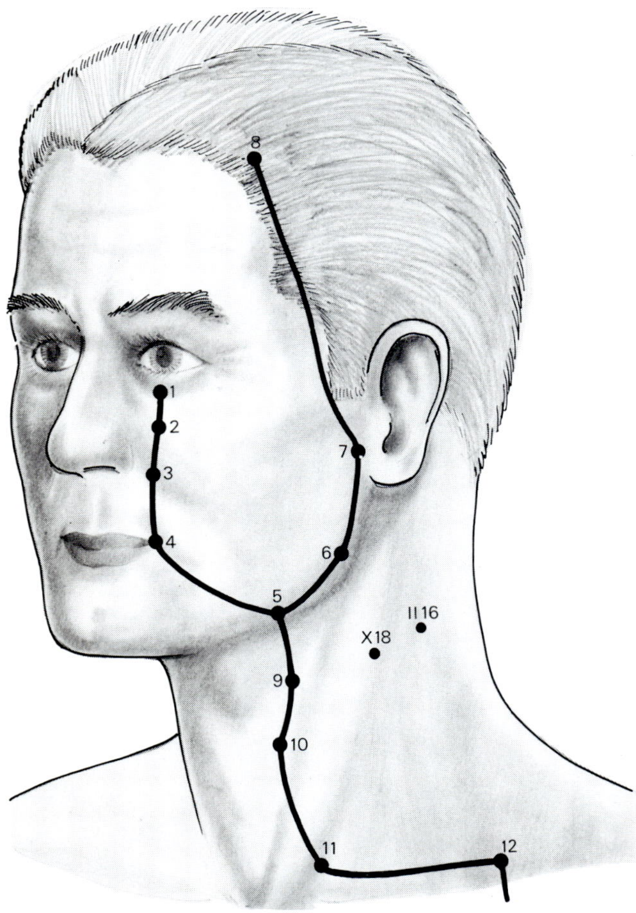
1
2
3
4
5
6
7
8
9
10
11
12
X18
II16

XI	1	On the cheek, immediately superior to the infra-orbital foramen, on the inferior border of the orbit, in line with the centre of the pupil with the eye looking straight ahead.
XI	2	On the cheek, in the depression of the infra-orbital foramen, 3 fen inferior to the inferior edge of the orbit.
XI	3	On the zygomatic bone, directly inferior to the infra-orbital foramen, at the level of the inferior border of the alum of the nose.
XI	4	4 fen lateral to, and level with, the angle of the mouth.
XI	5	On the inferior border of the mandible, anterior to the masseter, in the depression of the facial artery.
XI	6	4 fen anterior and superior to the angle of the mandible, in the depression between the two bellies of the masseter.
XI	7	In the depression which is inferior to the zygomatic arch and anterior to the condyle of the mandible. When the mouth is opened wide this depression disappears.
XI	8	On the head, $\frac{1}{2}$ ACI posterior and superior to the natural hair line, at the superior corner of the forehead.
XI	9	On the anterior surface of the neck, upon the carotid artery, at the anterior border of the sternocleidomastoid at the level of the laryngeal prominence, level with X 18 and II 16.
XI	10	On the anterior border of the sternocleidomastoid, at the level of the cricoid cartilage, approximately 1 ACI inferior to XI 9.
XI	11	Superior to the clavicle, between the two heads of the sternocleidomastoid, 2 ACI lateral to the median line.
XI	12	In the centre of the supraclavicular fossa, 4 ACI lateral to the median line and on the paramedian nipple line.

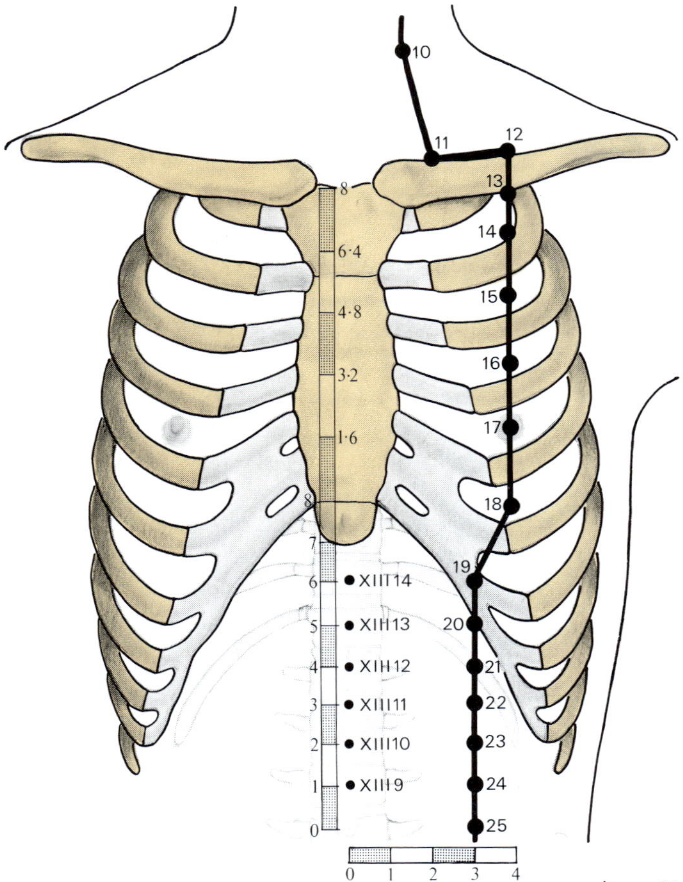
10
11
12
13
14
15
16
17
18
19
20
21
22
23
24
25
8
6·4
4·8
3·2
1·6
8
7
6
5
4
3
2
1
0
XIII 14
XIII 13
XIII 12
XIII 11
XIII 10
XIII 9
0 1 2 3 4

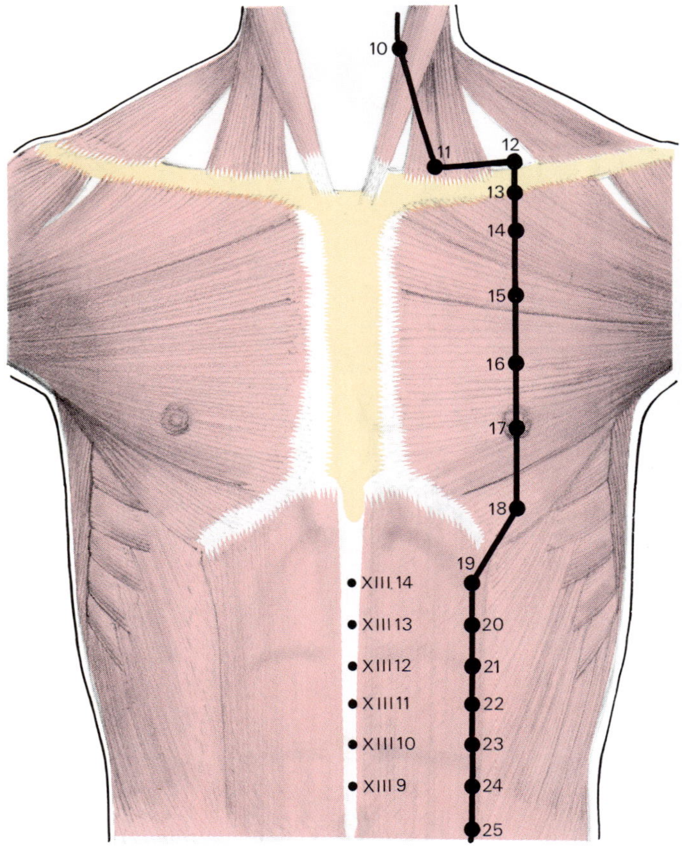
10
11
12
13
14
15
16
17
18
19
20
21
22
23
24
25
XIII 14
XIII 13
XIII 12
XIII 11
XIII 10
XIII 9

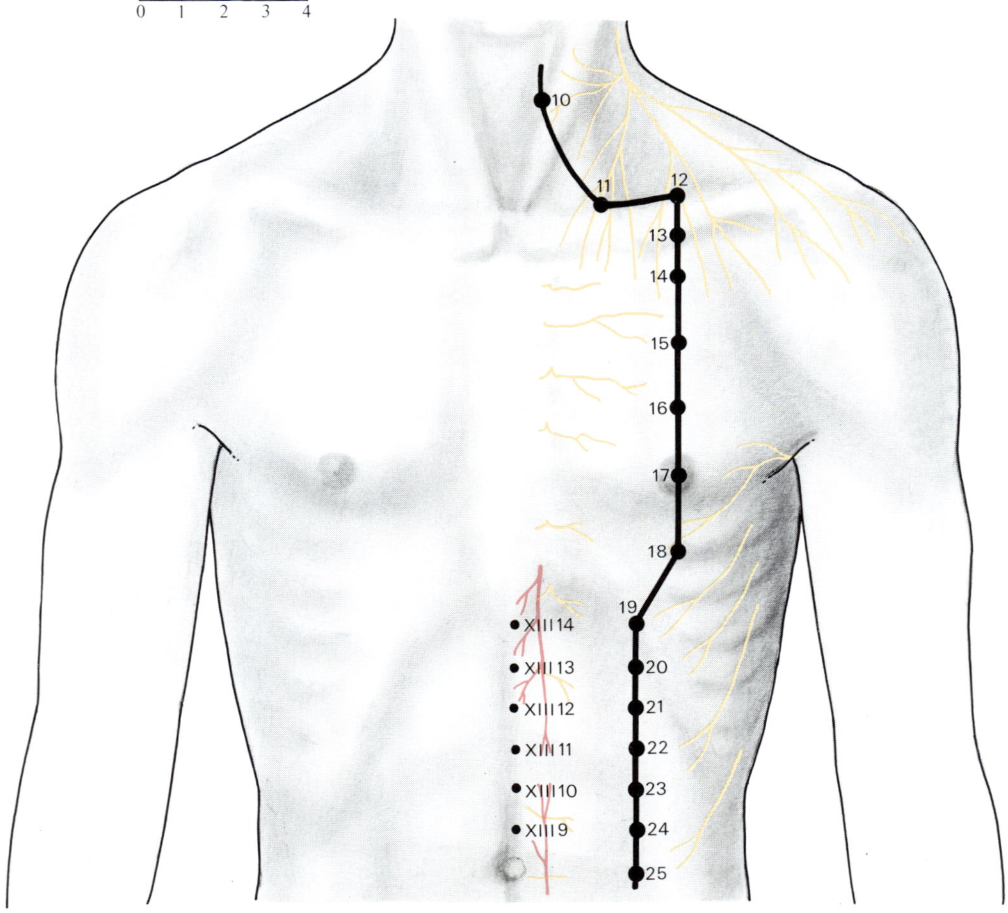
10
11
12
13
14
15
16
17
18
19
20
21
22
23
24
25
XIII 14
XIII 13
XIII 12
XIII 11
XIII 10
XIII 9

XI	**11**	Superior to the clavicle, between the two heads of the sternocleidomastoid, 2 ACI lateral to the median line.
XI	**12**	In the centre of the supraclavicular fossa, 4 ACI lateral to the median line and on the paramedian nipple line.
XI	**13**	On the inferior edge of the clavicle, 4 ACI lateral to the median line and on the paramedian nipple line.
XI	**14**	In the first intercostal space, 4 ACI lateral to the median line and on the paramedian nipple line.
XI	**15**	In the second intercostal space, 4 ACI lateral to the median line and on the paramedian nipple line.
XI	**16**	In the third intercostal space, 4 ACI lateral to the median line and on the paramedian nipple line.
XI	**17**	In the centre of the nipple
XI	**18**	In the fifth intercostal space, 4 ACI lateral to the median line and on the paramedian nipple line.
XI	**19**	On the thorax, 3 ACI lateral to the median line and 6 ACI superior to the level of the umbilicus, at the level of XIII 14.
XI	**20**	On the abdomen, 3 ACI lateral to the median line and 5 ACI superior to the level of the umbilicus, at the level of XIII 13.
XI	**21**	On the abdomen, 3 ACI lateral to the median line and 4 ACI superior to the level of the umbilicus, at the level of XIII 12.
XI	**22**	On the abdomen, 3 ACI lateral to the median line and 3 ACI superior to the level of the umbilicus, at the level of XIII 11.
XI	**23**	On the abdomen, 3 ACI lateral to the median line and 2 ACI superior to the level of the umbilicus, at the level of XIII 10.
XI	**24**	On the abdomen, 3 ACI lateral to the median line and 1 ACI superior to the level of the umbilicus, at the level of XIII 9.
XI	**25**	On the abdomen, 3 ACI lateral to the median line, at the level of the centre of the umbilicus, on the lateral edge of the rectus abdominis.

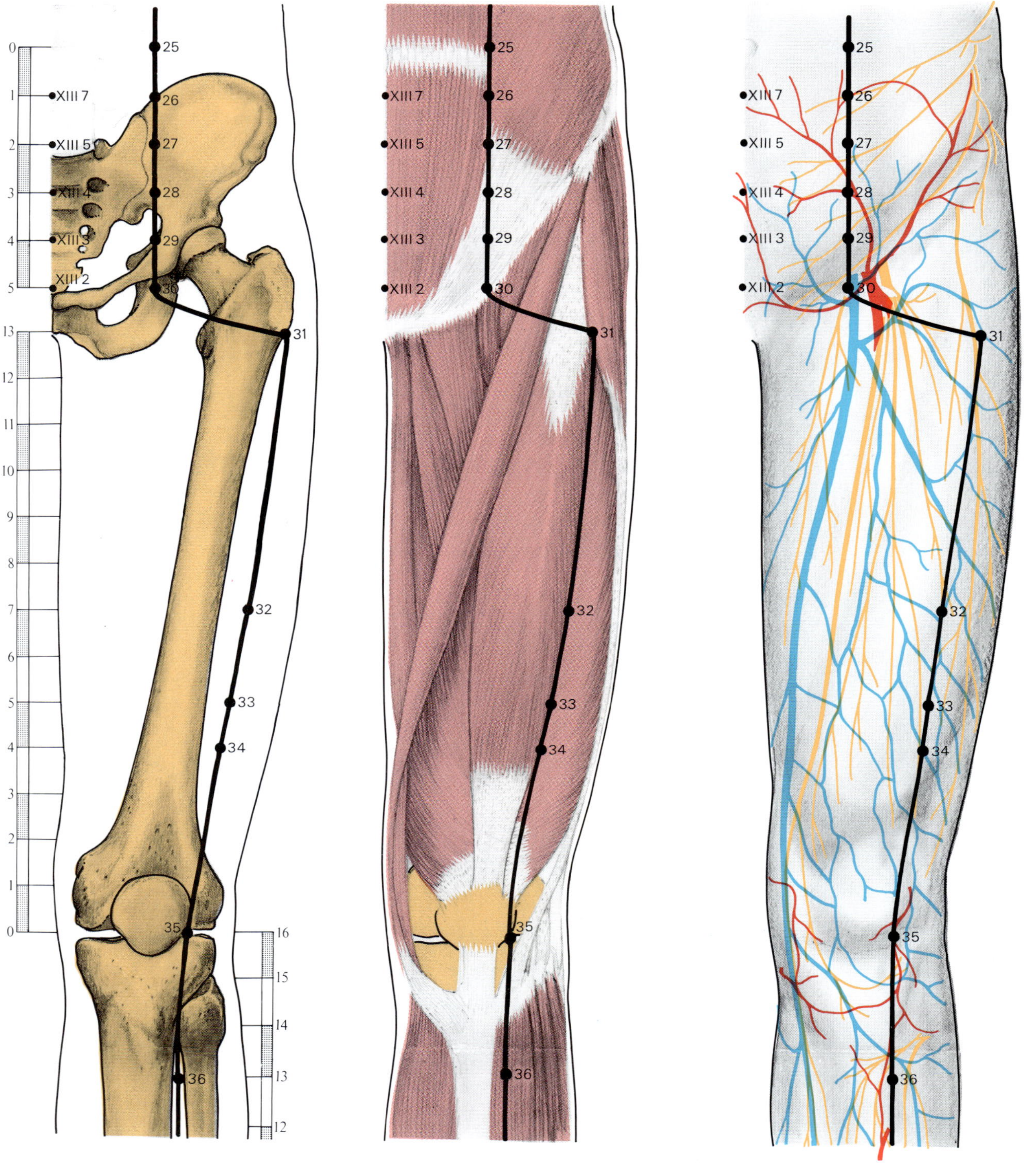
25
26
27
28
29
30
31
32
33
34
35
36
XIII 7
XIII 5
XIII 4
XIII 3
XIII 2
0
1
2
3
4
5
13
12
11
10
9
8
7
6
5
4
3
2
1
0
16
15
14
13
12
25
26
27
28
29
30
31
32
33
34
35
36
XIII 7
XIII 5
XIII 4
XIII 3
XIII 2
25
26
27
28
29
30
31
32
33
34
35
36
XIII 7
XIII 5
XIII 4
XIII 3
XIII 2

XI	**25**	On the abdomen, 3 ACI lateral to the median line, at the level of the centre of the umbilicus, on the lateral edge of the rectus abdominis.
XI	**26**	On the abdomen, 3 ACI lateral to the median line and 1 ACI inferior to the level of the umbilicus, at the level of XIII 7.
XI	**27**	On the abdomen, 3 ACI lateral to the median line and 2 ACI inferior to the level of the umbilicus, at the level of XIII 5.
XI	**28**	On the abdomen, 3 ACI lateral to the median line and 3 ACI inferior to the level of the umbilicus, at the level of XIII 4.
XI	**29**	On the abdomen, 3 ACI lateral to the median line and 4 ACI inferior to the level of the umbilicus, at the level of XIII 3.
XI	**30**	On the abdomen, 3 ACI lateral to the median line, at the level of the superior edge of the pubic symphysis, at the level of XIII 2.
XI	**31**	On the anterior surface of the thigh, 13 ACI proximal to the flexure of the knee, between the vastus lateralis and the rectus femoris.
XI	**32**	On the anterior surface of the thigh, 7 ACI proximal to the flexure of the knee, between the vastus lateralis and the rectus femoris.
XI	**33**	On the anterior surface of the thigh, 5 ACI proximal to the flexure of the knee, between the vastus lateralis and the rectus femoris.
XI	**34**	On the anterior surface of the thigh, 4 ACI proximal to the flexure of the knee, between the vastus lateralis and the rectus femoris.
XI	**35**	On the anterior surface of the knee, between the patella and the tibia, lateral to the patellar tendon. When the knee is flexed, a depression appears at this point.

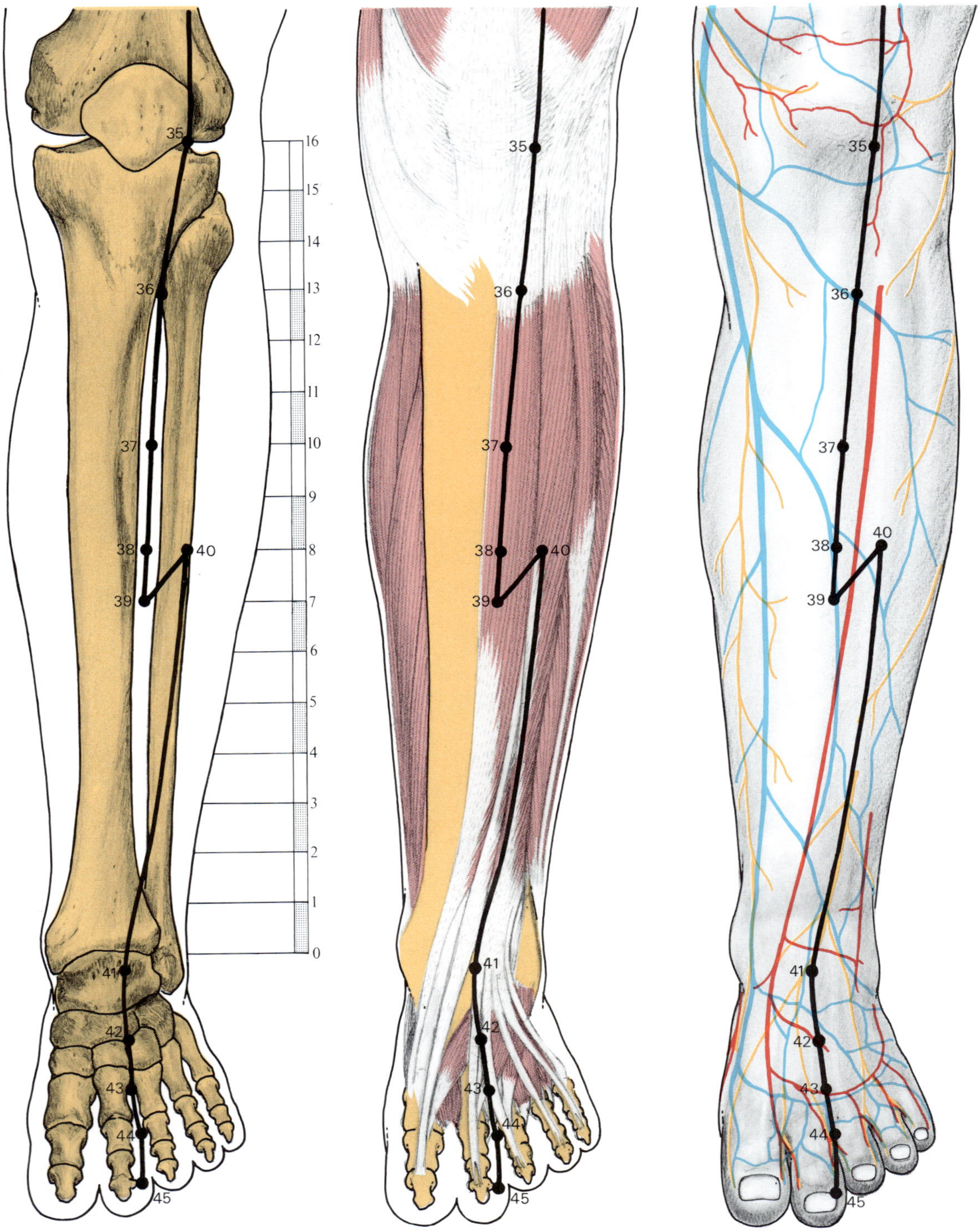
35
36
37
38
39
40
41
42
43
44
45
16
15
14
13
12
11
10
9
8
7
6
5
4
3
2
1
0

XI	35	On the anterior surface of the knee, between the patella and the tibia, lateral to the patellar tendon. When the knee is flexed, a depression appears at this point.
XI	36	On the anterior surface of the leg, 13 ACI proximal to the level of the prominence of the lateral malleolus, lateral to the edge of the tibia.
XI	37	On the anterior surface of the leg, 10 ACI proximal to the level of the prominence of the lateral malleolus, lateral to the edge of the tibia.
XI	38	On the anterior surface of the leg, 8 ACI proximal to the level of the prominence of the lateral malleolus, lateral to the edge of the tibia.
XI	39	On the anterior surface of the leg, 7 ACI proximal to the level of the prominence of the lateral malleolus, lateral to the edge of the tibia.
XI	40	On the anterolateral surface of the leg, 8 ACI proximal to the level of the prominence of the lateral malleolus, on the lateral edge of the tibialis anterior, at the level of XI 38.
XI	41	At the middle of the anterior flexure of the ankle, between the tendons of the extensor digitorum longus and the extensor hallucis longus.
XI	42	On the dorsal surface of the foot, in the concavity at the meeting of the navicular, lateral cuneiform and intermediate cuneiform bones.
XI	43	On the dorsal surface of the foot, in the angle between the second and third metatarsal bones.
XI	44	On the dorsal surface of the foot, between the second and third toes, just distal to the base of the proximal phalanx of the second toe.
XI	45	Lateral nail point of the second toe.

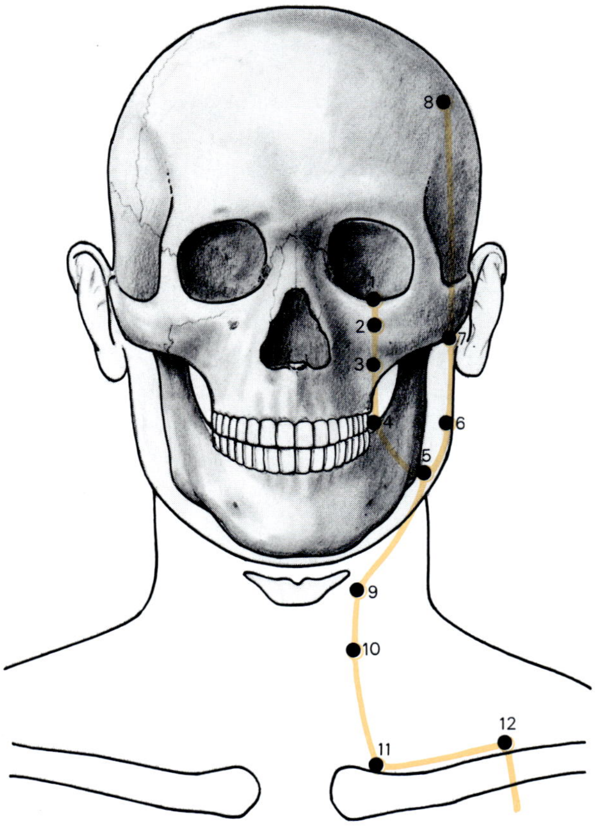
8
2
3
4
5
6
7
9
10
11
12

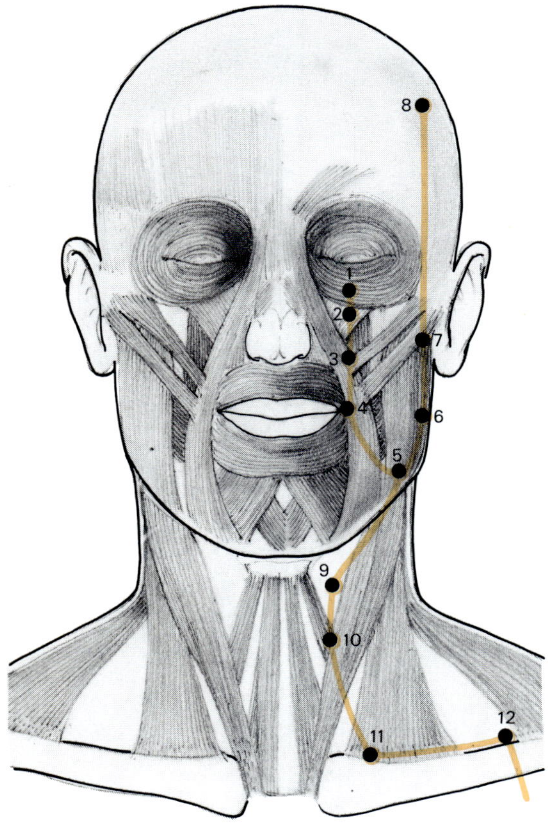
8
1
2
3
4
5
6
7
9
10
11
12

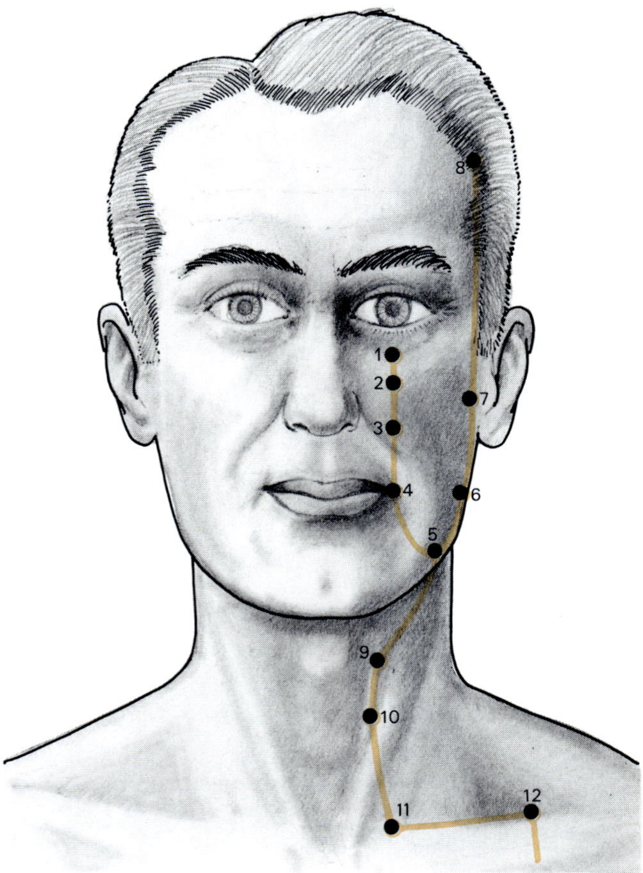
8
1
2
3
4
5
6
7
9
10
11
12

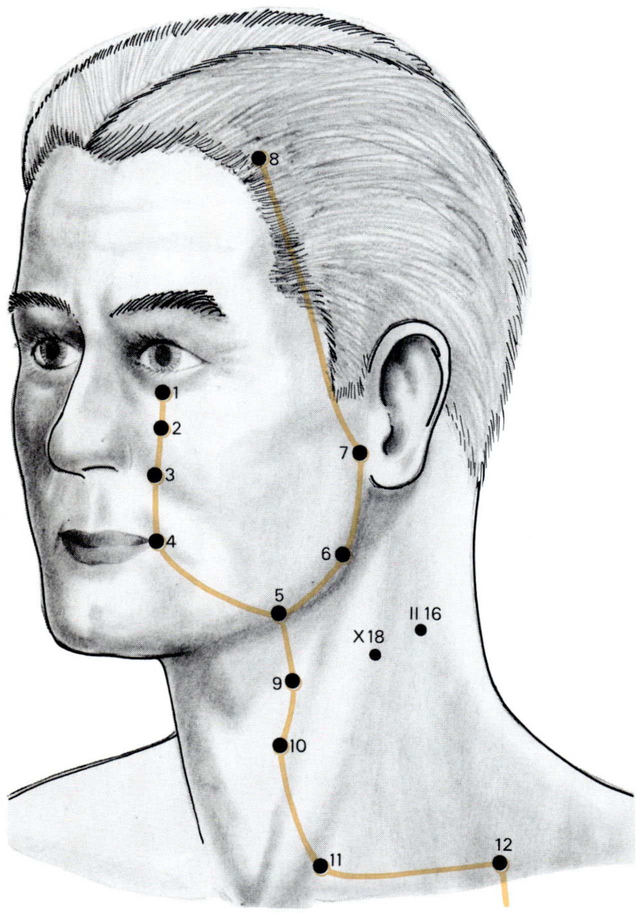
8
1
2
3
4
5
6
7
II 16
X18
9
10
11
12

XI **1** **Receive Tears** (Chengchi)

⊥ 1–3 Entry
△ X

On the cheek, immediately superior to the infra-orbital foramen, on the inferior border of the orbit, in line with the centre of the pupil with the eye looking straight ahead.

Point of Yang Qiao Mo

XI **2** **Four Whites** (Szupai)

⊥ 1–3
△ 3

On the cheek, in the depression of the infra-orbital foramen, 3 fen inferior to the inferior edge of the orbit.

Point of Yang Qiao Mo

XI **3** **Great Cheekbone** (Chuliao)

⊥ 1–3
△ 5

On the zygomatic bone, directly inferior to the infra-orbital foramen, at the level of the inferior border of the alum of the nose.

Point of Yang Qiao Mo

XI **4** **Earth Granary** (Titsang)

⊥ 1–3
△ 5
XP5

4 fen lateral to, and level with, the angle of the mouth.

Point of Yang Qiao Mo

XI **5** **Great Welcome** (Taying)

⊥ 3–5
△ 3–5

On the inferior border of the mandible, anterior to the masseter, in the depression of the facial artery.

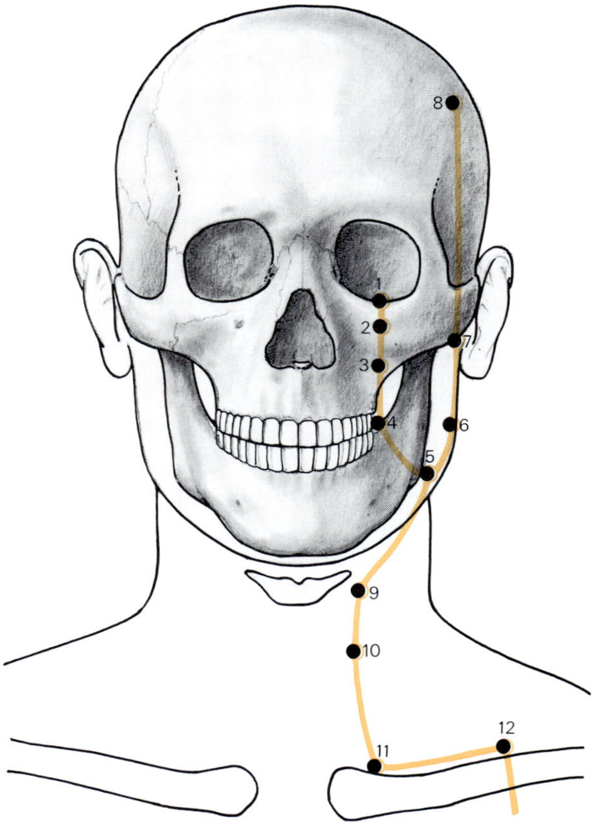
8
1
2
7
3
4
6
5
9
10
12
11

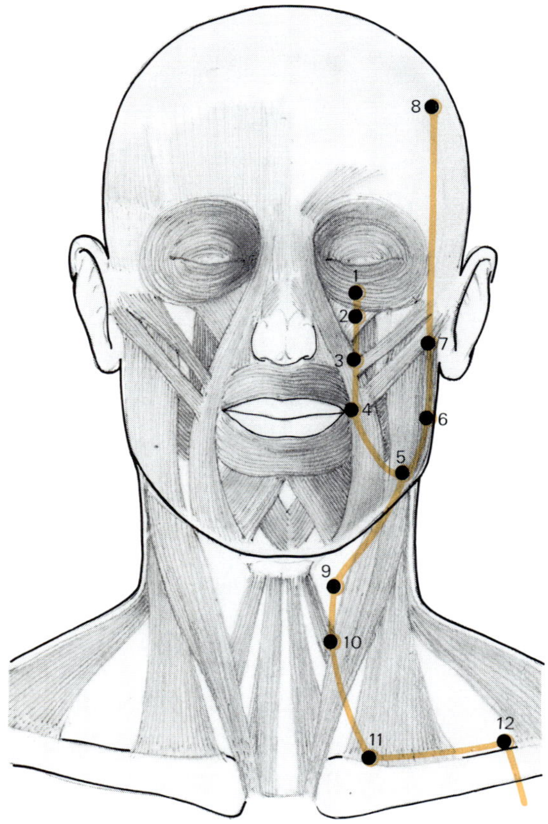
8
1
2
7
3
4
6
5
9
10
12
11

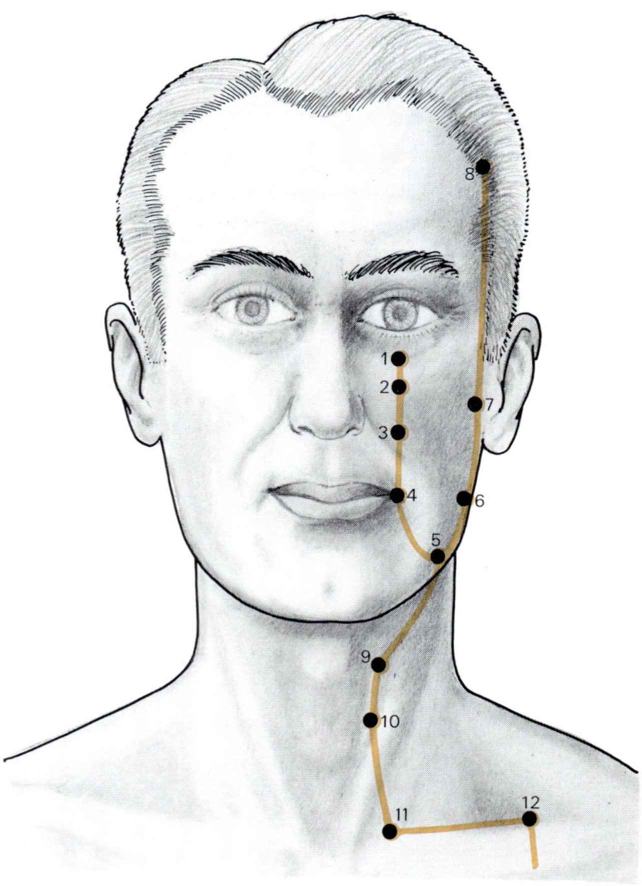
8
1
2
7
3
4
6
5
9
10
11
12

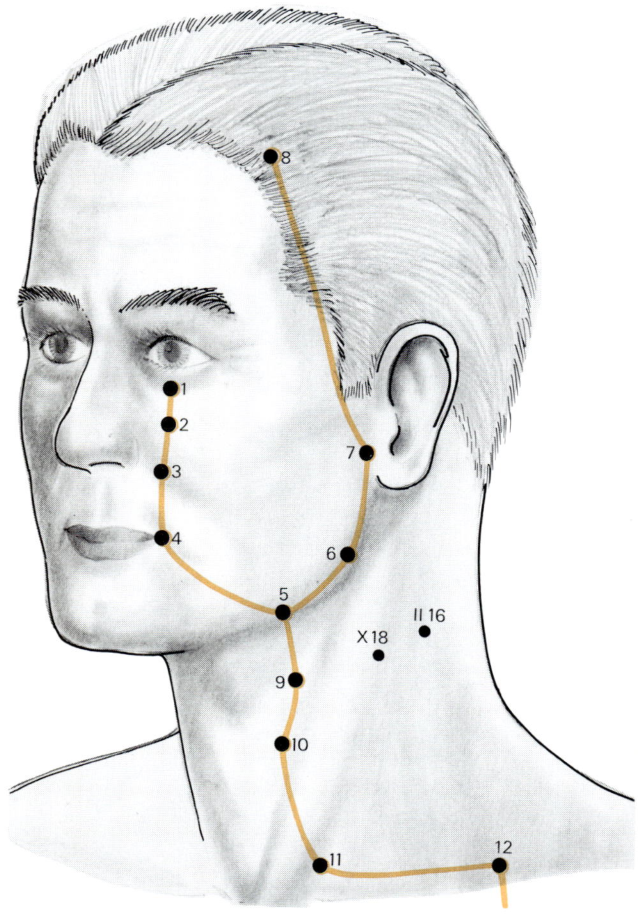
8
1
2
7
3
4
6
5
II 16
X 18
9
10
12
11

XI **6** **Mandible Wheel** (Chiache)

⊥ 3
△ 7

4 fen anterior and superior to the angle of the mandible, in the depression between the two bellies of the masseter.

XI **7** **Lower Passage** (Hsiakuan)

⊥ 3
△ X

In the depression which is inferior to the zygomatic arch and anterior to the condyle of the mandible. When the mouth is opened wide this depression disappears.

XI **8** **Head Tied** (Touwei)

⊥ 3
△ X

On the head, $\frac{1}{2}$ ACI posterior and superior to the natural hair line, at the superior corner of the forehead.

XI **9** **People Welcome** (Jenying)

⊥ 1–3
△ X

On the anterior surface of the neck, upon the carotid artery, at the anterior border of the sternocleidomastoid at the level of the laryngeal prominence, level with X 18 and II 16.

Sea of Energy
Window of the Sky

XI **10** **Water Rushing Out** (Shuitu)

⊥ 1–3
△ X

On the anterior border of the sternocleidomastoid, at the level of the cricoid cartilage, approximately 1 ACI inferior to XI 9.

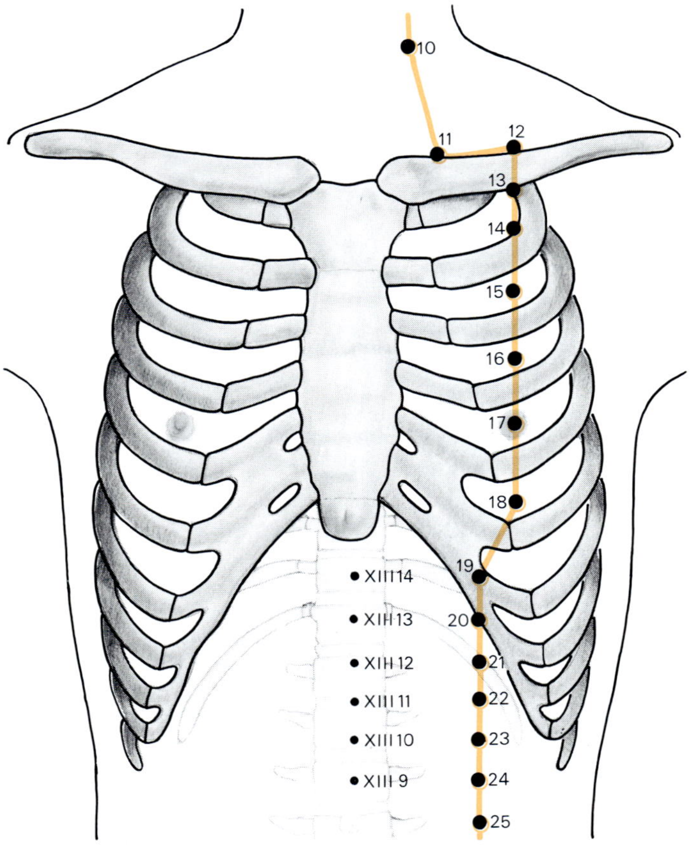
10
11
12
13
14
15
16
17
18
19
20
21
22
23
24
25
XIII 14
XIII 13
XIII 12
XIII 11
XIII 10
XIII 9

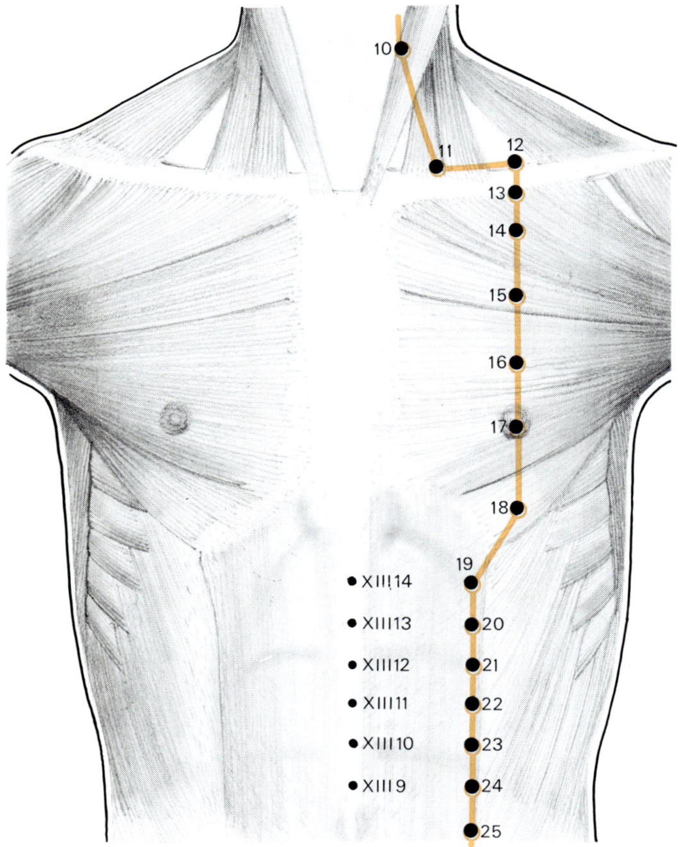
10
11
12
13
14
15
16
17
18
19
20
21
22
23
24
25
XIII 14
XIII 13
XIII 12
XIII 11
XIII 10
XIII 9

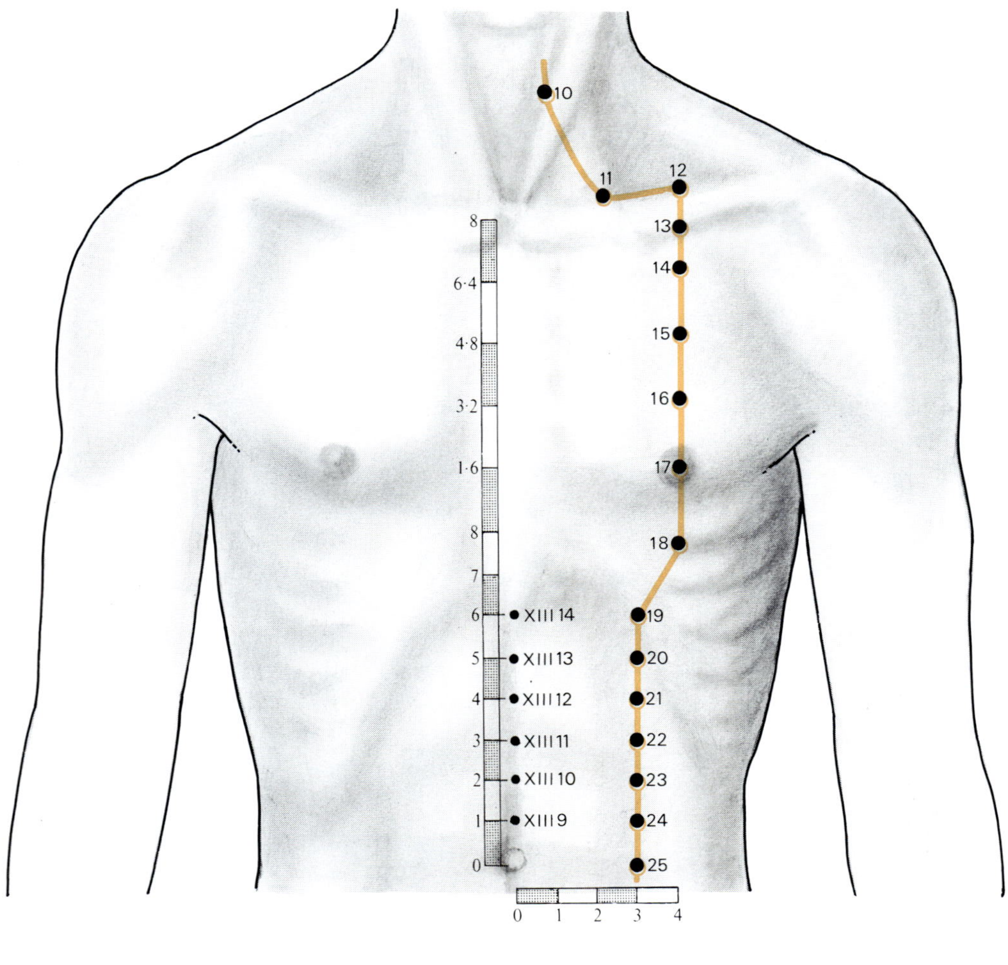
10
11
12
13
14
15
16
17
18
19
20
21
22
23
24
25
XIII 14
XIII 13
XIII 12
XIII 11
XIII 10
XIII 9
8
6·4
4·8
3·2
1·6
8
7
6
5
4
3
2
1
0
0 1 2 3 4

XI **11** **Ch'i Cottage** (Chishe)

⊥ 3
△ 3

Superior to the clavicle, between the two heads of the sternocleidomastoid, 2 ACI lateral to the median line.

XI **12** **Broken Bowl** (Chuehpen)

⊥ 3
△ 3

In the centre of the supraclavicular fossa, 4 ACI lateral to the median line and on the paramedian nipple line.

Point of Yin Qiao Mo

XI **13** **Ch'i Door** (Chihu)

⊥ 3
△ 5

On the inferior edge of the clavicle, 4 ACI lateral to the median line and on the paramedian nipple line.

XI **14** **Storehouse** (Kufang)

⊥ 3
△ 5

In the first intercostal space, 4 ACI lateral to the median line and on the paramedian nipple line.

XI **15** **Room Screen** (Wuyi)

⊥ 3
△ 5

In the second intercostal space, 4 ACI lateral to the median line and on the paramedian nipple line.

XI **16** **Breast Window** (Yingchuang)

⊥ 3
△ 5

In the third intercostal space, 4 ACI lateral to the median line and on the paramedian nipple line.

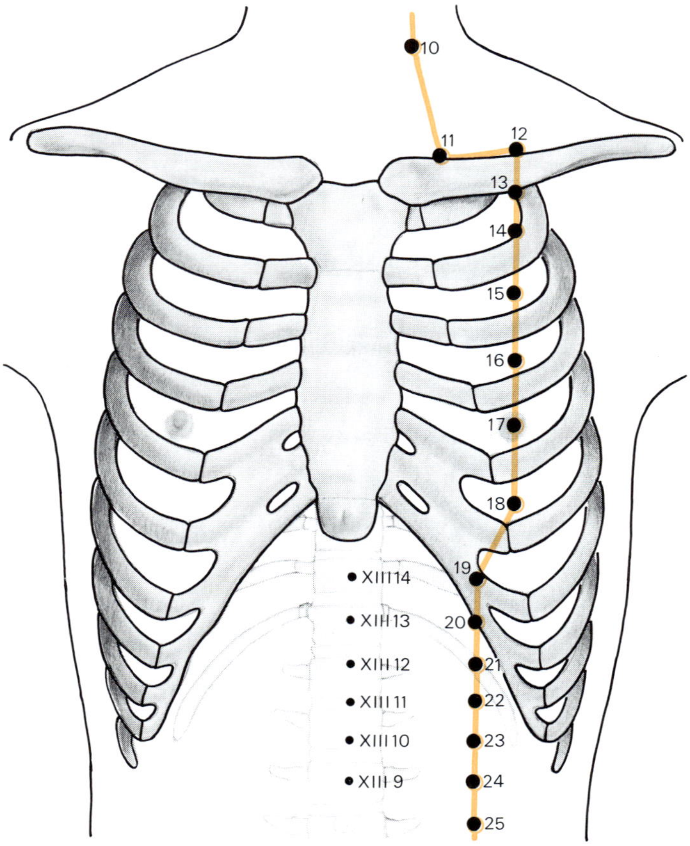
10
11
12
13
14
15
16
17
18
19
20
21
22
23
24
25
XIII 14
XIII 13
XIII 12
XIII 11
XIII 10
XIII 9

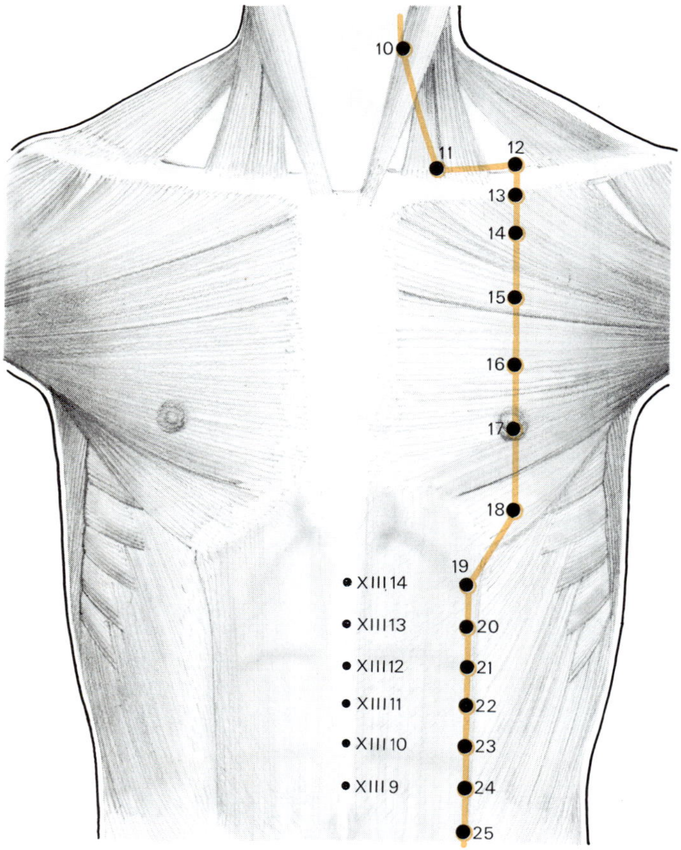
10
11
12
13
14
15
16
17
18
19
20
21
22
23
24
25
XIII 14
XIII 13
XIII 12
XIII 11
XIII 10
XIII 9

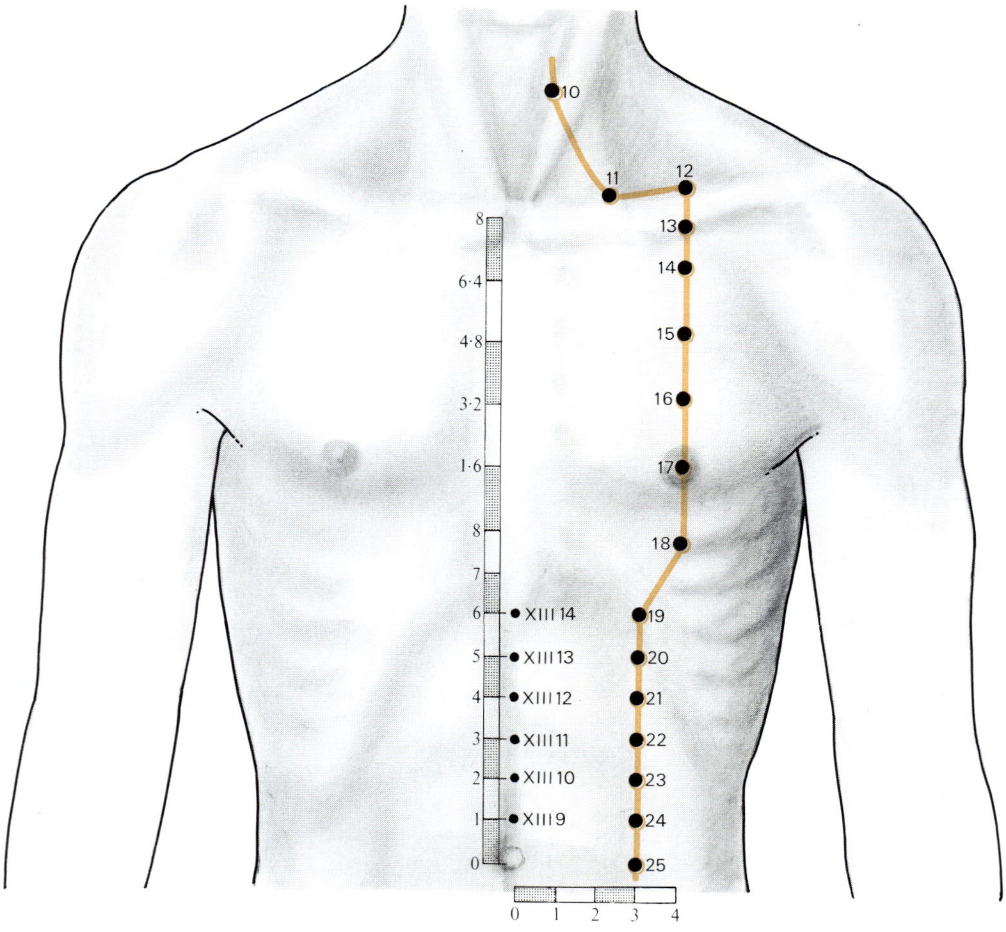
10
11
12
13
14
15
16
17
18
19
20
21
22
23
24
25
XIII 14
XIII 13
XIII 12
XIII 11
XIII 10
XIII 9
8
6·4
4·8
3·2
1·6
8
7
6
5
4
3
2
1
0
0 1 2 3 4

XI	**17**	**Centre Of The Breasts** (Juchung)
⊥	X	
△	X	
		In the centre of the nipple.

XI	**18**	**Root Of The Breasts** (Juken)
⊥	3	
△	3–5	
		In the fifth intercostal space, 4 ACI lateral to the median line and on the paramedian nipple line.

XI	**19**	**Not At Ease** (Pujung)
⊥	5	
△	3–7	
		On the thorax, 3 ACI lateral to the median line and 6 ACI superior to the level of the umbilicus, at the level of XIII 14.

XI	**20**	**Receiving Fullness** (Chengman)
⊥	5	
△	3–7	
		On the abdomen, 3 ACI lateral to the median line and 5 ACI superior to the level of the umbilicus, at the level of XIII 13.

XI	**21**	**Bridge Gate** (Liangmen)
⊥	7	
△	5–15	
		On the abdomen, 3 ACI lateral to the median line and 4 ACI superior to the level of the umbilicus, at the level of XIII 12.

XI	**22**	**Border Gate** (Kuanmen)
⊥	8	
△	5–15	
		On the abdomen, 3 ACI lateral to the median line and 3 ACI superior to the level of the umbilicus, at the level of XIII 11.

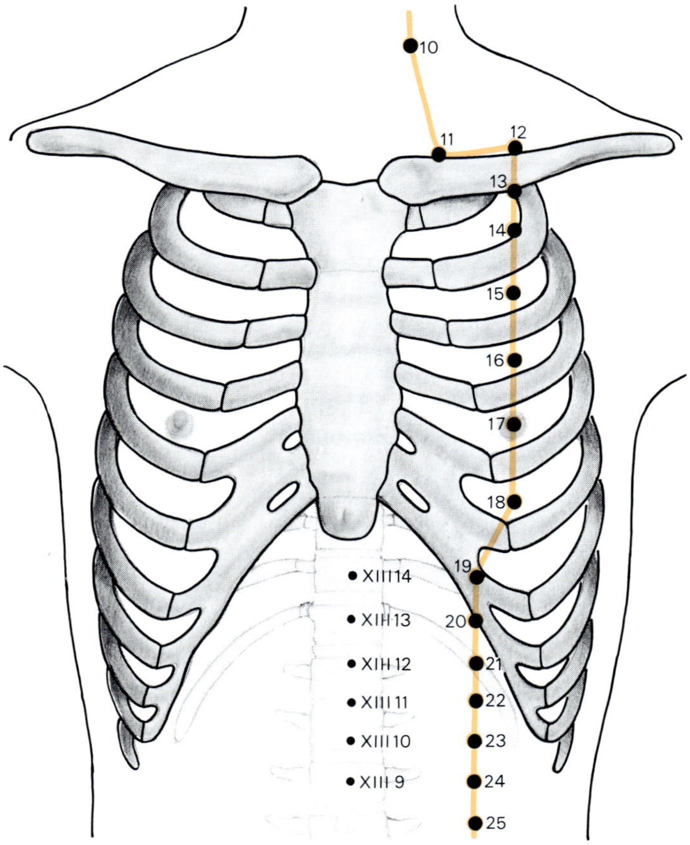
10
11
12
13
14
15
16
17
18
19
20
21
22
23
24
25
XIII 14
XIII 13
XIII 12
XIII 11
XIII 10
XIII 9

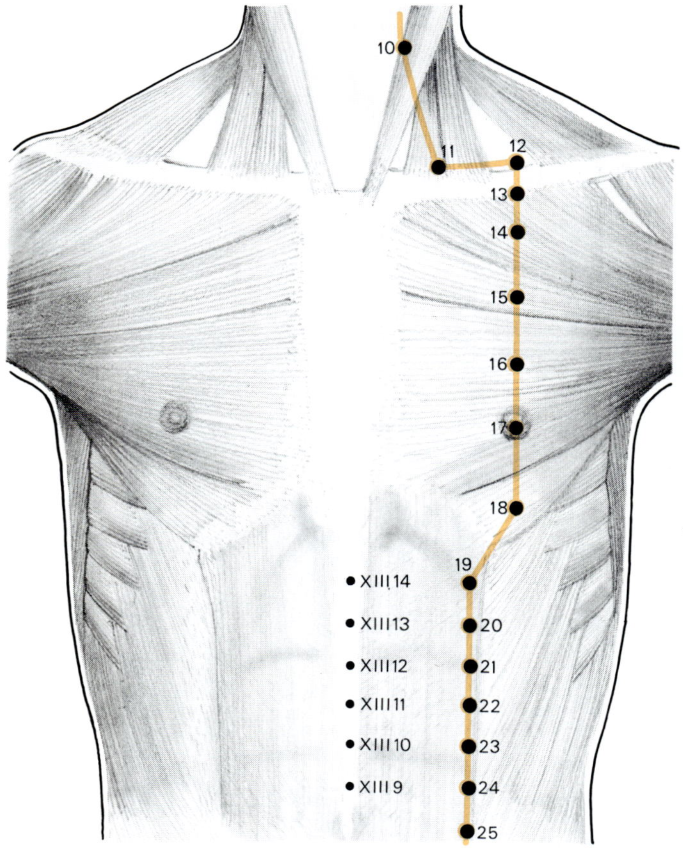
10
11
12
13
14
15
16
17
18
19
20
21
22
23
24
25
XIII 14
XIII 13
XIII 12
XIII 11
XIII 10
XIII 9

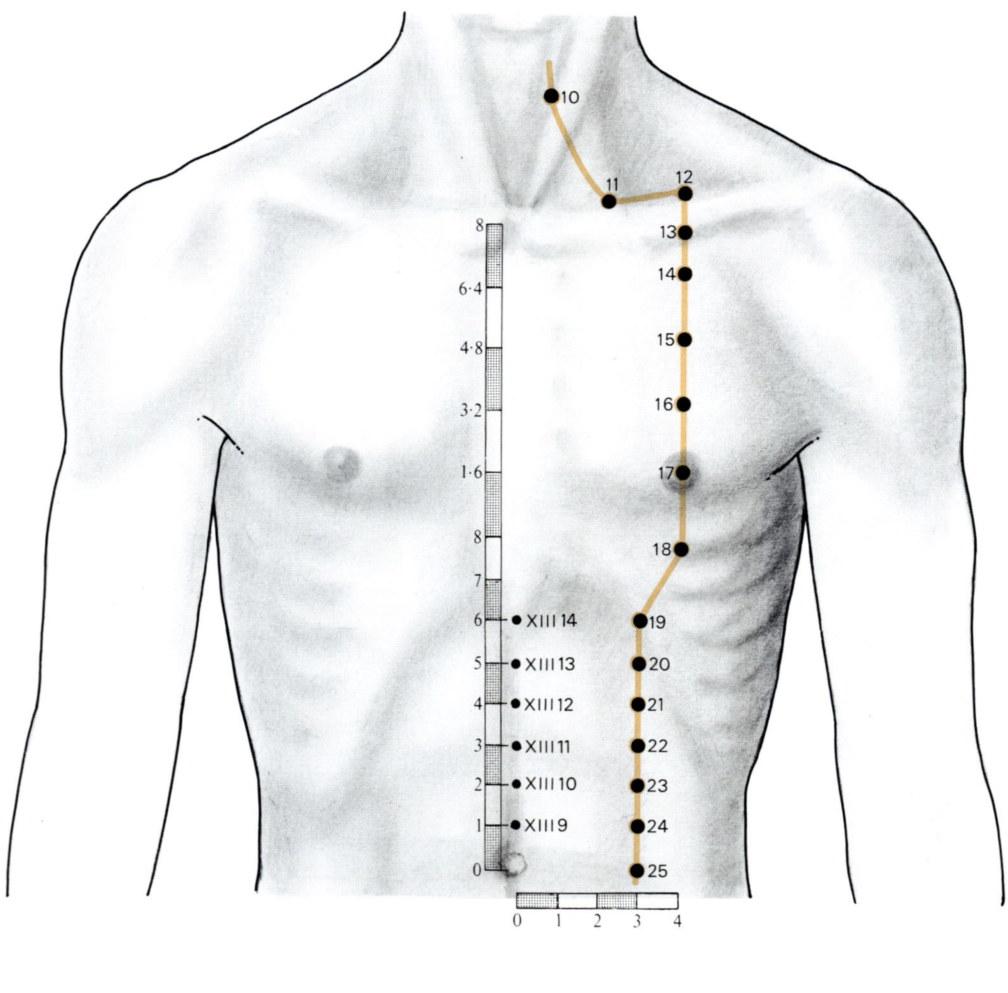
10
11
12
13
14
15
16
17
18
19
20
21
22
23
24
25
XIII 14
XIII 13
XIII 12
XIII 11
XIII 10
XIII 9
8
6·4
4·8
3·2
1·6
8
7
6
5
4
3
2
1
0
0 1 2 3 4

XI **23** **Great Oneness** (Taiyi)

⊥ 8
△ 5–10

On the abdomen, 3 ACI lateral to the median line and 2 ACI superior to the level of the umbilicus, at the level of XIII 10.

XI **24** **Lubrication Food Gate** (Huajoumen)

⊥ 8
△ 5–15

On the abdomen, 3 ACI lateral to the median line and 1 ACI superior to the level of the umbilicus, at the level of XIII 9.

XI **25** **Heavenly Pivot** (Tienshu)

⊥ 5
△ 5–20

On the abdomen, 3 ACI lateral to the median line, at the level of the centre of the umbilicus, on the lateral edge of the rectus abdominis.

Alarm Point of X
A Point of the pattern to release the 7 Dragons on the 7 Internal Demons.

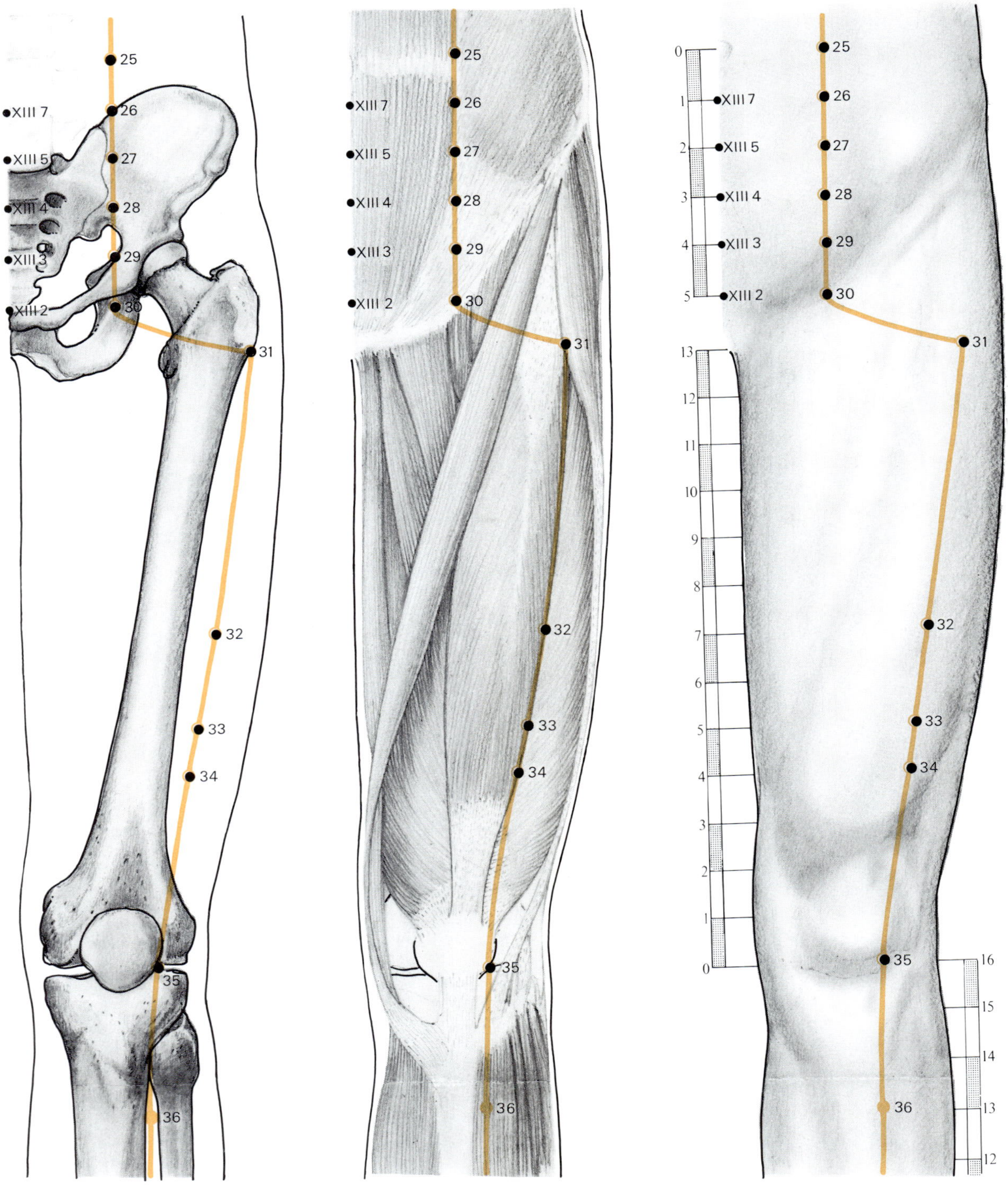
25
26
27
28
29
30
31
32
33
34
35
36
XIII 7
XIII 5
XIII 4
XIII 3
XIII 2
25
26
27
28
29
30
31
32
33
34
35
36
XIII 7
XIII 5
XIII 4
XIII 3
XIII 2
0
1
2
3
4
5
XIII 7
XIII 5
XIII 4
XIII 3
XIII 2
25
26
27
28
29
30
31
13
12
11
10
9
8
7
6
5
4
3
2
1
0
32
33
34
35
36
16
15
14
13
12

XI **26** **Outside Mound** (Wailing)

⊥ 8–10
△ 5

On the abdomen, 3 ACI lateral to the median line and 1 ACI inferior to the level of the umbilicus, at the level of XIII 7.

XI **27** **Great Might** (Tachu)

⊥ 8–10
△ 5–10

On the abdomen, 3 ACI lateral to the median line and 2 ACI inferior to the level of the umbilicus, at the level of XIII 5.

XI **28** **Water Path** (Shuitao)

⊥ 8
△ 5–10

On the abdomen, 3 ACI lateral to the median line and 3 ACI inferior to the level of the umbilicus, at the level of XIII 4.

XI **29** **The Return** (Kueilai)

⊥ 5
△ 5–10

On the abdomen, 3 ACI lateral to the median line and 4 ACI inferior to the level of the umbilicus, at the level of XIII 3.

XI **30** **Ch'i Rushing** (Chichung)

⊥ 3
△ 7

On the abdomen, 3 ACI lateral to the median line, at the level of the superior edge of the pubic symphysis, at the level of XIII 2.

Point of Chong Mo
Sea of Nourishment
First Aid: food poisoning

XI **31** **Thigh Border** (Pikuan)

⊥ 6
△ 3–7

On the anterior surface of the thigh, 13 ACI proximal to the flexure of the knee, between the vastus lateralis and the rectus femoris.

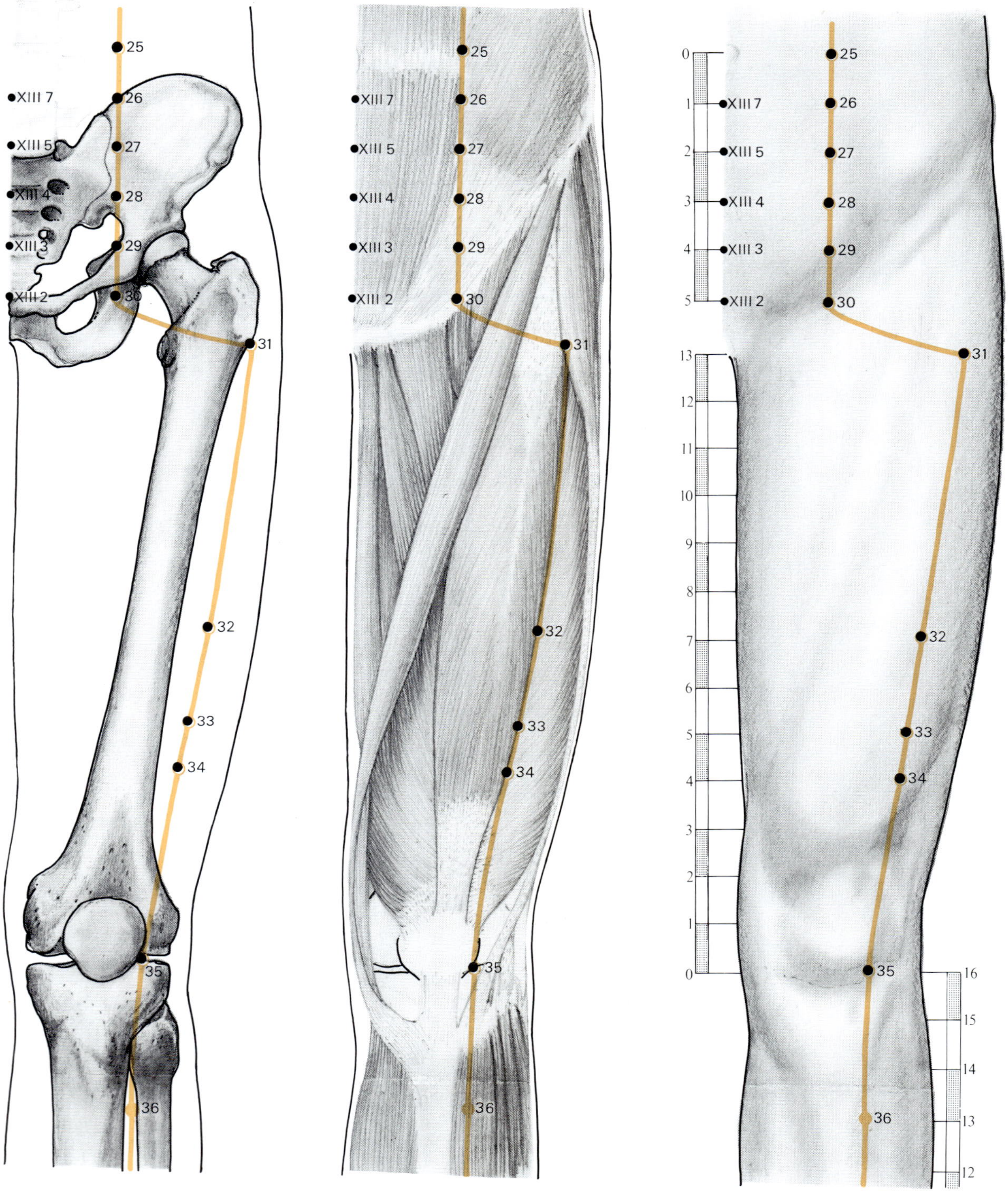
25
XIII 7
26
XIII 5
27
XIII 4
28
XIII 3
29
XIII 2
30
31
32
33
34
35
36

XI **32** **Prostrate Hare** (Futu)

⊥ 6
△ 3–7

On the anterior surface of the thigh, 7 ACI proximal to the flexure of the knee, between the vastus lateralis and the rectus femoris.

A point of the pattern to release the 7 Dragons on the 7 Internal Demons

XI **33** **Yin Market** (Yinshih)

⊥ 4
△ 3–5

On the anterior surface of the thigh, 5 ACI proximal to the flexure of the knee, between the vastus lateralis and the rectus femoris.

XI **34** **Beam Mound** (Liangchiu)

⊥ 4
△ 3–5

On the anterior surface of the thigh, 4 ACI proximal to the flexure of the knee, between the vastus lateralis and the rectus femoris.

XI **35** **Calf Nose** (Tupi)

⊥ 3
△ 3

On the anterior surface of the knee, between the patella and the tibia, lateral to the patellar tendon. When the knee is flexed, a depression appears at this point.

XI **36** **Leg Three Miles** (Tsu sanli)

⊥ 5–8 Earth
△ 7–20 Horary 7 a.m.–9 a.m.
XP8

On the anterior surface of the leg, 13 ACI proximal to the level of the prominence of the lateral malleolus, lateral to the edge of the tibia.

Point for acupuncture blackout
Point of Ho (Autumn)
Sea of Nourishment
Centre Reunion Particular Point of Energy
Greater Assembling Point of the stomach and abdomen
A Centre of Energy
A point of the pattern to release the 7 Dragons on the 7 Internal Demons (Master point between XI 36 and XI 37).
First Aid: fainting, indigestion

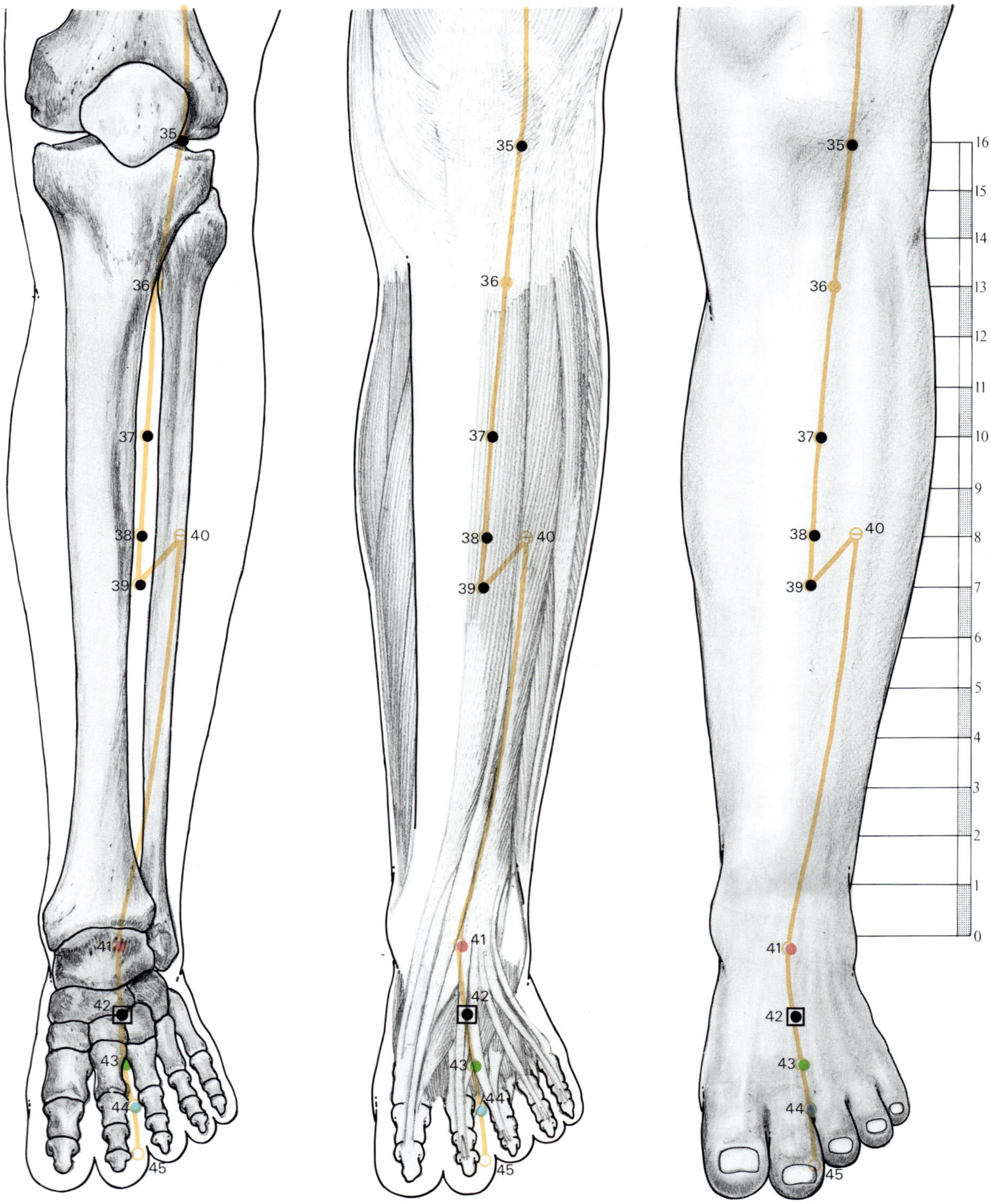
35
36
37
38
40
39
41
42
43
44
45
16
15
14
13
12
11
10
9
8
7
6
5
4
3
2
1
0

XI **37** **Upper Great Void** (Shangchuhsu)

⊥ 5
△ 3–7

On the anterior surface of the leg, 10 ACI proximal to the level of the prominence of the lateral malleolus, lateral to the edge of the tibia.

Sea of Blood

XI **38** **Branch Opening** (Tiaokou)

⊥ 5
△ 3–7

On the anterior surface of the leg, 8 ACI proximal to the level of the prominence of the lateral malleolus, lateral to the edge of the tibia.

XI **39** **Lower Great Void** (Hsiachuhsu)

⊥ 5
△ 3–7

On the anterior surface of the leg, 7 ACI proximal to the level of the prominence of the lateral malleolus, lateral to the edge of the tibia.

Sea of Blood

XI **40** **Abundant Splendour** (Fenglung)

⊖ ⊥ 3 Junction
△ 3–5

On the anterolateral surface of the leg. 8 ACI proximal to the level of the prominence of the lateral malleolus, on the lateral edge of the tibialis anterior, at the level of XI 38.

XI **41** **Released Stream** (Chiehhsi)

● ⊥ 5 Fire
△ 3–7 Tonification

At the middle of the anterior flexure of the ankle, between the tendons of the extensor digitorum longus and the extensor hallucis longus.

Point of Ching (late Summer)
A point of the pattern to release the 7 Dragons on the 7 Internal Demons.

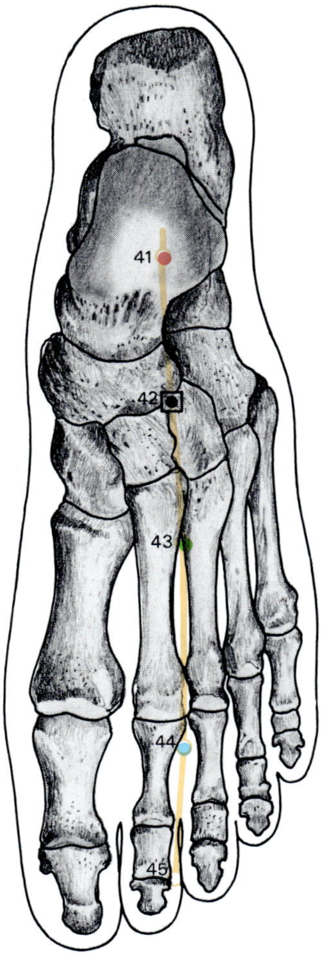
41
42
43
44
45

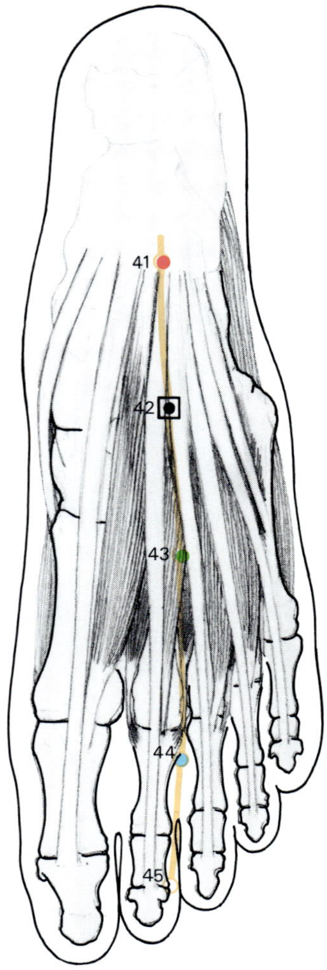
41
42
43
44
45

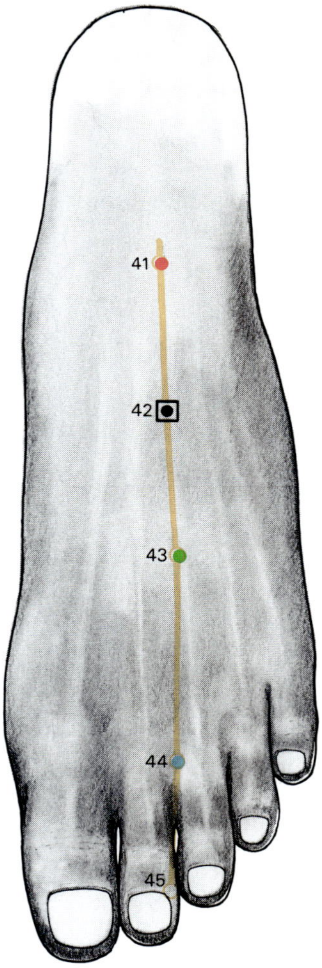
41
42
43
44
45

XI **42** **Rushing Yang** (Chungyang)

□ ⊥ 3 Source
△ 3–5 Exit

On the dorsal surface of the foot, in the concavity at the meeting of the navicular, lateral cuneiform and intermediate cuneiform bones.

XI **43** **Sinking Valley** (Hsienku)

● ⊥ 3 Wood
△ 3

On the dorsal surface of the foot, in the angle between the second and third metatarsal bones.

Point of Yu (Summer)

XI **44** **Inner Courtyard** (Neiting)

● ⊥ 3 Water
△ 3

On the dorsal surface of the foot, between the second and third toes, just distal to the base of the proximal phalanx of the second toe.

Point of Yung (Spring)

XI **45** **Hard Bargain** (Litui)

○ ⊥ 1 Metal
△ 3 Sedation
XP6

Lateral nail point of the second toe.

Point of Cheng (Winter)
First Aid: hangover, indigestion, toothache

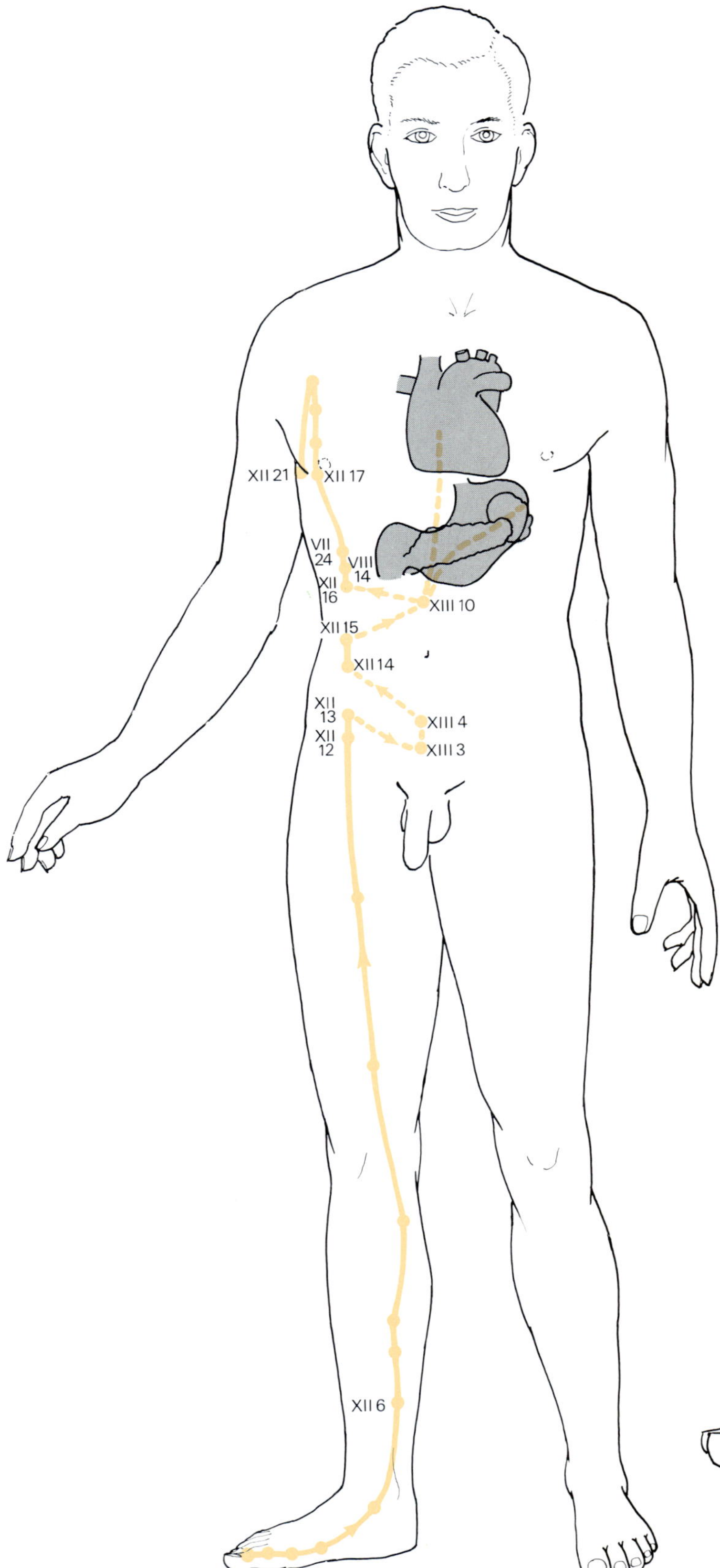

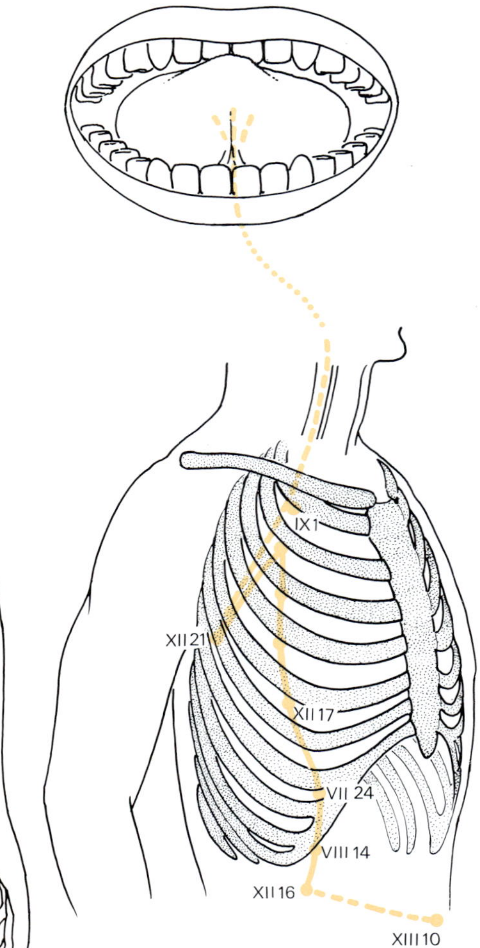

Author's Note: There is a deep pathway connection between XII 21 and I 1 which is not shown on these diagrams.

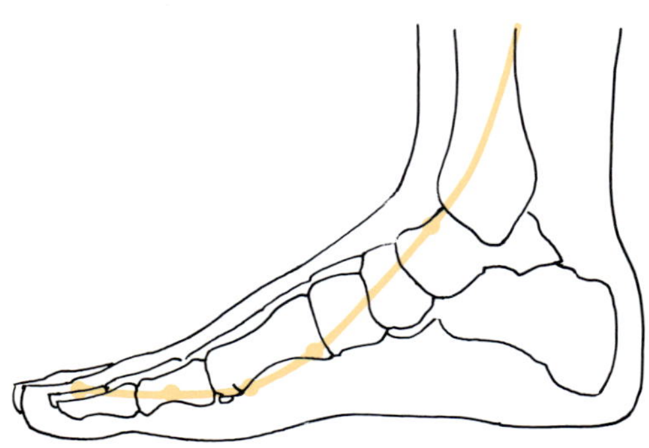

The spleen meridian begins as the superficial pathway at the medial nail point of the big toe. It runs along the medial edge of the foot, in the line where the plantar skin meets the dorsal skin, to the head of the first metatarsal bone. It passes anterior to the medial malleolus, and up the medial surface of the leg to connect with the kidney and liver meridians, 4 ACI superior to the medial malleolus, at XII 6.

The meridian continues up the posterior border of the tibia to the gastrocnemius, past the medial side of the patella to the vastus medialis and up to the inguinal region of the abdomen at XII 12 and XII 13. Here the pathway goes deep and joins the median line, at XIII 3 and XIII 4. It returns laterally to become briefly superficial as it follows up the abdomen in line with the nipple through XII 14 and XII 15. Again as a deep pathway, it travels to the median line, at XIII 10, and from there enters the spleen, the pancreas and the stomach. From XIII 10, the meridian returns to the line of the nipple, at XII 16, and becomes superficial. It rises up the thorax, passing VIII 14 and VII 24, and diverges laterally to XII 17 and ascends as the superficial pathway to arrive at the second intercostal space. Here it turns inferiorly and laterally to a point in the sixth intercostal space, in the axillary line, ending at the exit point, XII 21. From XII 21 the pathway becomes deep and crosses the inner surface of the chest wall, passing IX 1, ascends the oesophagus and disperses throughout the tongue.

A branch leaves from XIII 10 and penetrates the diaphragm to enter the heart. Here it connects with the heart meridian.

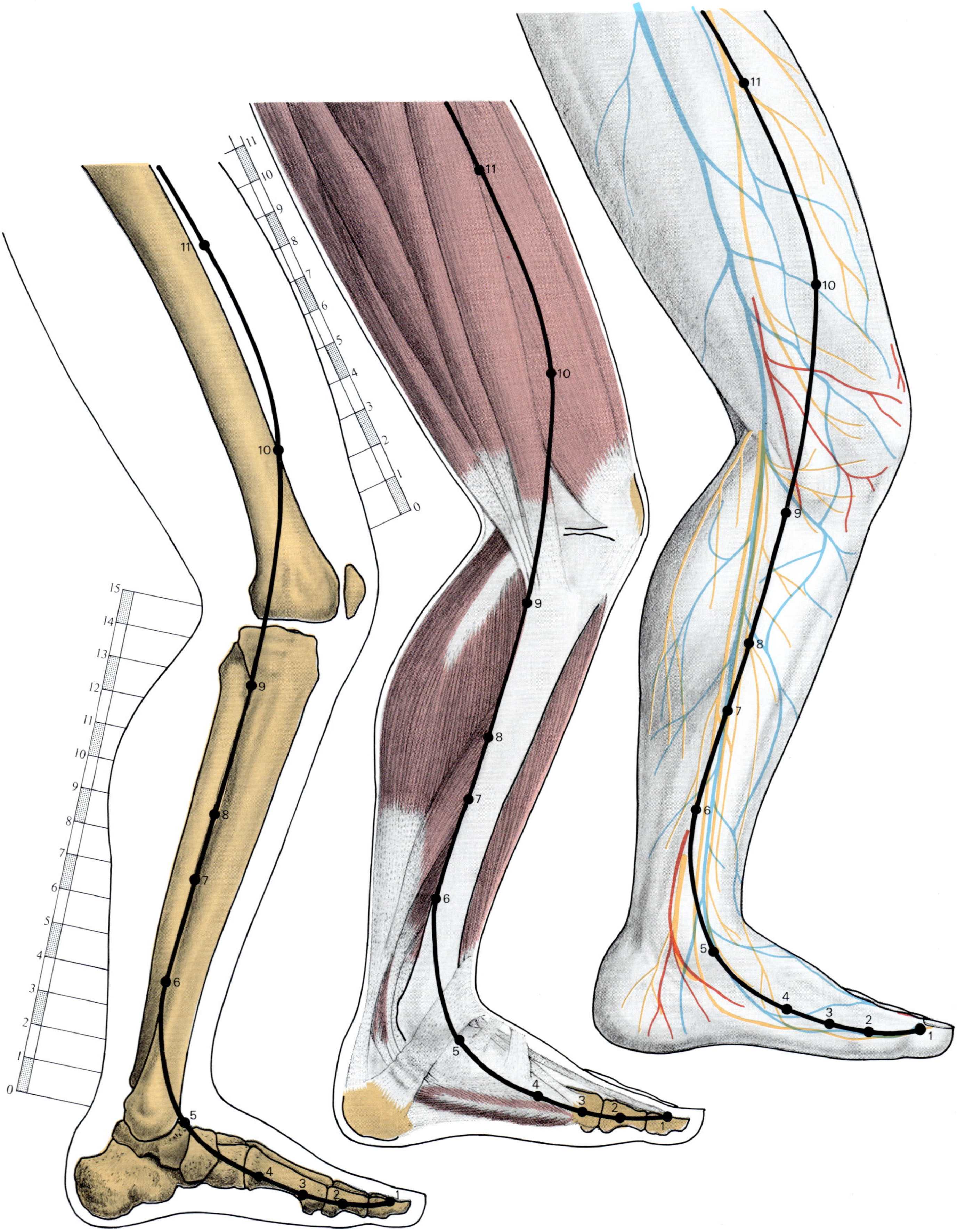
11
10
9
8
7
6
5
4
3
2
1
15
14
13
12
11
10
9
8
7
6
5
4
3
2
1
0
11
10
9
8
7
6
5
4
3
2
1
0

XII 1 Medial nail point of the big toe.

XII 2 On the medial edge of the big toe, just distal to the base of the proximal phalanx.

XII 3 On the medial edge of the foot, just proximal to the head of the first metatarsal bone.

XII 4 On the medial edge of the foot, just distal to the proximal end of the first metatarsal bone.

XII 5 In the hollow anterior to the medial malleolus, posterior to the tendon of the tibialis anterior.

XII 6 On the medial surface of the leg, 4 ACI proximal to the prominence of the medial malleolus, posterior to the edge of the tibia.

XII 7 On the medial surface of the leg, 7 ACI proximal to the prominence of the medial malleolus, posterior to the edge of the tibia.

XII 8 On the medial surface of the leg, 9 ACI proximal to the prominence of the medial malleolus, posterior to the edge of the tibia.

XII 9 On the medial surface of the leg, 13 ACI proximal to the prominence of the medial malleolus, on the posterior edge of the tibia.

XII 10 On the anterior surface of the thigh, 3 ACI proximal to the flexure of the knee, in the middle of the belly of the vastus medialis.

XII 11 On the anterior surface of the thigh, 9 ACI proximal to the flexure of the knee, on the anterior border of the sartorius.

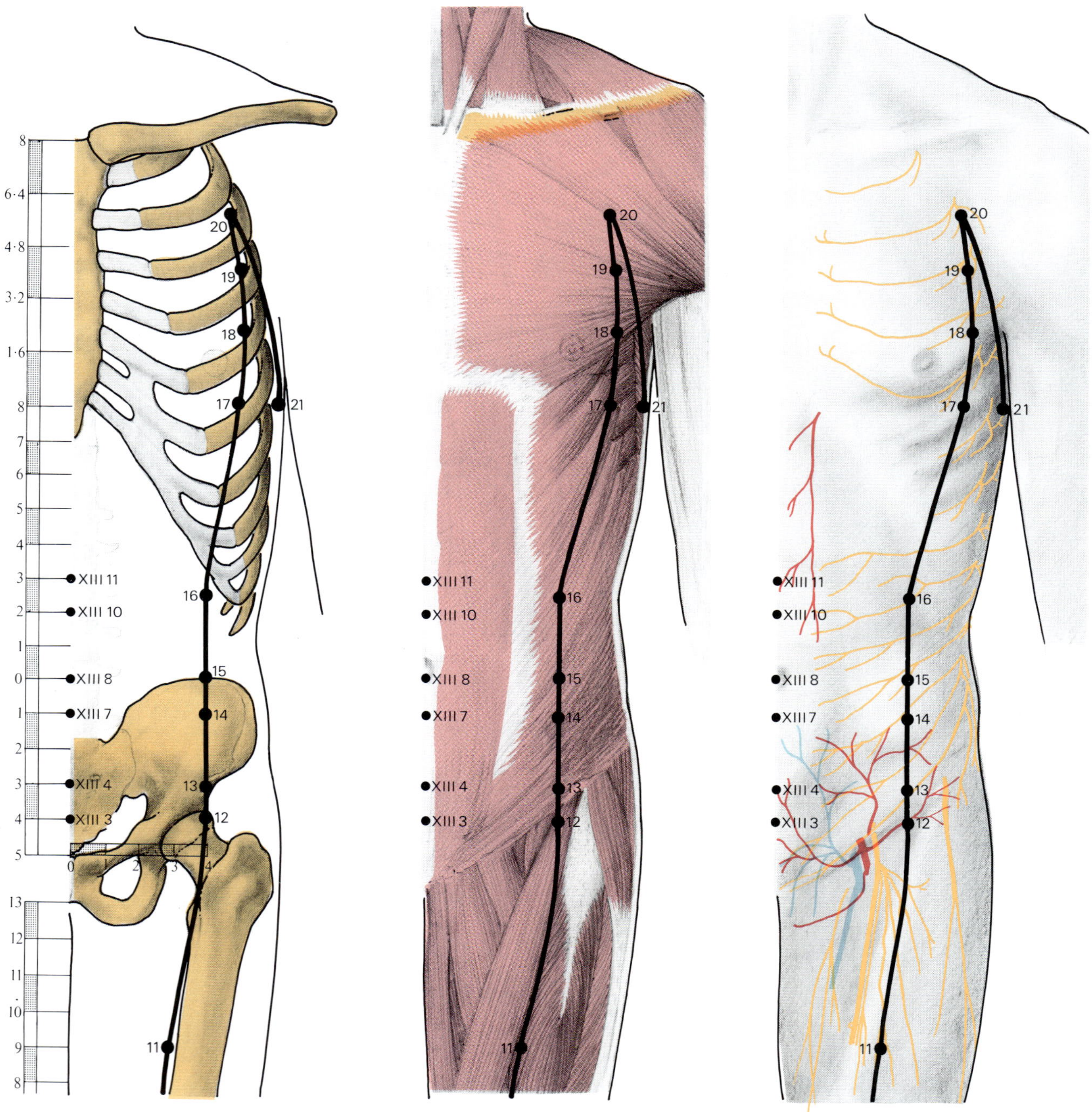
20
19
18
17
21
16
15
14
13
12
11
XIII 11
XIII 10
XIII 8
XIII 7
XIII 4
XIII 3
8
6·4
4·8
3·2
1·6
8
7
6
5
4
3
2
1
0
1
2
3
4
5
0
1
2
3
4
13
12
11
10
9
8

XII	**11**	On the anterior surface of the thigh, 9 ACI proximal to the flexure of the knee, on the anterior border of the sartorius.
XII	**12**	On the flexure of the groin, 4 ACI lateral to the median line and 4 ACI inferior to the level of the umbilicus, on a level with XIII 3.
XII	**13**	On the abdomen, 4 ACI lateral to the median line and 3 ACI inferior to the level of the umbilicus, on a level with XIII 4.
XII	**14**	On the abdomen, 4 ACI lateral to the median line and 1 ACI inferior to the level of the umbilicus, on a level with XIII 7.
XII	**15**	On the abdomen, 4 ACI lateral to the median line, at the level of the centre of the umbilicus and XIII 8.
XII	**16**	On the abdomen, 4 ACI lateral to the median line and $2\frac{1}{2}$ ACI superior to the level of the umbilicus, at a level half-way between XIII 10 and XIII 11, on the paramedian nipple line.
XII	**17**	On the thorax, in the fifth intercostal space, 6 ACI lateral to the median line.
XII	**18**	On the thorax, in the fourth intercostal space, 6 ACI lateral to the median line.
XII	**19**	On the thorax, in the third intercostal space, 6 ACI lateral to the median line.
XII	**20**	On the thorax, in the second intercostal space, 6 ACI lateral to the median line.
XII	**21**	On the thorax, in the sixth intercostal space, on the mid-axillary line.

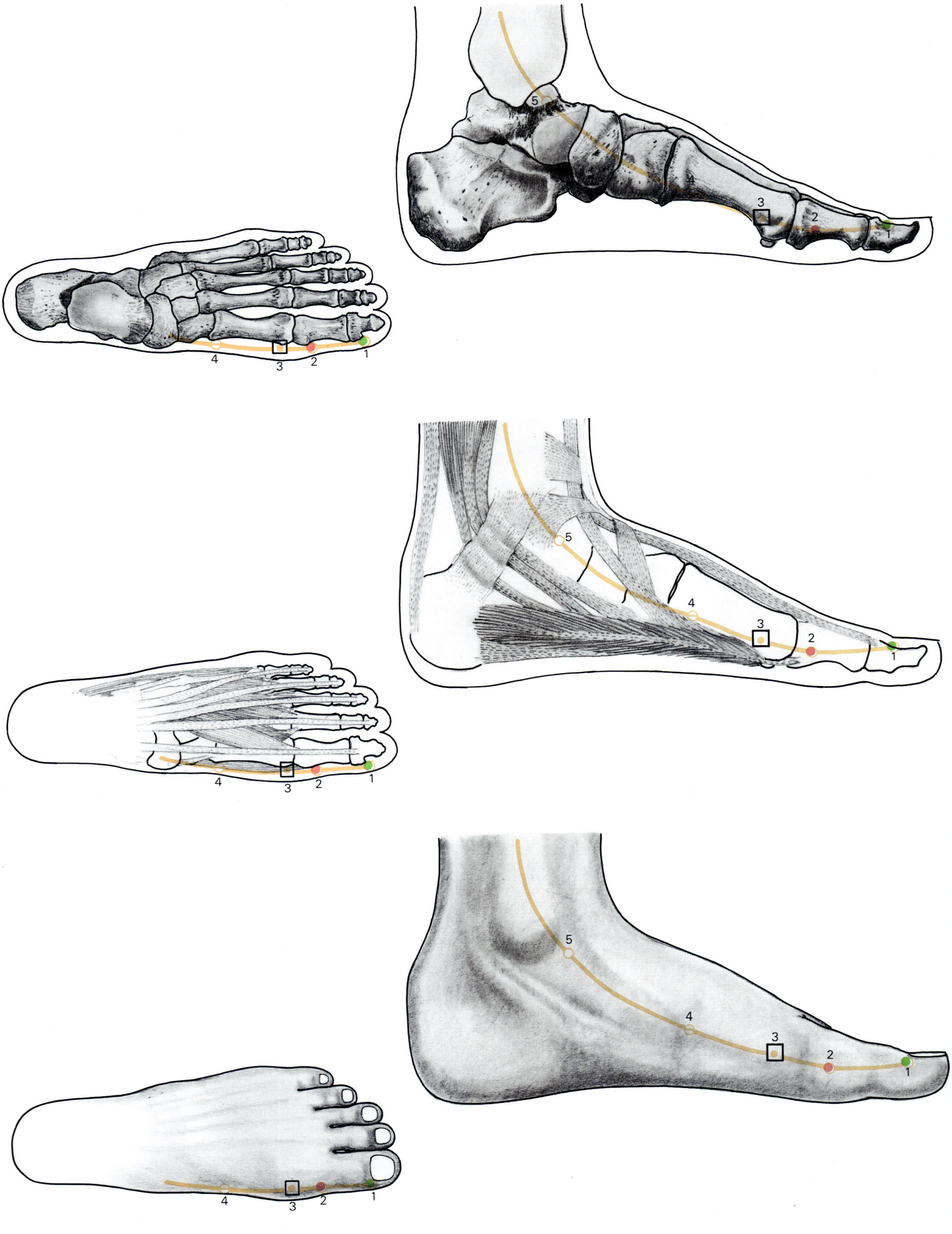
5
4
3
2
1

XII **1** **Retired White** (Yinpai)

⊥ 1 Wood
△ X Entry
XP1

Medial nail point of the big toe.

Point of Cheng (Winter)

XII **2** **Great Capital** (Tatu)

⊥ 3 Fire
△ 3–5 Tonification
XP1

On the medial edge of the big toe, just distal to the base of the proximal phalanx.

Point of Yung (Spring)
First Aid: fractures, sprains

XII **3** **Supreme White** (Taipai)

⊥ 3 Earth
△ 3–5 Horary 9 a.m.–11 a.m.
□ Source

On the medial edge of the foot, just proximal to the head of the first metatarsal bone.

Point of Yu (Summer)

XII **4** **Prince's Grandson** (Kungsun)

⊖ ⊥ 3 Junction
△ 3

On the medial edge of the foot, just distal to the proximal end of the first metatarsal bone.

Master Point of Chong Mo
Coupled Point of Yin Wei Mo

XII **5** **Merchant Mound** (Shangchiu)

○ ⊥ 3 Metal
△ 3–7 Sedation

In the hollow anterior to the medial malleolus, posterior to the tendon of the tibialis anterior.

Point of Ching (late Summer)
Reunion of veins

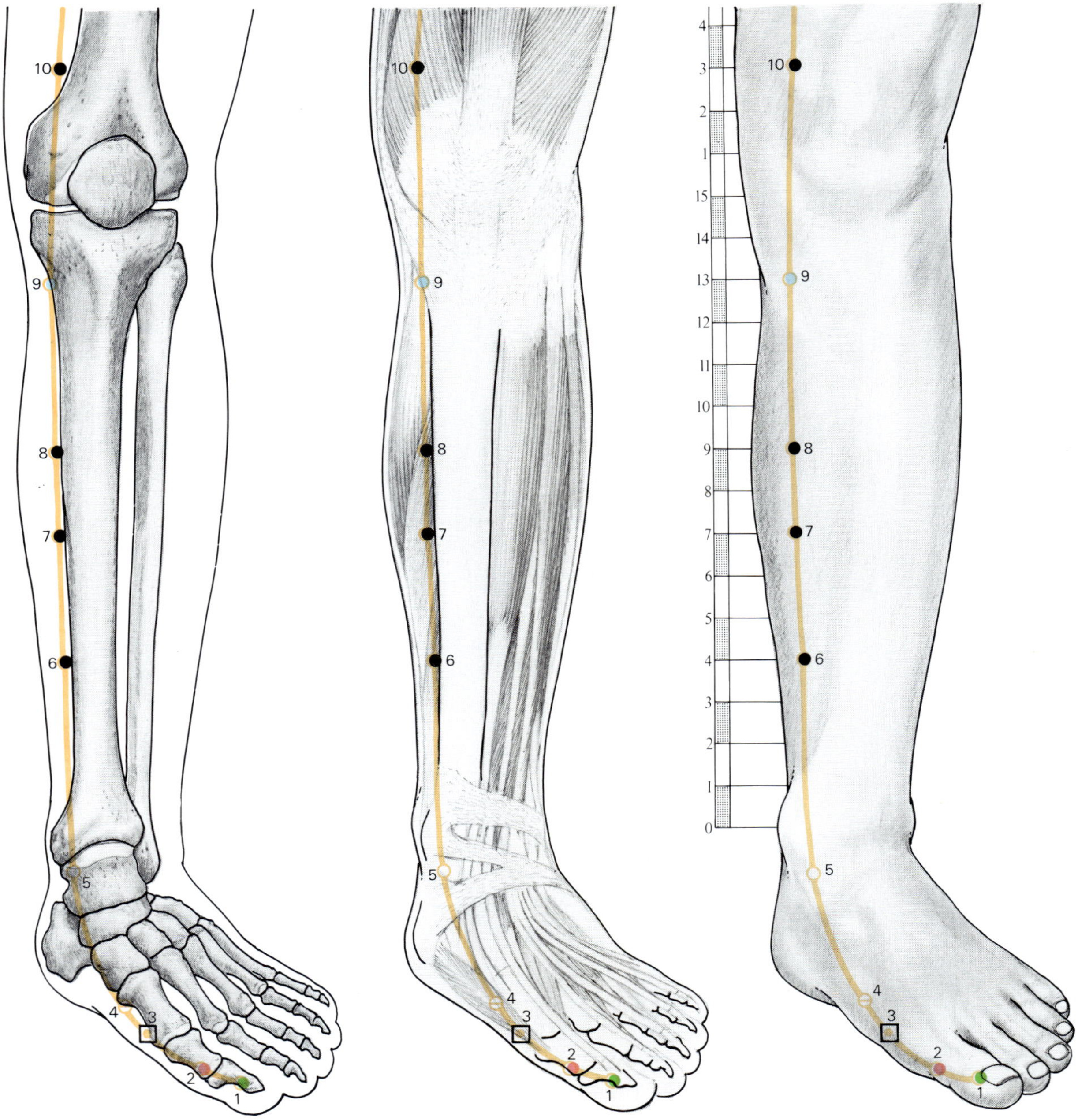
10
9
8
7
6
5
4
3
2
1
10
9
8
7
6
5
4
3
2
1
10
9
8
7
6
5
4
3
2
1

XII **6** **Three Yin Crossing** (Sanyinchiao)

⊥ 4
△ 3–10
XP9

On the medial surface of the leg, 4 ACI proximal to the prominence of the medial malleolus, posterior to the edge of the tibia.

A Centre of Energy
Meeting Point of the three lower Yin meridians (IV—VIII—XII)

XII **7** **Leaky Valley** (Louku)

⊥ 4
△ X

On the medial surface of the leg, 7 ACI proximal to the prominence of the medial malleolus, posterior to the edge of the tibia.

XII **8** **Earth Motivator** (Tichi)

⊥ 4
△ 3–7

On the medial surface of the leg, 9 ACI proximal to the prominence of the medial malleolus, posterior to the edge of the tibia.

XII **9** **Yin Mound Spring** (Yinlingchuan)

⊥ 5–8 Water
△ X

On the medial surface of the leg, 13 ACI proximal to the prominence of the medial malleolus, on the posterior edge of the tibia.

Point of Ho (Autumn)

XII **10** **Sea Of Blood** (Hsuehhai)

⊥ 3–5
△ 3–10

On the anterior surface of the thigh, 3 ACI proximal to the flexure of the knee, in the middle of the belly of the vastus medialis.

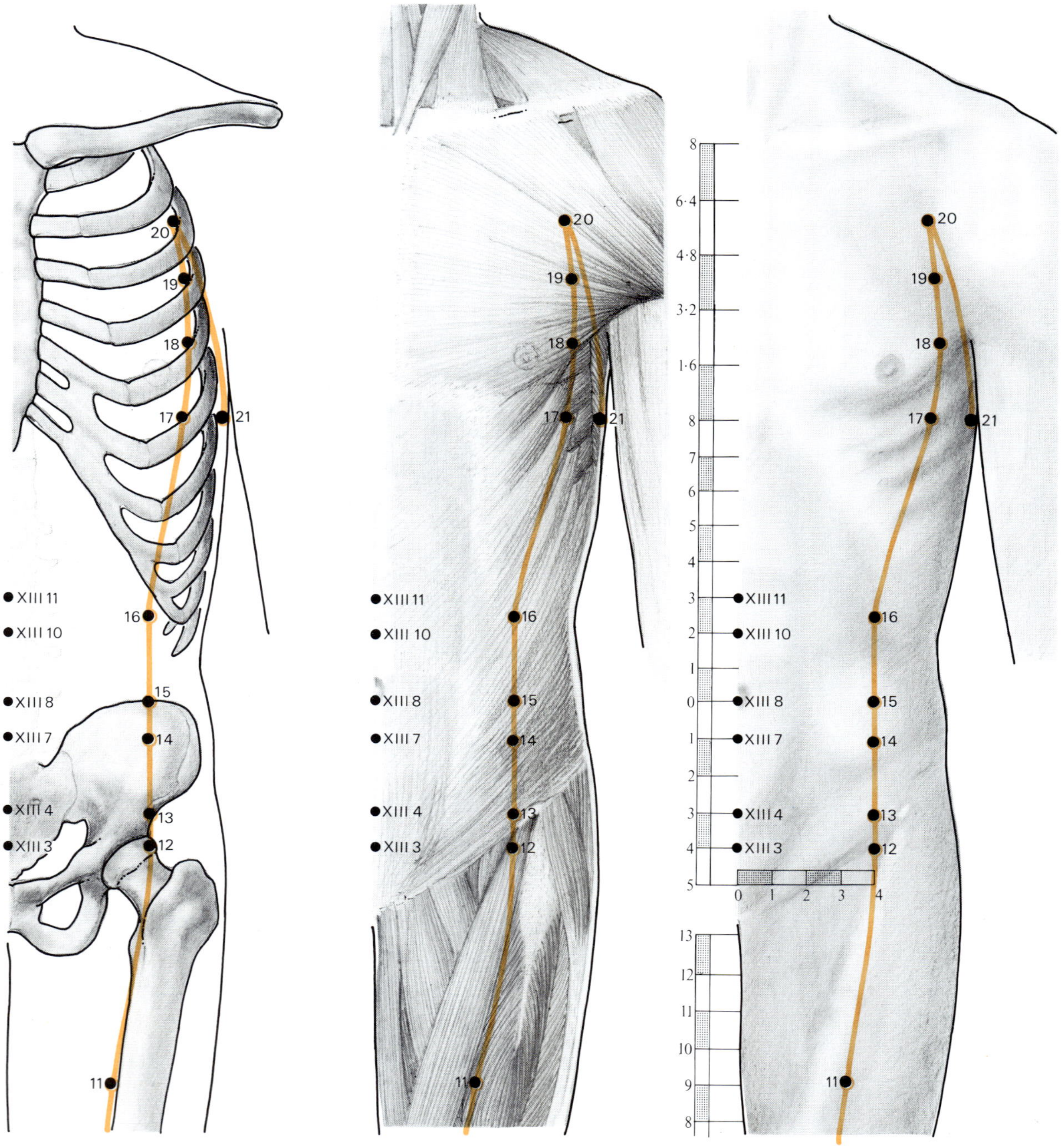
20
19
18
17
21
16
15
14
13
12
11
XIII 11
XIII 10
XIII 8
XIII 7
XIII 4
XIII 3
8
6·4
4·8
3·2
1·6
8
7
6
5
4
3
2
1
0
1
2
3
4
5
0
1
2
3
4
13
12
11
10
9
8

XII **11** **Basket Gate** (Chimen)

⊥ 5
△ 3

On the anterior surface of the thigh, 9 ACI proximal to the flexure of the knee, on the anterior border of the sartorius.

Point of Yin Wei Mo

XII **12** **Rushing Gate** (Chungmen)

⊥ 7
△ 5

On the flexure of the groin, 4 ACI lateral to the median line and 4 ACI inferior to the level of the umbilicus, on a level with XIII 3.

XII **13** **Official Residence** (Fushe)

⊥ 7
△ 5–10

On the abdomen, 4 ACI lateral to the median line and 3 ACI inferior to the level of the umbilicus, on a level with XIII 4.

Point of Yin Wei Mo

XII **14** **Abdomen Knot** (Fuchieh)

⊥ 7
△ 5–15

On the abdomen, 4 ACI lateral to the median line and 1 ACI inferior to the level of the umbilicus, on a level with XIII 7.

XII **15** **Great Horizontal** (Taheng)

⊥ 10
△ 5–10

On the abdomen, 4 ACI lateral to the median line, at the level of the centre of the umbilicus and XIII 8.

Point of Yin Wei Mo

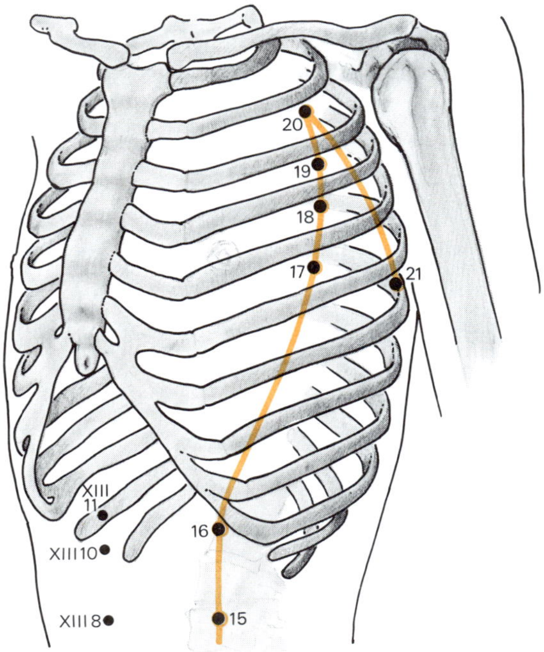
20
19
18
17
21
XIII
11
16
XIII10
XIII8
15

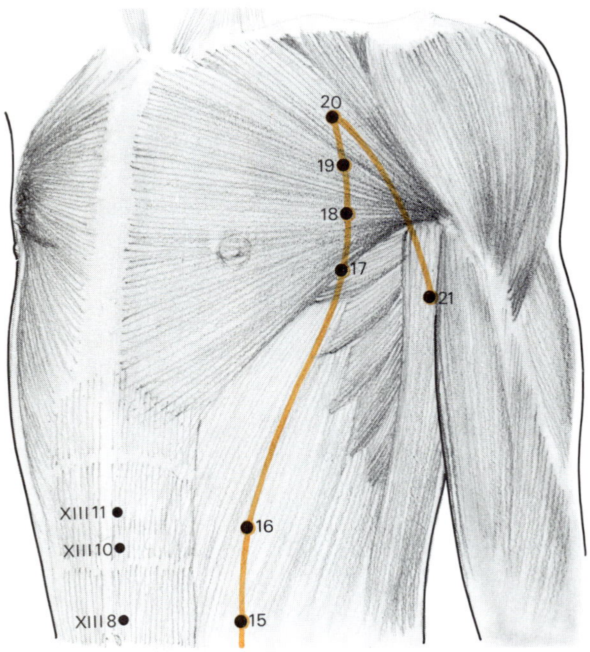
20
19
18
17
21
XIII11
16
XIII10
XIII8
15

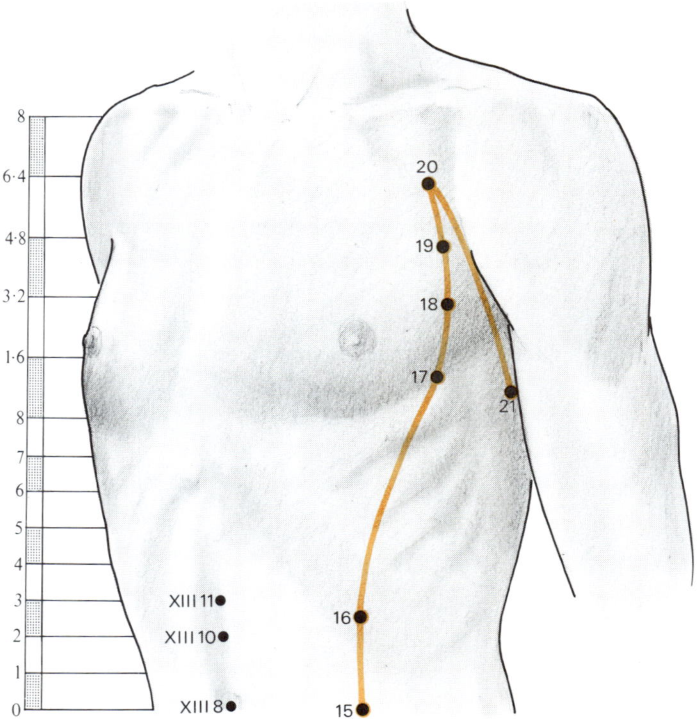
8
6·4
4·8
3·2
1·6
8
7
6
5
4
3
2
1
0
20
19
18
17
21
XIII11
XIII10
16
XIII8
15

XII **16** **Abdomen Sorrow** (Fuai)

⊥ 7
△ 5–10

On the abdomen, 4 ACI lateral to the median line and $2\frac{1}{2}$ ACI superior to the level of the umbilicus, at a level half-way between XIII 10 and XIII 11, on the paramedian nipple line.

Point of Yin Wei Mo

XII **17** **Food Drain** (Shihtou)

⊥ 3
△ 5

On the thorax, in the fifth intercostal space, 6 ACI lateral to the median line.

XII **18** **Heavenly Stream** (Tienhsi)

⊥ 3
△ 5

On the thorax, in the fourth intercostal space, 6 ACI lateral to the median line.

XII **19** **Chest Region** (Hsiunghsiang)

⊥ 3
△ 5

On the thorax, in the third intercostal space, 6 ACI lateral to the median line.

XII **20** **Encircling Glory** (Choujung)

⊥ 3
△ 5

On the thorax, in the second intercostal space, 6 ACI lateral to the median line.

XII **21** **Great Enveloping** (Tapao)

⊥ 3 Exit
△ 3–7

On the thorax, in the sixth intercostal space, on the mid-axillary line.

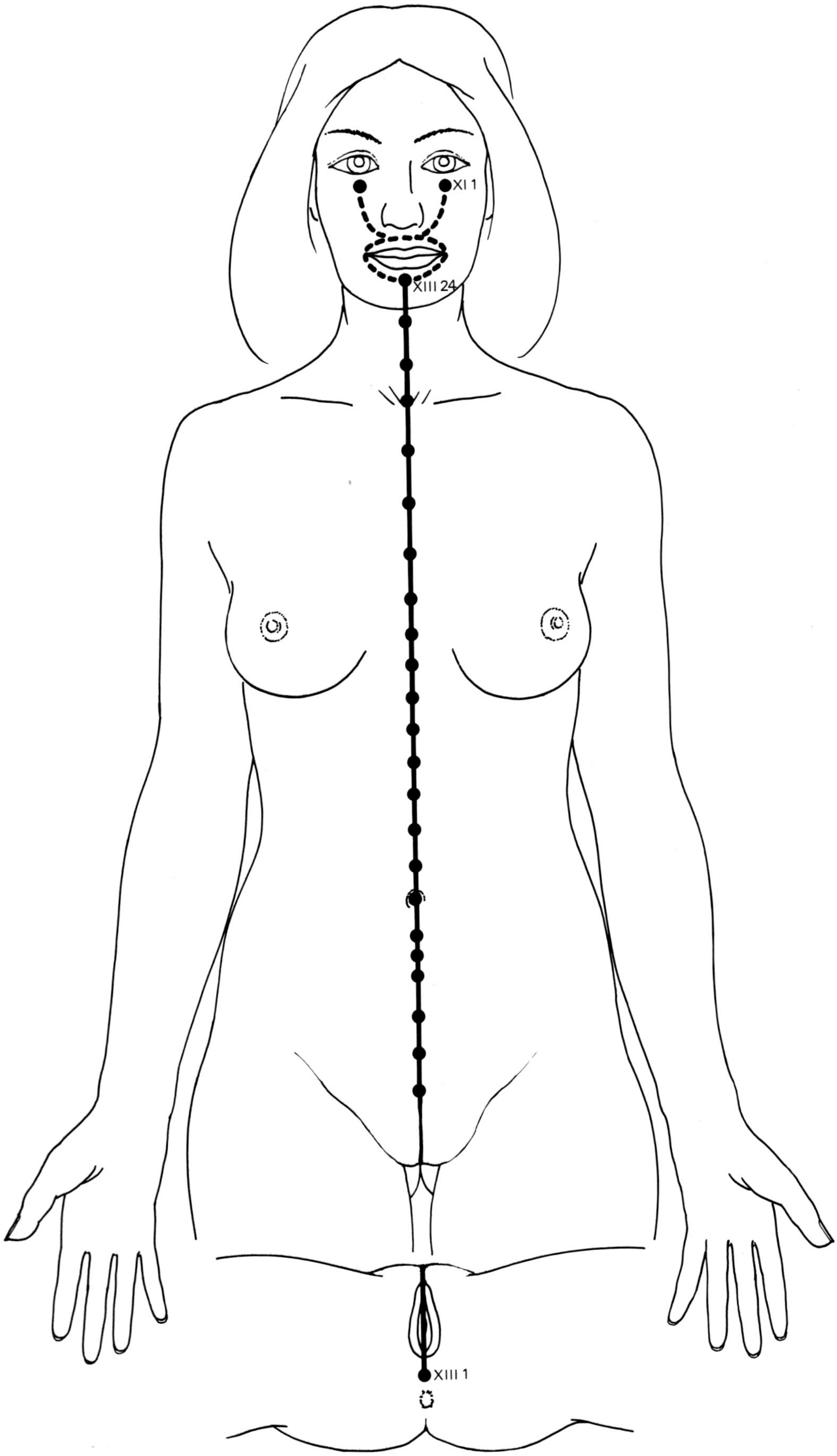
XI 1
XIII 24
XIII 1

The conception vessel begins on the perineum, at XIII 1, and travels up the anterior median line of the abdomen, thorax and neck, over the chin on to the lower lip, where it ends at XIII 24.

From XIII 24, bilateral deep branches go around the angle of the mouth to the gums, under the upper lip. From the gums bilateral branches ascend the cheeks to the optic foramen where they meet XI 1.

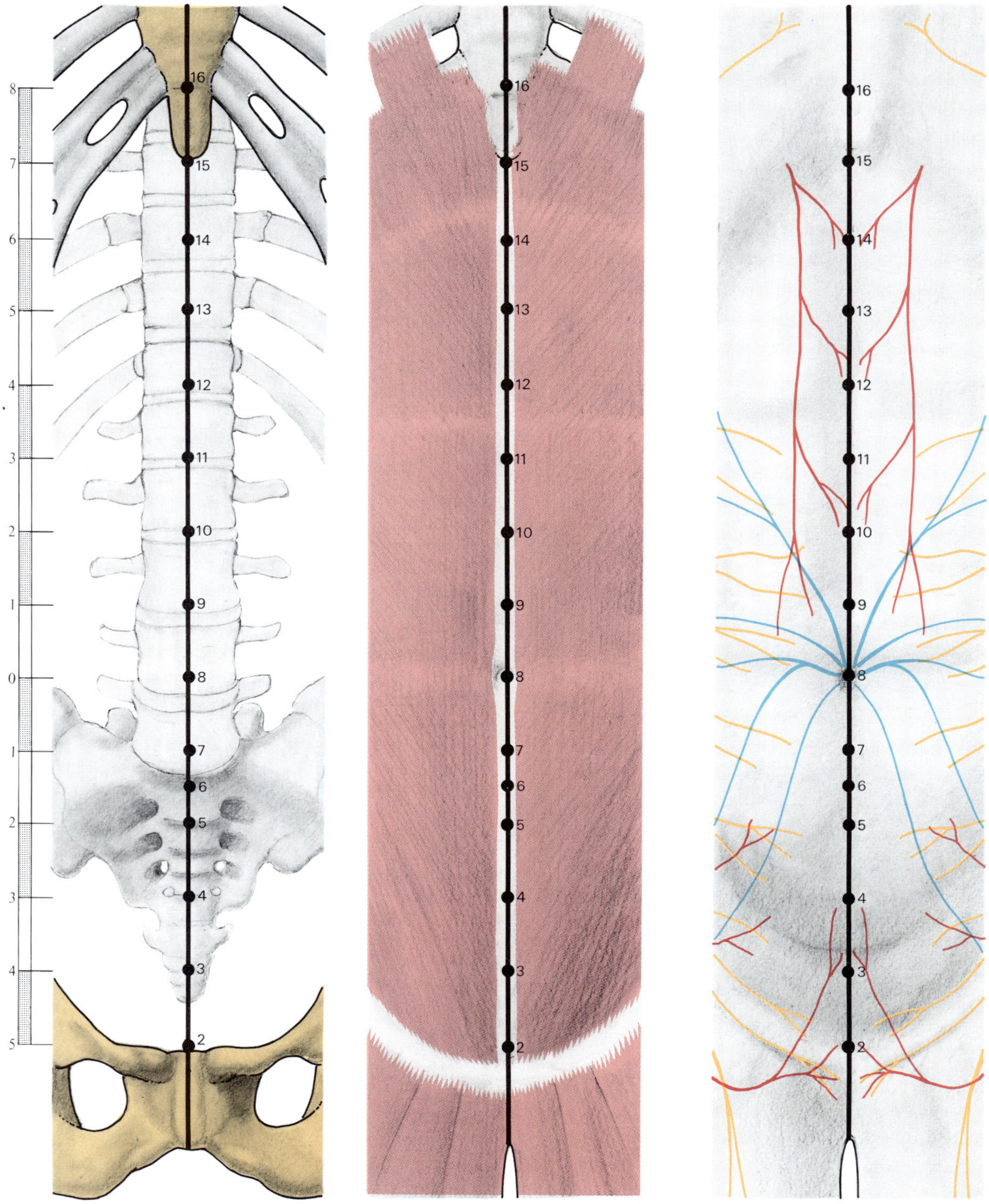
8
7
6
5
4
3
2
1
0
1
2
3
4
5
16
15
14
13
12
11
10
9
8
7
6
5
4
3
2

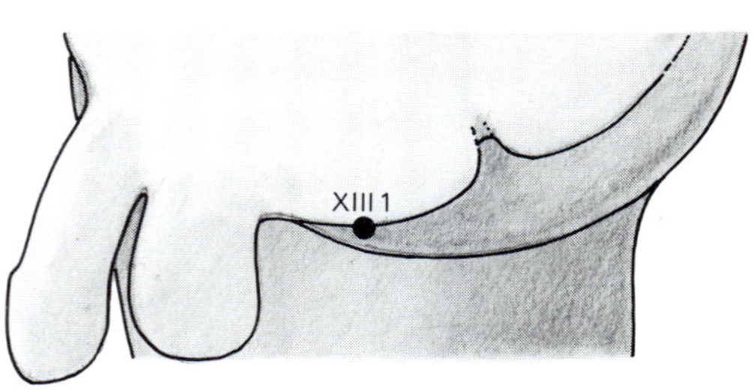
XIII 1

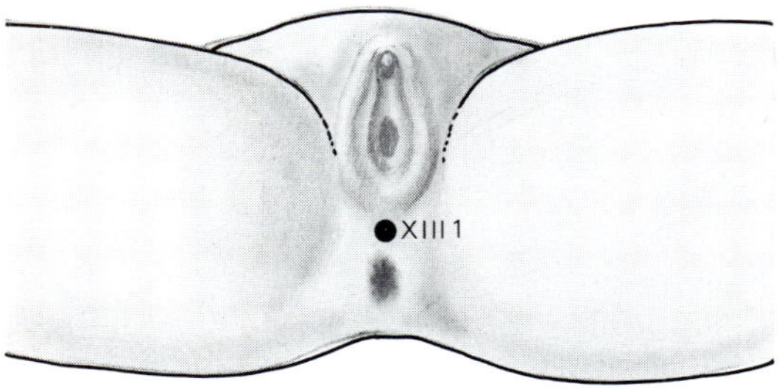
XIII 1

XIII	1	On the centre of the perineum.
XIII	2	On the anterior median line, just superior to the superior edge of the pubic symphysis, 5 ACI inferior to the umbilicus.
XIII	3	On the anterior median line, 4 ACI inferior to the umbilicus.
XIII	4	On the anterior median line, 3 ACI inferior to the umbilicus.
XIII	5	On the anterior median line, 2 ACI inferior to the umbilicus.
XIII	6	On the anterior median line, $1\frac{1}{2}$ ACI inferior to the umbilicus.
XIII	7	On the anterior median line, 1 ACI inferior to the umbilicus.
XIII	8	In the centre of the umbilicus.
XIII	9	On the anterior median line, 1 ACI superior to the umbilicus.
XIII	10	On the anterior median line, 2 ACI superior to the umbilicus.
XIII	11	On the anterior median line, 3 ACI superior to the umbilicus.
XIII	12	On the anterior median line, 4 ACI superior to the umbilicus.
XIII	13	On the anterior median line, 5 ACI superior to the umbilicus.
XIII	14	On the anterior median line, 6 ACI superior to the umbilicus.
XIII	15	On the anterior median line, 7 ACI superior to the umbilicus, inferior to the xiphoid process.

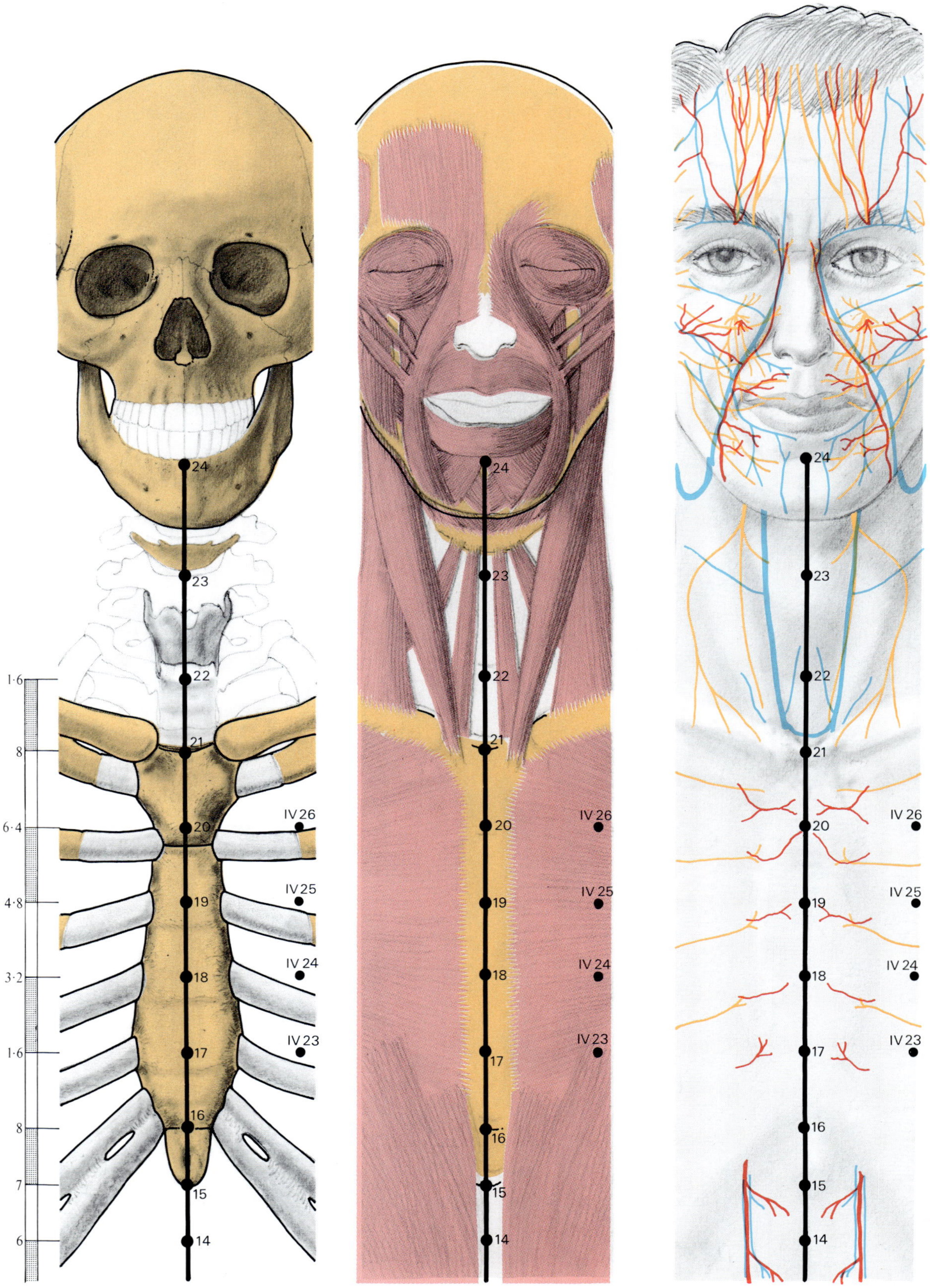
24
23
22
21
20
19
18
17
16
15
14
IV 26
IV 25
IV 24
IV 23
1·6
8
6·4
4·8
3·2
1·6
8
7
6

XIII	**14**	On the anterior median line, 6 ACI superior to the umbilicus.
XIII	**15**	On the anterior median line, 7 ACI superior to the umbilicus, inferior to the xiphoid process.
XIII	**16**	On the anterior median line, 8 ACI superior to the umbilicus, at the xiphisternal joint.
XIII	**17**	On the anterior median line, 1.6 ACI superior to XIII 16, at the level of the fourth intercostal space, and level with IV 23.
XIII	**18**	On the anterior median line, 1.6 ACI superior to XIII 17, at the level of the third intercostal space, and level with IV 24.
XIII	**19**	On the anterior median line, 1.6 ACI superior to XIII 18, at the level of the second intercostal space, and level with IV 25.
XIII	**20**	On the anterior median line, 1.6 ACI superior to XIII 19, at the level of the first intercostal space, and level with IV 26.
XIII	**21**	On the anterior median line, in the suprasternal notch.
XIII	**22**	On the anterior median line, 1.6 ACI superior to XIII 21, inferior to the cricoid cartilage.
XIII	**23**	On the anterior median line, directly inferior to the hyoid bone.
XIII	**24**	On the anterior median line, in the depression between the point of the chin and the lower lip.

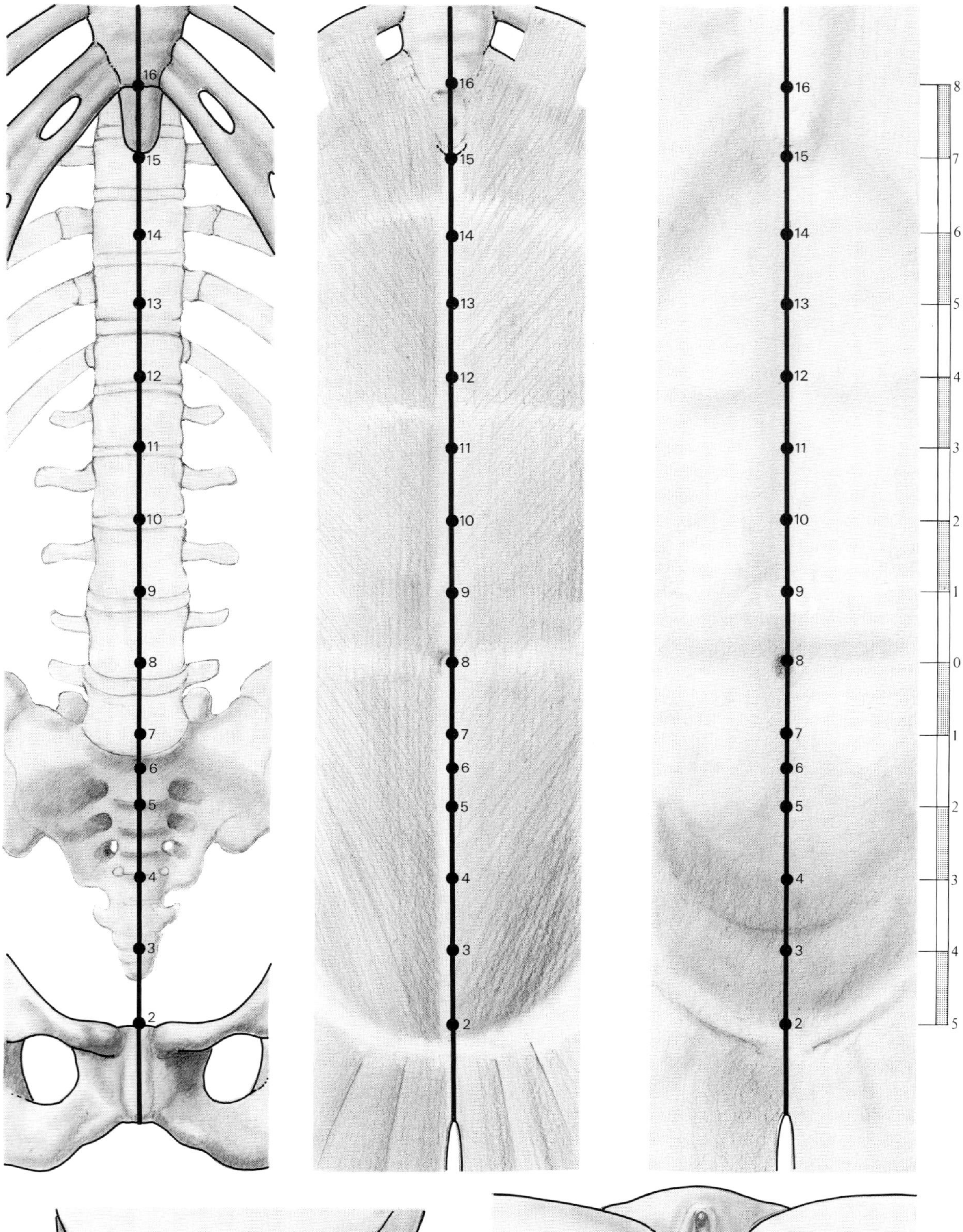
16
15
14
13
12
11
10
9
8
7
6
5
4
3
2
16
15
14
13
12
11
10
9
8
7
6
5
4
3
2
16
15
14
13
12
11
10
9
8
7
6
5
4
3
2
8
7
6
5
4
3
2
1
0
1
2
3
4
5

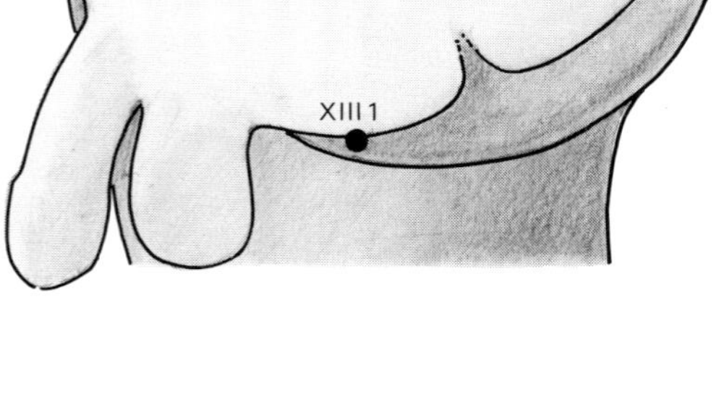
XIII 1

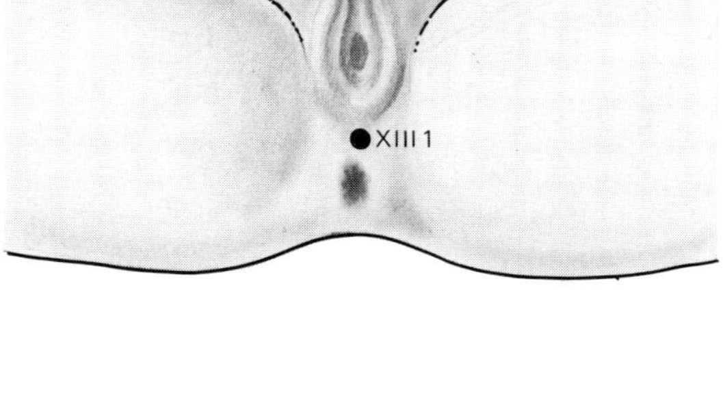
XIII 1

XIII **1** **Meeting Of Yin** (Huiyin)

⊥ 10 Entry
△ X General Junction Point

On the centre of the perineum.

Point of Ren Mo
Point of Chong Mo
First Aid: drowning, resuscitation

XIII **2** **Crooked Bone** (Chuku)

⊥ 5
△ 7

On the anterior median line, just superior to the superior edge of the pubic symphysis, 5 ACI inferior to the umbilicus.

Point of Ren Mo

XIII **3** **Utmost Middle** (Chungchi)

⊥ 8
△ 5–15

On the anterior median line, 4 ACI inferior to the umbilicus.

Point of Ren Mo
Alarm Point of III
A Centre of Energy
First Aid: urine retention

XIII **4** **First Gate** (Kuanyuan)

⊥ 10–15
△ 7–15

On the anterior median line, 3 ACI inferior to the umbilicus.

Point of Ren Mo
Alarm Point of II
A Centre of Energy

XIII **5** **Stone Gate** (Shihmen)

⊥ 7–8
△ 7–15

On the anterior median line, 2 ACI inferior to the umbilicus.

Point of Ren Mo
Alarm Point of VI (Main Alarm Point for whole Three Heater)
Main Centre of Energy

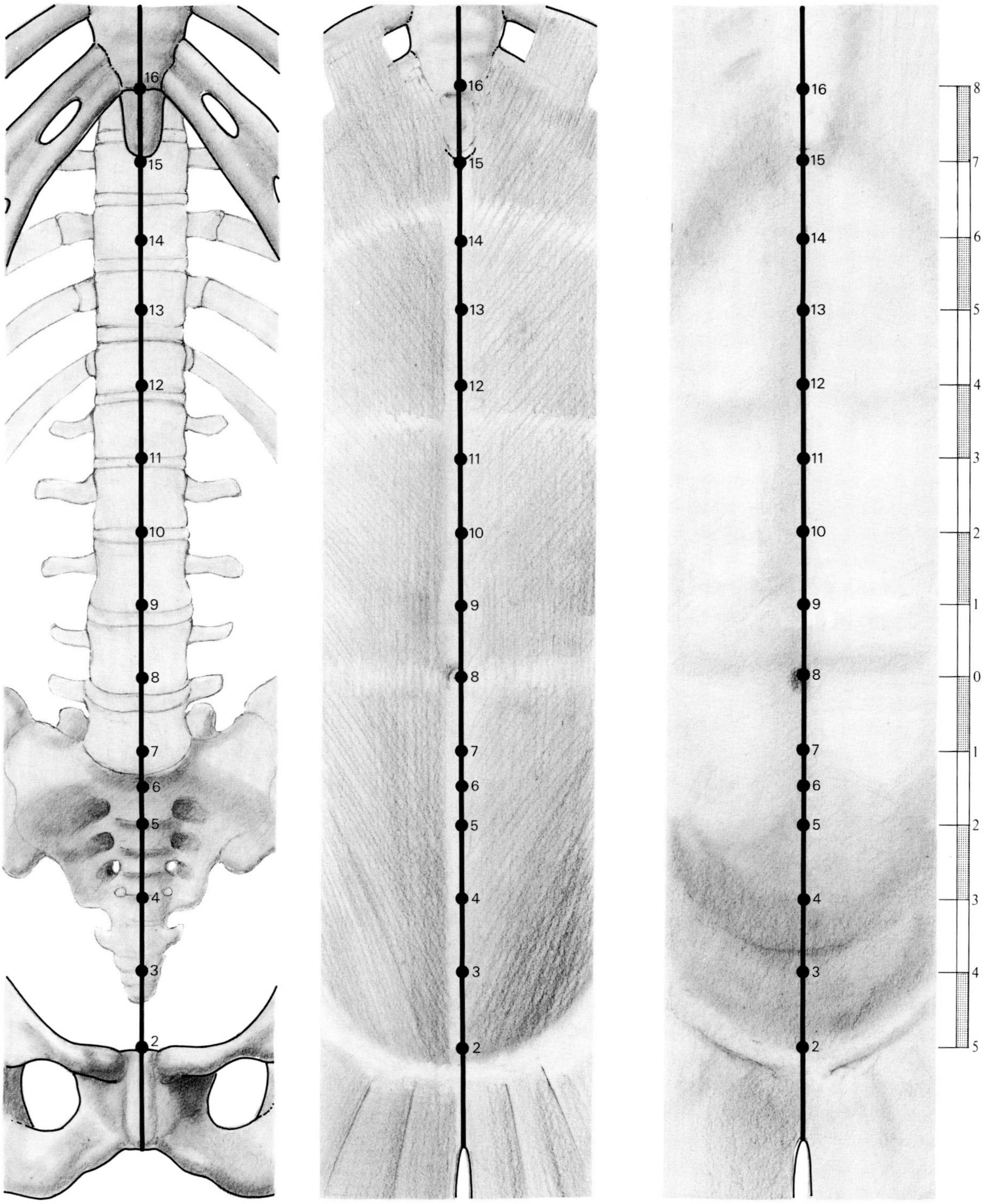
16
15
14
13
12
11
10
9
8
7
6
5
4
3
2
8
7
6
5
4
3
2
1
0
1
2
3
4
5

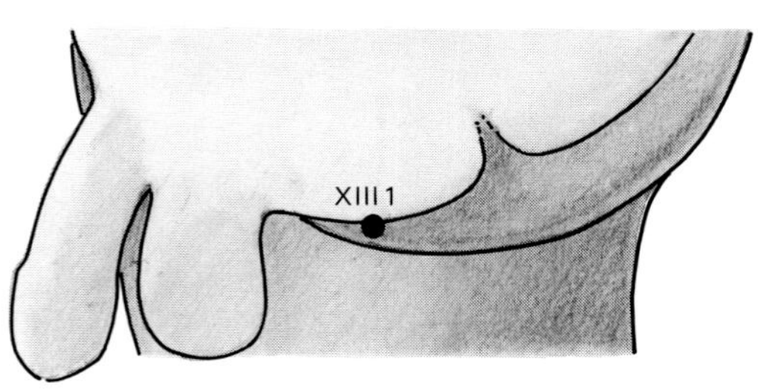
XIII 1

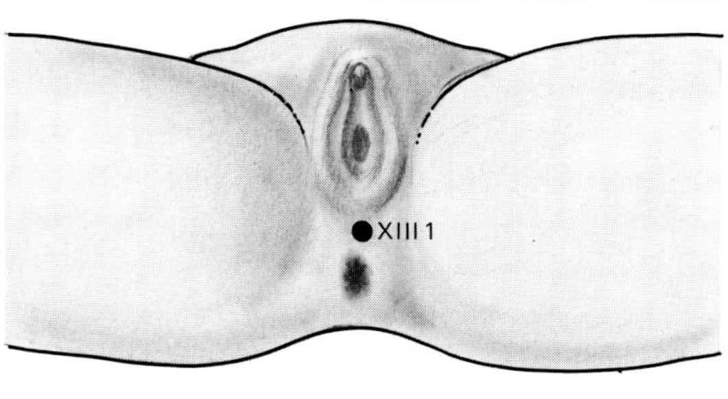
XIII 1

XIII **6** **Sea Of Ch'i** (Chihai)

⊥ 8
△ 7–15

On the anterior median line, $1\frac{1}{2}$ ACI inferior to the umbilicus.

Point of Ren Mo
Main Centre of Energy

XIII **7** **Yin Crossing** (Yinchiao)

⊥ 8
△ 7

On the anterior median line, 1 ACI inferior to the umbilicus.

Point of Ren Mo
Alarm Point of VI (Lower Chou)

XIII **8** **Spirit Deficiency** (Shenchueh)

⊥ X
△ 3–30
(on salt)

In the centre of the umbilicus.

Point of Ren Mo

XIII **9** **Water Division** (Shuifen)

⊥ 5
△ 5–15

On the anterior median line, 1 ACI superior to the umbilicus.

Point of Ren Mo

XIII **10** **Lower Duct** (Hsiawan)

⊥ 8
△ 7–15

On the anterior median line, 2 ACI superior to the umbilicus.

Point of Ren Mo

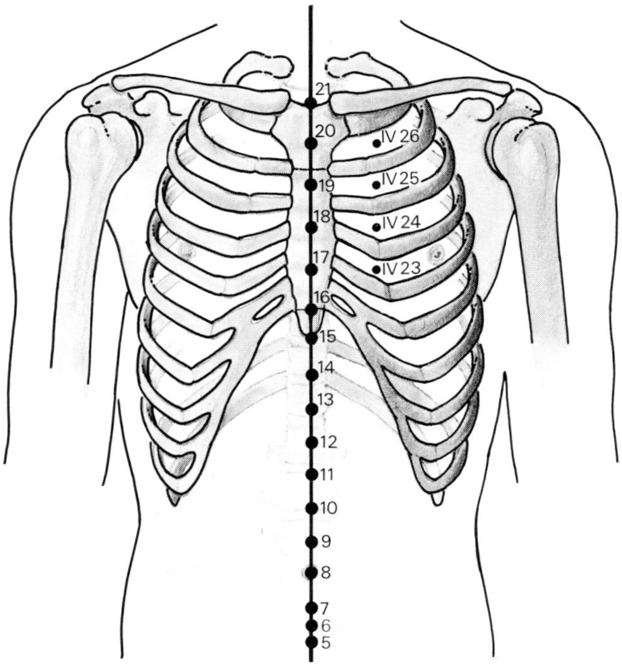
21
20
IV 26
19
IV 25
18
IV 24
17
IV 23
16
15
14
13
12
11
10
9
8
7
6
5

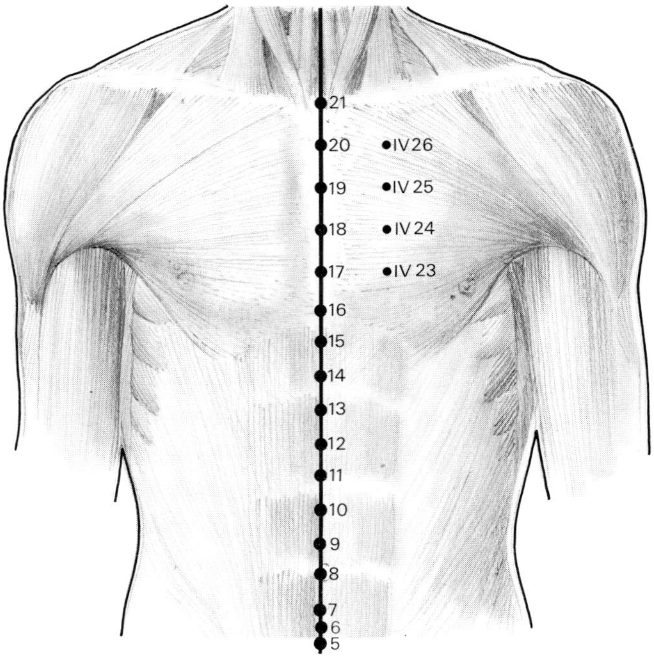
21
20
IV 26
19
IV 25
18
IV 24
17
IV 23
16
15
14
13
12
11
10
9
8
7
6
5

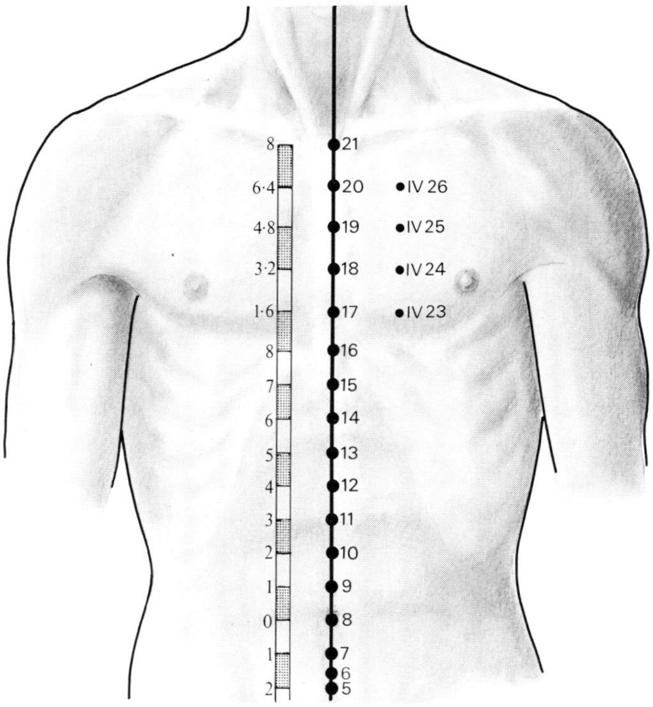
8
6·4
4·8
3·2
1·6
8
7
6
5
4
3
2
1
0
1
2
21
20
IV 26
19
IV 25
18
IV 24
17
IV 23
16
15
14
13
12
11
10
9
8
7
6
5

XIII **11** **Established Mile** (Chienli)

⊥ 5–8
△ 5–15

On the anterior median line, 3 ACI superior to the umbilicus.

Point of Ren Mo

XIII **12** **Middle Duct** (Chungwan)

⊥ 3–8
△ 7–15

On the anterior median line, 4 ACI superior to the umbilicus.

Point of Ren Mo
Alarm Point of XI and VI (Middle Chou)
Assembling Point of hollow organs
A Centre of Energy
Meeting Point of the five Yang Organs

XIII **13** **Upper Duct** (Shangwan)

⊥ 5–8
△ 7–15

On the anterior median line, 5 ACI superior to the umbilicus.

Point of Ren Mo

XIII **14** **Great Deficiency** (Chuchueh)

⊥ 6
△ 7–15

On the anterior median line, 6 ACI superior to the umbilicus.

Point of Ren Mo
Alarm Point of I
First Aid: sea and travel sickness

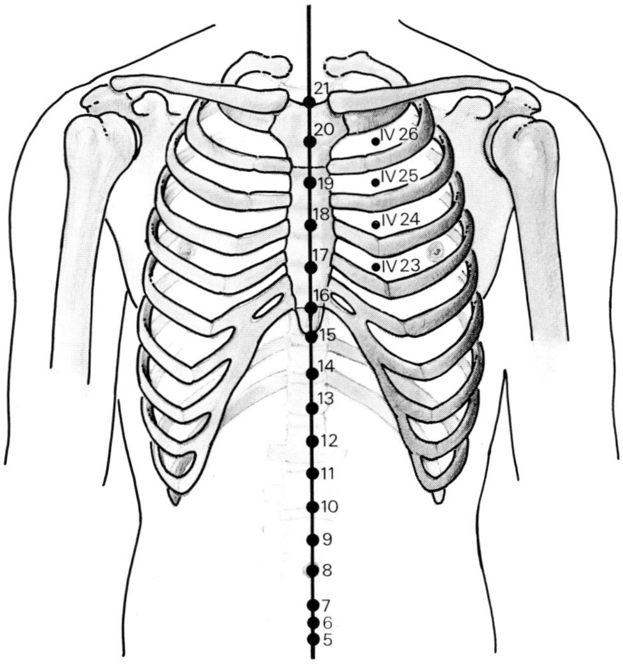
21
20
IV 26
19
IV 25
18
IV 24
17
IV 23
16
15
14
13
12
11
10
9
8
7
6
5

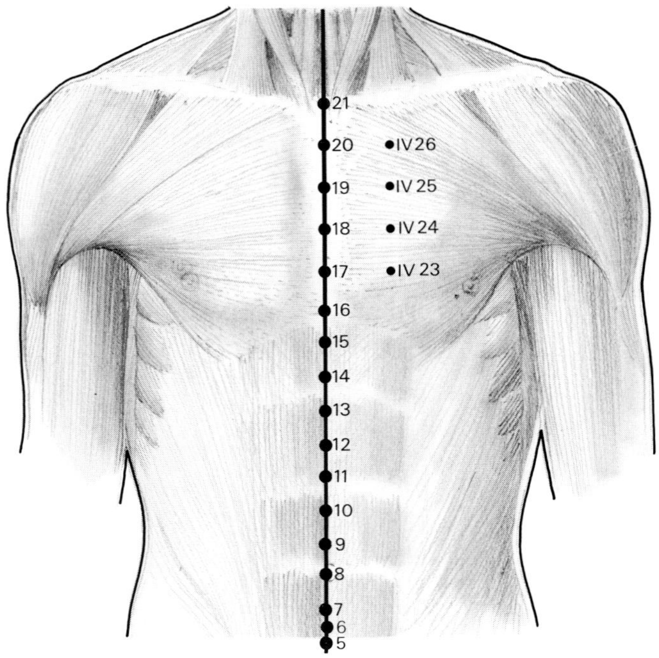
21
20
IV 26
19
IV 25
18
IV 24
17
IV 23
16
15
14
13
12
11
10
9
8
7
6
5

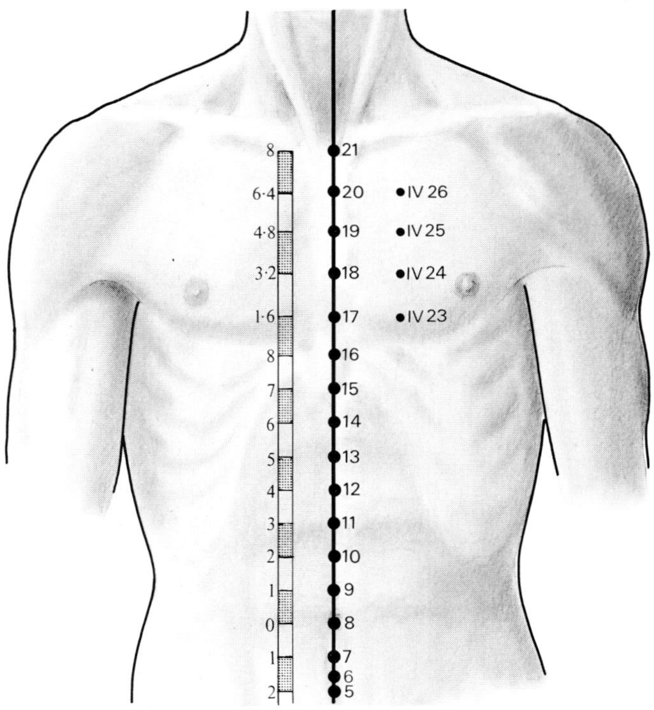
8
6·4
4·8
3·2
1·6
8
7
6
5
4
3
2
1
0
1
2
21
20
IV 26
19
IV 25
18
IV 24
17
IV 23
16
15
14
13
12
11
10
9
8
7
6
5

XIII **15** **Dove Tail** (Chiuwei)

⊥ 3–5
△ 3–5

On the anterior median line, 7 ACI superior to the umbilicus, inferior to the tip of the xiphoid process.

Point of Ren Mo
Alarm Point of V
A point of the pattern to release the 7 Dragons on the 7 Internal Demons (Master point below XIII 15).

XIII **16** **Middle Hall** (Chungting)

⊥ 3
△ 5

On the anterior median line, 8 ACI superior to the umbilicus, at the xiphisternal joint.

Point of Ren Mo

XIII **17** **Within The Breast** (Shanchung)

⊥ X
△ 3

On the anterior median line, 1.6 ACI superior to XIII 16, at the level of the fourth intercostal space, and level with IV 23.

Point of Ren Mo
Sea of Energy
Alarm Point of VI (Upper Chou)
Assembling Point of Ch'i Energy
Centre Reunion Particular Point of breath energy

XIII **18** **Jade Court** (Yutang)

⊥ 3
△ 5

On the anterior median line, 1.6 ACI superior to XIII 17, at the level of the third intercostal space, and level with IV 24.

Point of Ren Mo

XIII **19** **Purple Palace** (Tzukung)

⊥ 3
△ 5

On the anterior median line, 1.6 ACI superior to XIII 18, at the level of the second intercostal space, and level with IV 25.

Point of Ren Mo

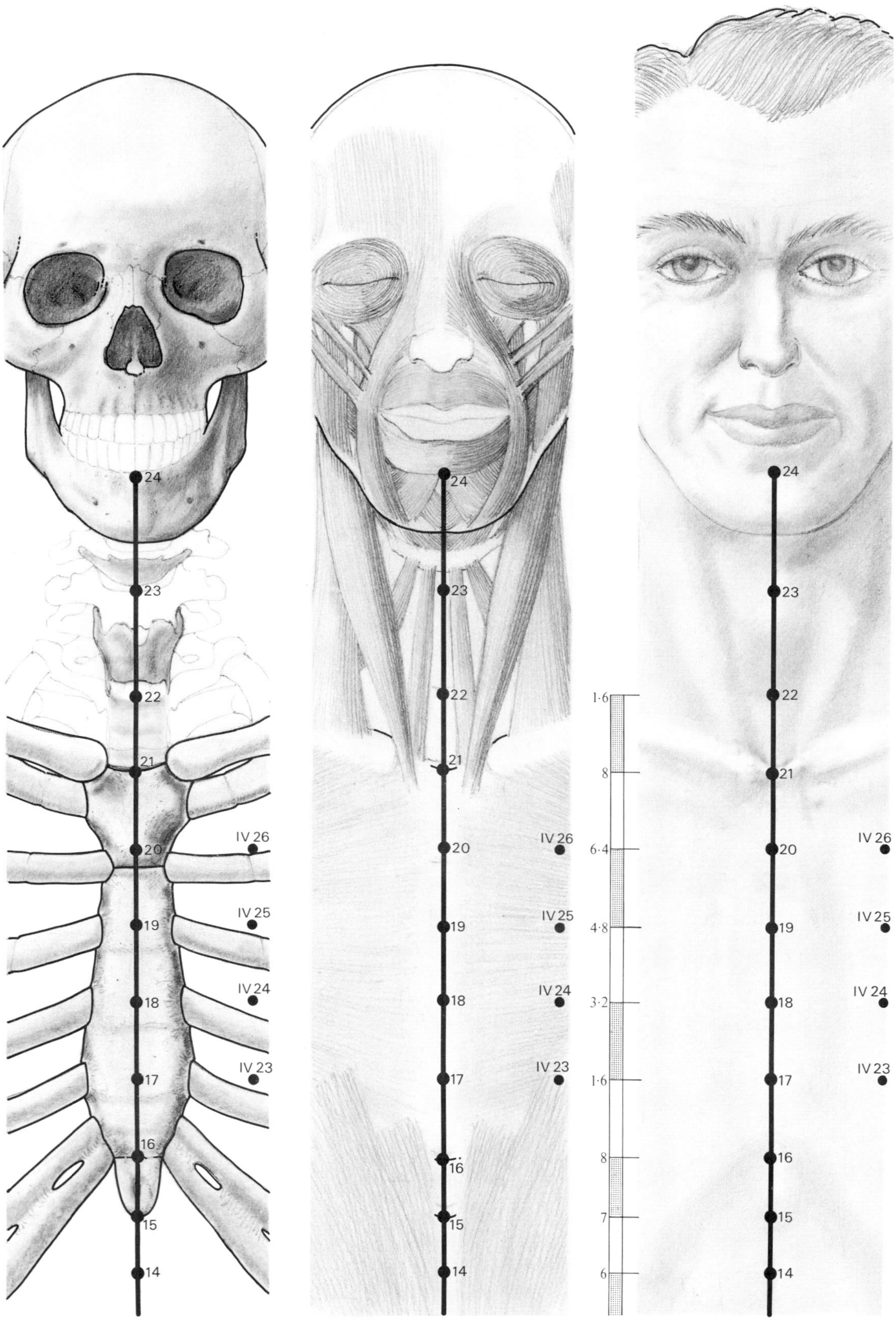
24
23
22
21
20
19
18
17
16
15
14
IV 26
IV 25
IV 24
IV 23
1·6
8
6·4
4·8
3·2
1·6
8
7
6

XIII **20** **Flower Covering** (Huakai)

⊥ 3
△ 3

On the anterior median line, 1.6 ACI superior to XIII 19, at the level of the first intercostal space, and level with IV 26.

Point of Ren Mo

XIII **21** **Pearl Jade** (Hsuanchi)

⊥ 3
△ 5

On the anterior median line, in the suprasternal notch.

Point of Ren Mo

XIII **22** **Heaven Rushing Out** (Tientu)

⊥ 3
△ 3–7

On the anterior median line, 1.6 ACI superior to XIII 21, inferior to the cricoid cartilage.

Point of Ren Mo
Point of Yin Wei Mo
Window of the Sky

XIII **23** **Angle Spring** (Lienchuan)

⊥ 3
△ 3–7

On the anterior median line, directly inferior to the hyoid bone.

Point of Ren Mo
Point of Yin Wei Mo
Point of Chong Mo

XIII **24** **Receiving Fluid** (Chengchiang)

⊥ 1–3 Exit
△ 3–7

On the anterior median line, in the depression between the point of the chin and the lower lip.

Point of Ren Mo

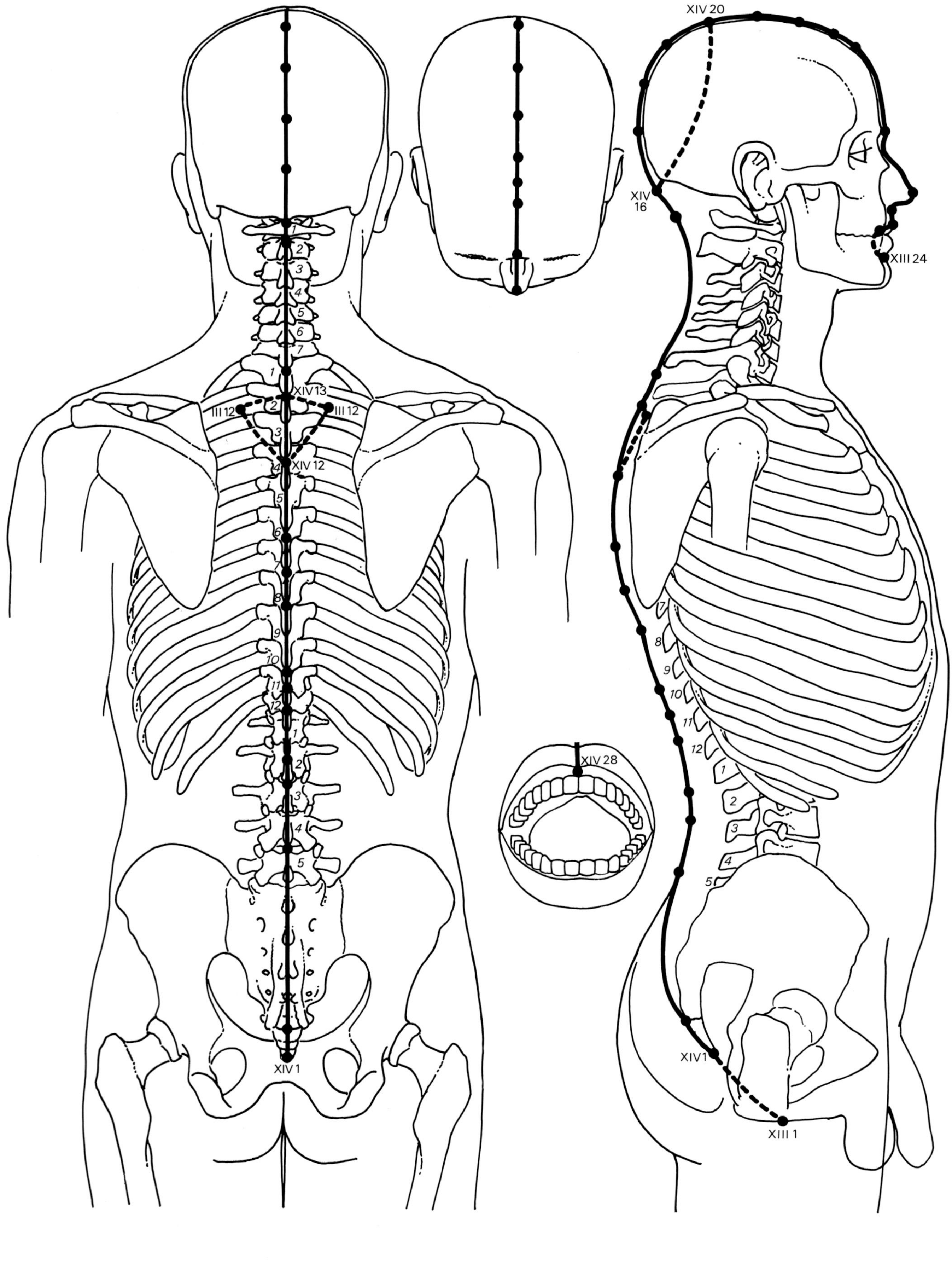
XIV 13
III 12
III 12
XIV 12
XIV 1
XIV 20
XIV 16
XIII 24
XIV 28
XIV 1
XIII 1

The governor vessel begins at the tip of the coccyx, at XIV 1. A deep branch extends to the perineum to meet XIII 1. The main pathway ascends the median line of the spine to the atlas bone, over the head in the median line and down the forehead and nose to the upper lip. It ends on the mid-point of the upper gum, at XIV 28. A deep branch goes to the lower lip to meet XIII 24 and the stomach meridian.

In the depression inferior to the third thoracic vertebra, at XIV 12, deep bilateral branches ascend laterally to III 12 and then turn medially to the depression inferior to the first thoracic vertebra to rejoin the main pathway at XIV 13. Between the atlas and the occipital bone, at XIV 16, a branch leaves the main pathway to enter the brain. It emerges and rejoins the main pathway at the mid-point of the sagittal fissure, XIV 20.

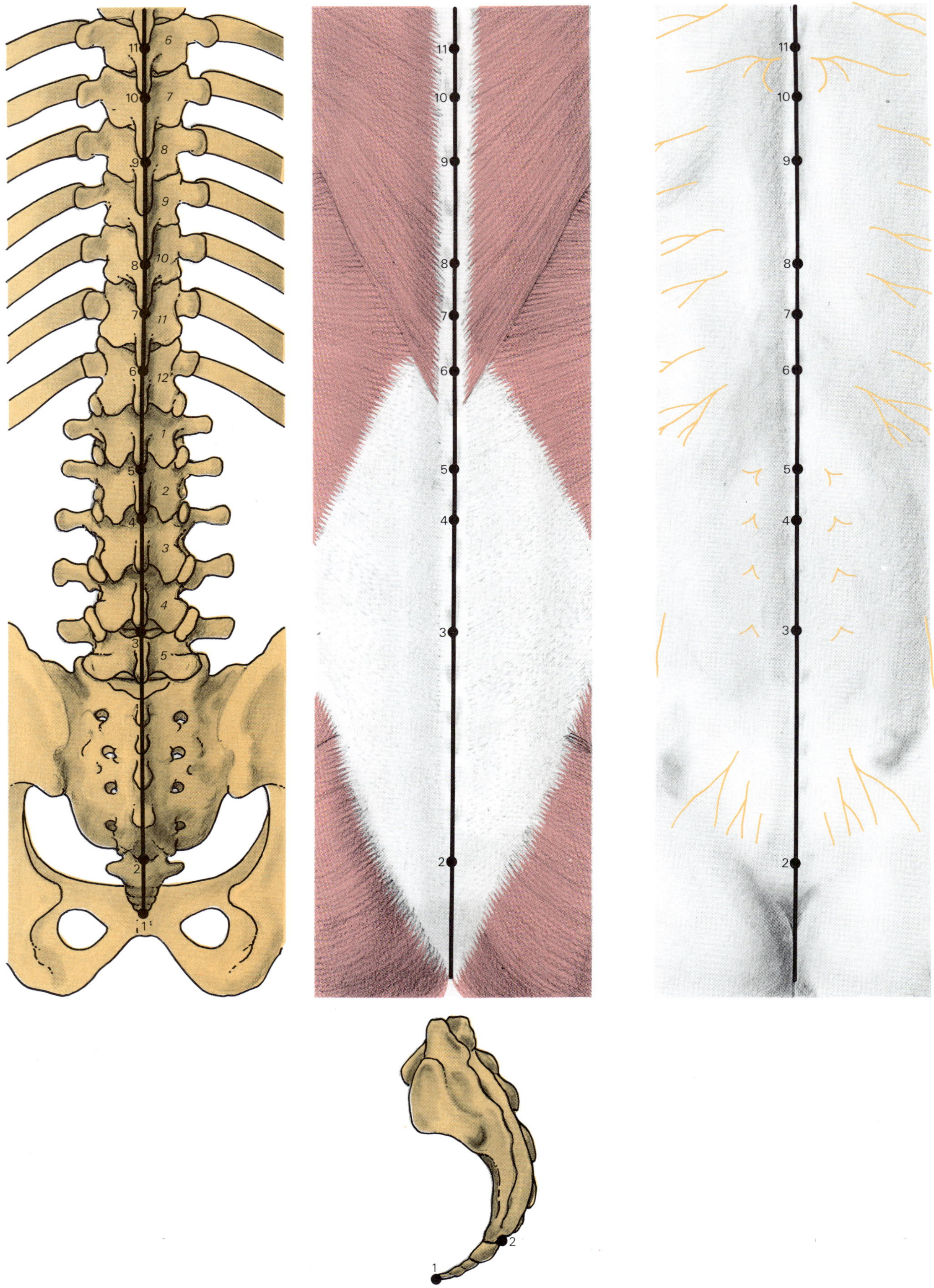
11
6
10
7
9
8
9
8
10
7
11
6
12
1
5
2
4
3
4
3
5
2
1

XIV	1	On the posterior median line, at the tip of the coccyx.
XIV	2	On the posterior median line, at the sacrococcygeal articulation.
XIV	3	On the posterior median line, in the depression between the fourth and fifth lumbar vertebrae.
XIV	4	On the posterior median line, in the depression between the second and third lumbar vertebrae.
XIV	5	On the posterior median line, in the depression between the first and second lumbar vertebrae.
XIV	6	On the posterior median line, in the depression between the eleventh and twelfth thoracic vertebrae.
XIV	7	On the posterior median line, in the depression between the tenth and eleventh thoracic vertebrae.
XIV	8	On the posterior median line, in the depression between the ninth and tenth thoracic vertebrae.
XIV	9	On the posterior median line, in the depression between the seventh and eighth thoracic vertebrae.
XIV	10	On the posterior median line, in the depression between the sixth and seventh thoracic vertebrae.
XIV	11	On the posterior median line, in the depression between the fifth and sixth thoracic vertebrae.

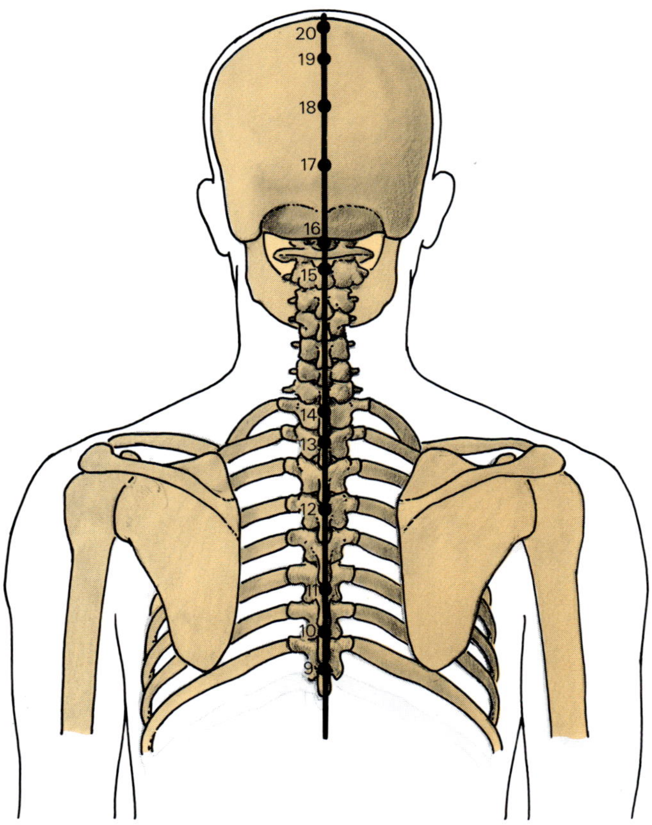
20
19
18
17
16
15
14
13
12
10
9

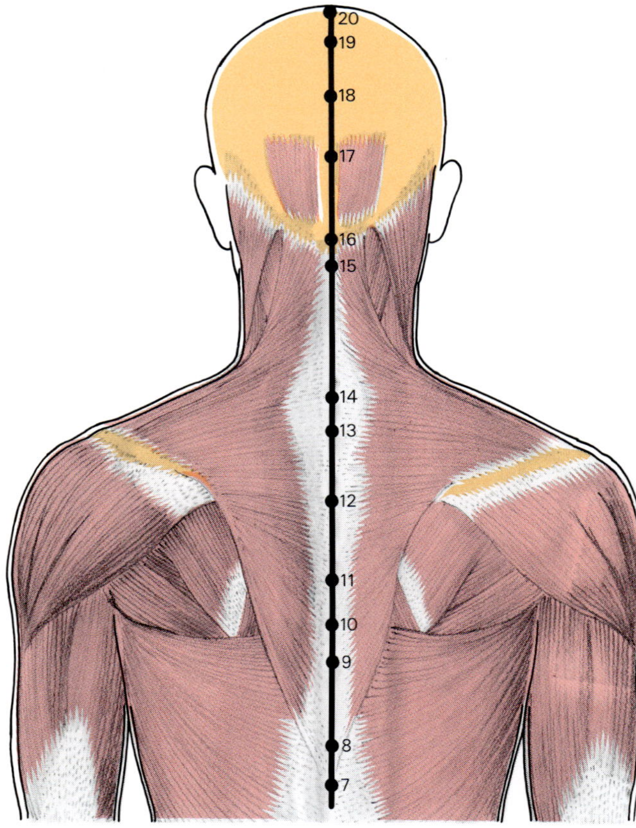
20
19
18
17
16
15
14
13
12
11
10
9
8
7

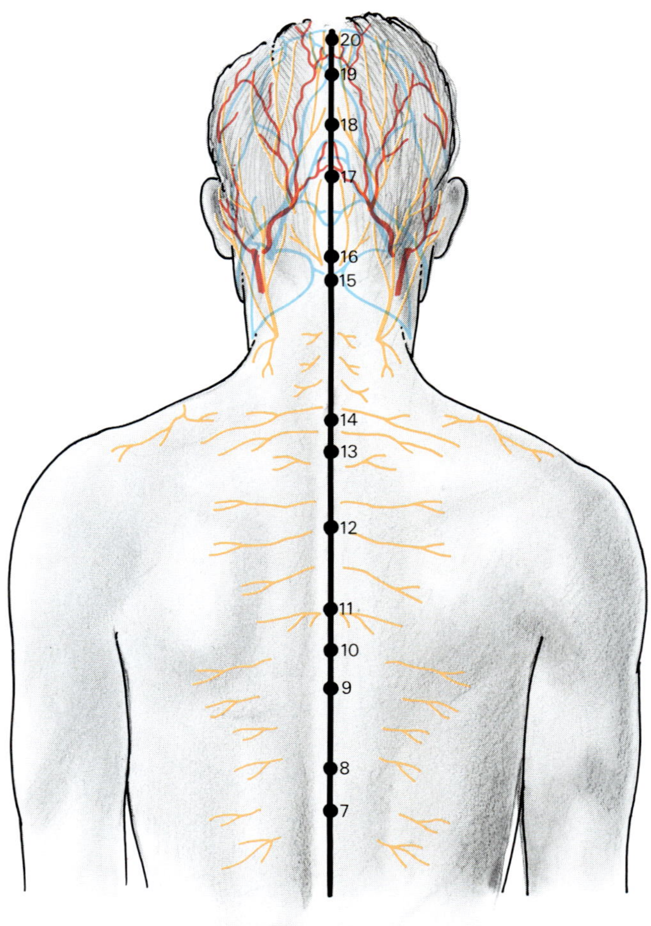
20
19
18
17
16
15
14
13
12
11
10
9
8
7

XIV **10**	On the posterior median line, in the depression between the sixth and seventh thoracic vertebrae.
XIV **11**	On the posterior median line, in the depression between the fifth and sixth thoracic vertebrae.
XIV **12**	On the posterior median line, in the depression between the third and fourth thoracic vertebrae.
XIV **13**	On the posterior median line, in the depression between the first and second thoracic vertebrae.
XIV **14**	On the posterior median line, in the depression between the seventh cervical and the first thoracic vertebrae.
XIV **15**	On the posterior median line, in the depression between the first and second cervical vertebrae.
XIV **16**	On the median line of the head, just inferior to the base of the occipital bone, $\frac{1}{2}$ ACI superior to XIV 15.
XIV **17**	On the median line of the head, $2\frac{1}{2}$ ACI superior to XIV 15.
XIV **18**	On the median line of the head, 4 ACI superior to XIV 15.
XIV **19**	On the median line of the head, $5\frac{1}{2}$ ACI superior to XIV 15.
XIV **20**	On the median line of the head, 7 ACI superior to XIV 15.

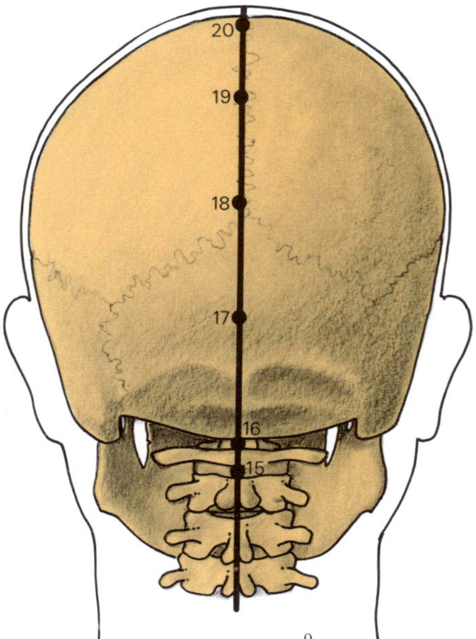
20
19
18
17
16
15

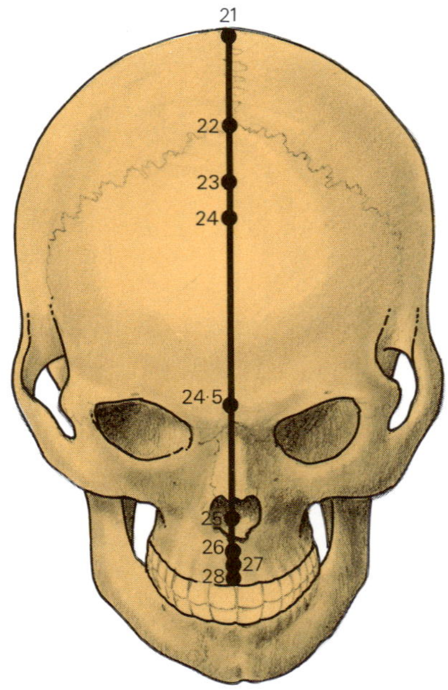
21
22
23
24
24·5
25
26
27
28

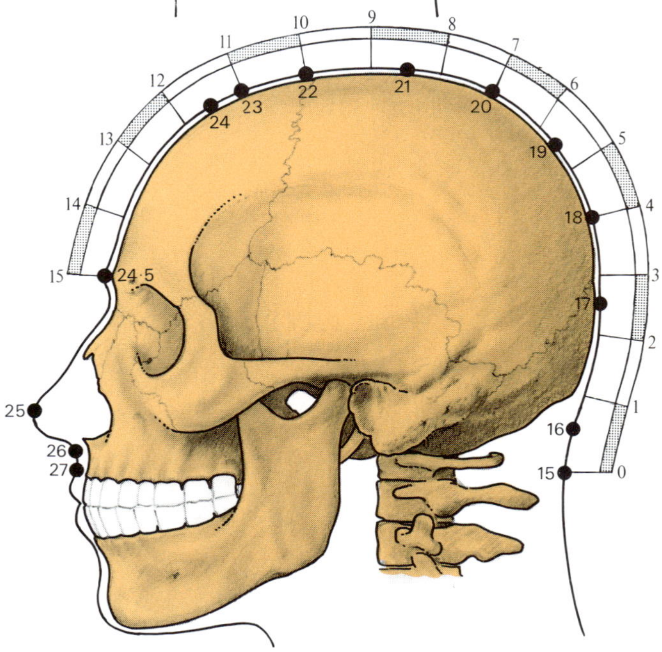
10
9
8
11
7
12
6
13
5
14
4
15
3
2
1
0
21
22
23
24
20
19
18
17
16
15
24·5
25
26
27

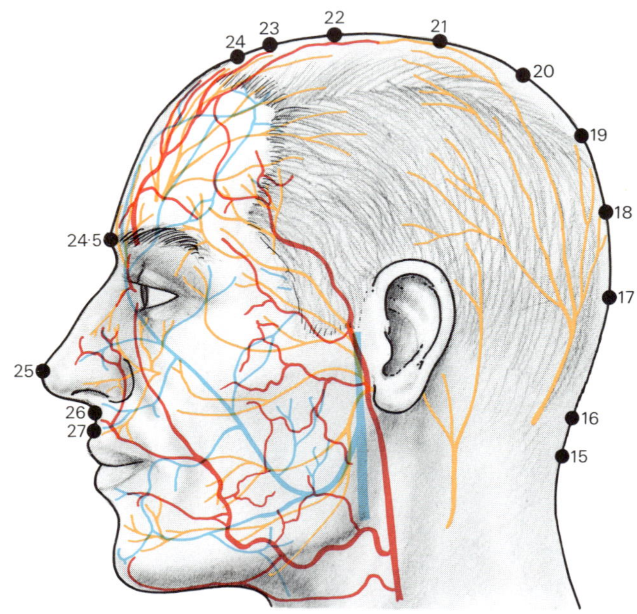
24
23
22
21
20
19
18
17
16
15
24·5
25
26
27

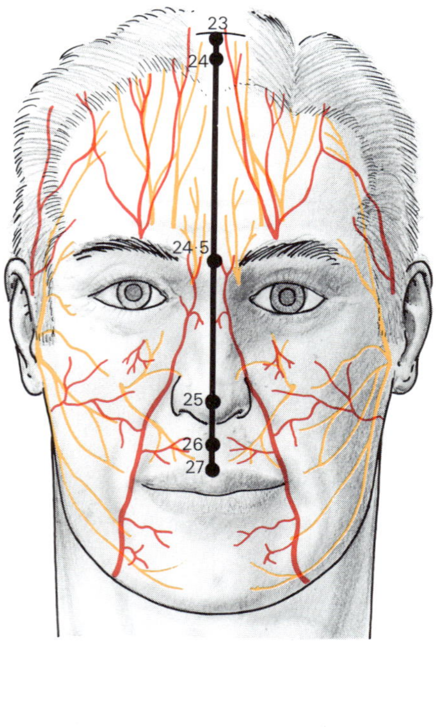
23
24
24·5
25
26
27

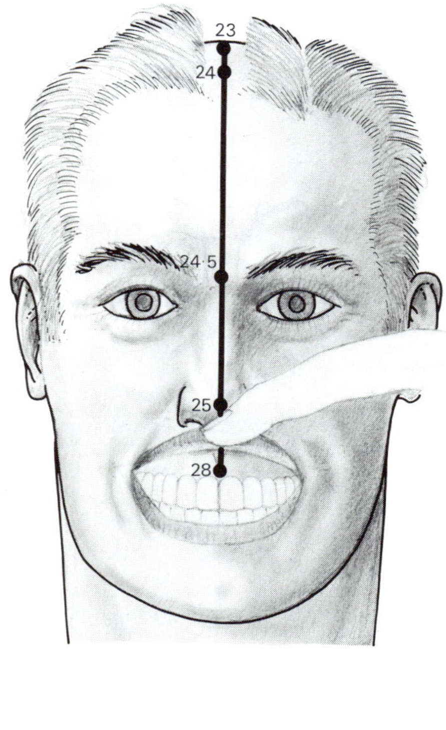
23
24
24·5
25
28

XIV	**15**	On the posterior median line, in the depression between the first and second cervical vertebrae.
XIV	**16**	On the median line of the head, just inferior to the base of the occipital bone, $\frac{1}{2}$ ACI superior to XIV 15.
XIV	**17**	On the median line of the head, $2\frac{1}{2}$ ACI superior to XIV 15.
XIV	**18**	On the median line of the head, 4 ACI superior to XIV 15.
XIV	**19**	On the median line of the head, $5\frac{1}{2}$ ACI superior to XIV 15.
XIV	**20**	On the median line of the head, 7 ACI superior to XIV 15.
XIV	**21**	On the median line of the head, $8\frac{1}{2}$ ACI superior to XIV 15.
XIV	**22**	On the median line of the head, 10 ACI superior to XIV 15.
XIV	**23**	On the median line of the head, 11 ACI superior to XIV 15.
XIV	**24**	On the median line of the head, $11\frac{1}{2}$ ACI superior to XIV 15.
XIV	**24.5**	On the anterior median line, between the medial extremities of the eyebrows, 15 ACI superior to XIV 15.
XIV	**25**	On the median line of the nose, at the inferior edge of the alar cartilage, just superior to the tip of the nose.
XIV	**26**	On the anterior median line, inferior to the nose, in the centre of the philtrum.
XIV	**27**	On the anterior median line, inferior to XIV 26, at the superior edge of the upper lip.
XIV	**28**	On the upper gum, just inferior to the insertion of the frenulum of the upper lip.

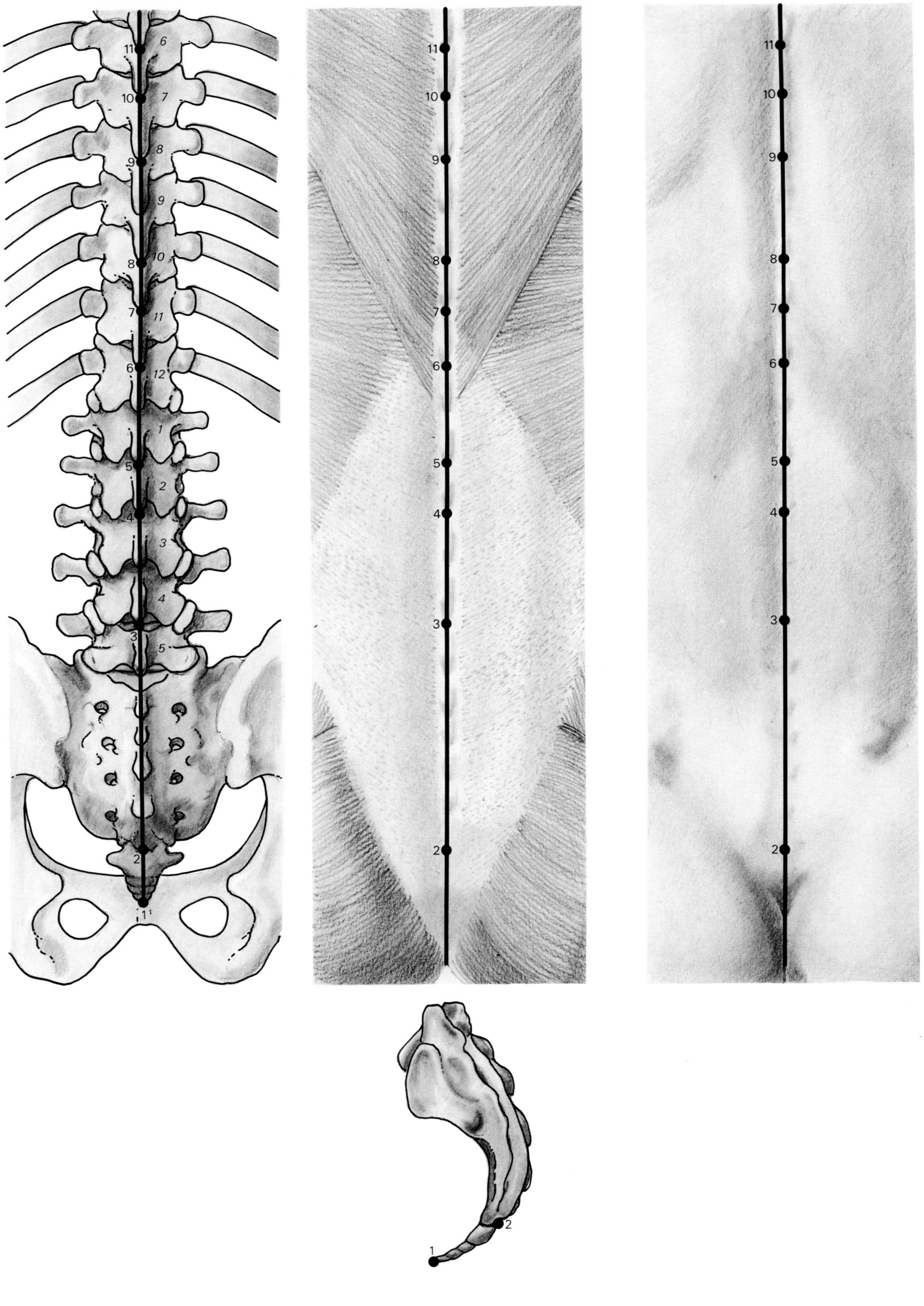
11
10
9
8
7
6
5
4
3
2
1
6
7
8
9
10
11
12
1
2
3
4
5

XIV **1** **Long Strength** (Changchiang)

⊥ 3 Entry
△ 5–15 General Junction Point

On the posterior median line at the tip of the coccyx.

Point of Du Mo

XIV **2** **Loins Correspondence** (Yaoshu)

⊥ 3–5
△ 5–15

On the posterior median line at the sacrococcygeal articulation.

Point of Du Mo
Independent Associated Point of the Renal Area

XIV **3** **Loins Yang Border** (Yao yangkuan)

⊥ 3–5
△ 5–15

On the posterior median line, in the depression between the fourth and fifth lumbar vertebrae.

Point of Du Mo
First Aid: concussion, fractures, insensibility, spinal injury, sprains

XIV **4** **Gate Of Life** (Mingmen)

⊥ 3
△ 7–15

On the posterior median line, in the depression between the second and third lumbar vertebrae.

Point of Du Mo
Point of Chong Mo

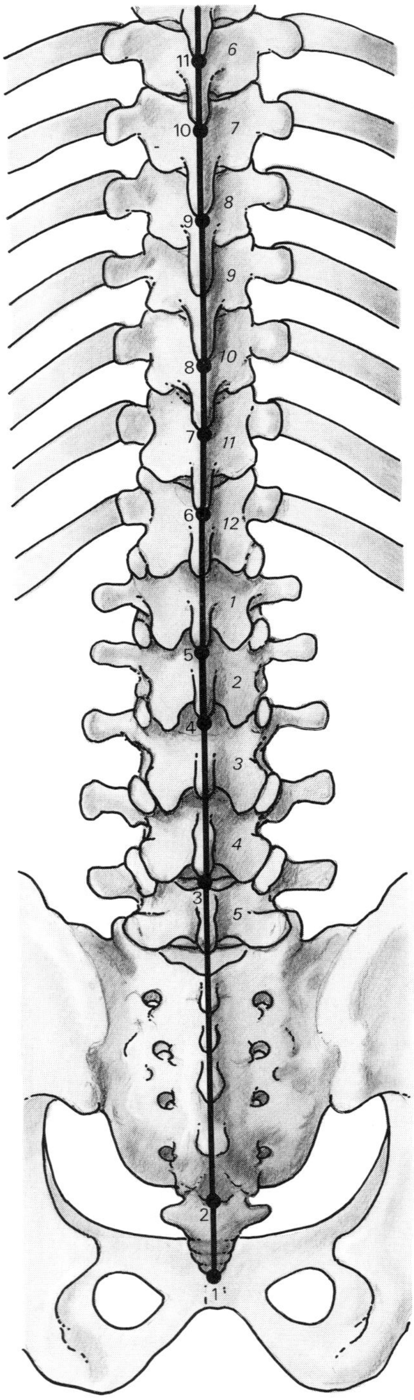
11
6
10
7
8
9
9
8
10
7
11
6
12
1
5
2
4
3
4
3
5
2
1

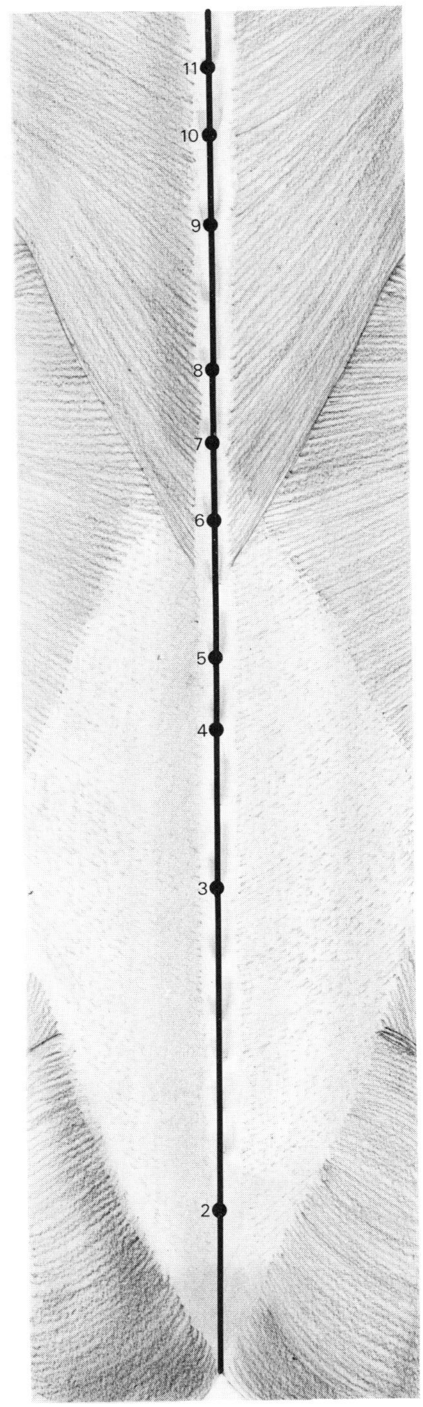
11
10
9
8
7
6
5
4
3
2

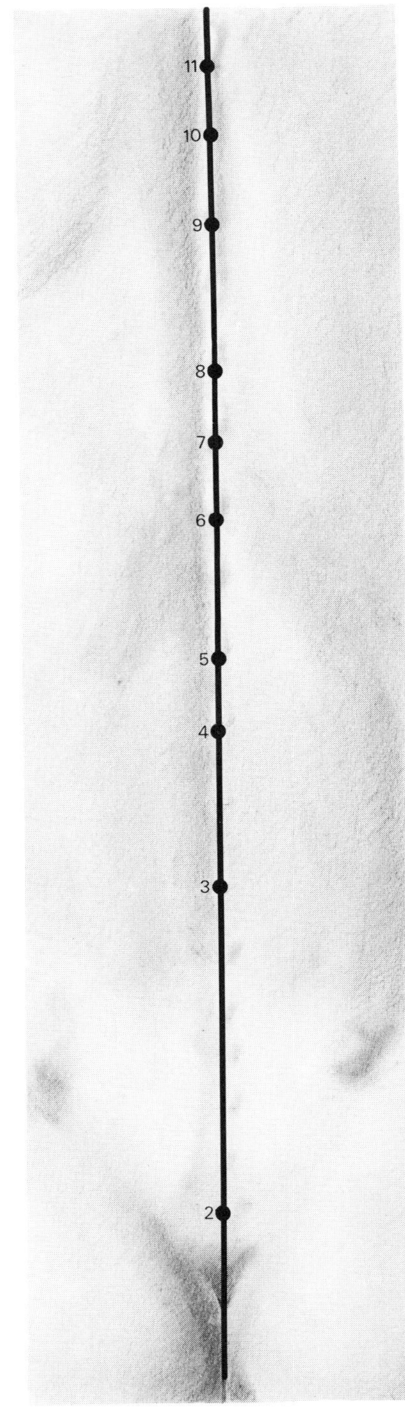
11
10
9
8
7
6
5
4
3
2

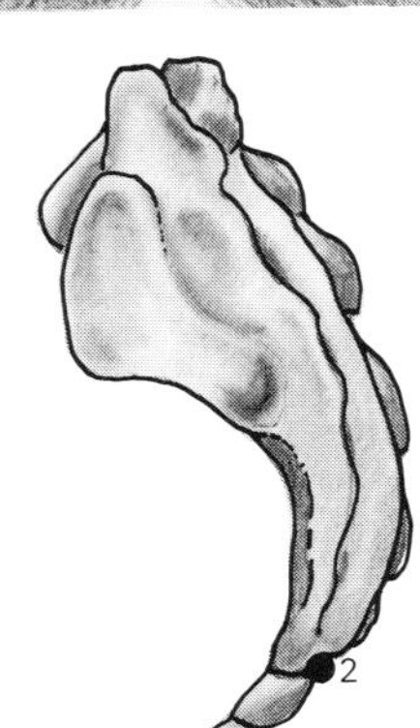
2
1

XIV **5** **Suspended Pivot** (Hsuanshu)

⊥ 3
△ 7–15

On the posterior median line, in the depression between the first and second lumbar vertebrae.

Point of Du Mo

XIV **6** **Middle Of The Spine** (Chichung)

⊥ 3
△ X

On the posterior median line, in the depression between the eleventh and twelfth thoracic vertebrae.

Point of Du Mo

XIV **7** **Middle Pivot** (Chungshu)

⊥ X
△ X

On the posterior median line, in the depression between the tenth and eleventh thoracic vertebrae.

Point of Du Mo

XIV **8** **Contracted Muscle** (Chinso)

⊥ 4
△ 3

On the posterior median line, in the depression between the ninth and tenth thoracic vertebrae.

Point of Du Mo.

XIV **9** **Utmost Yang** (Chihyang)

⊥ 5
△ 7

On the posterior median line, in the depression between the seventh and eighth thoracic vertebrae.

Point of Du Mo

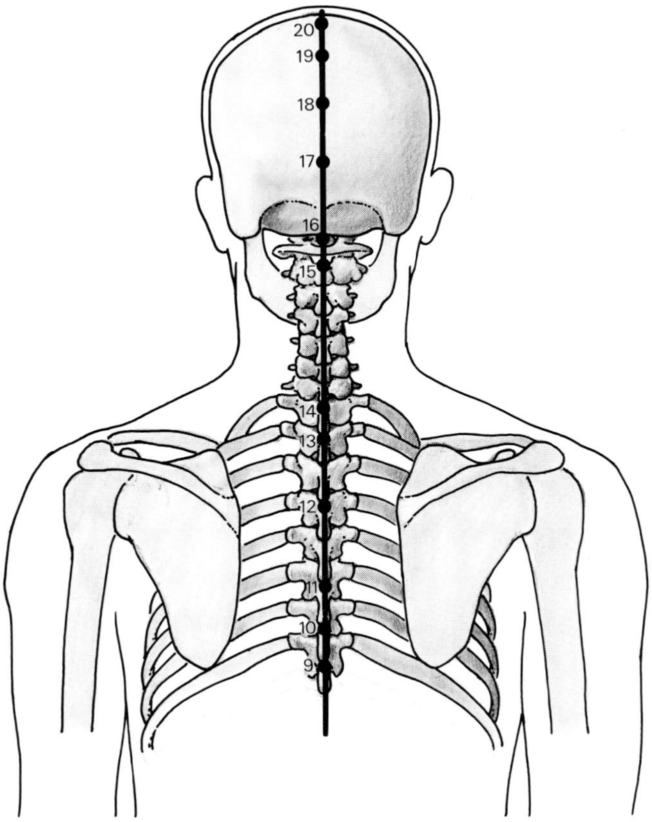
20
19
18
17
16
15
14
13
12
11
10
9

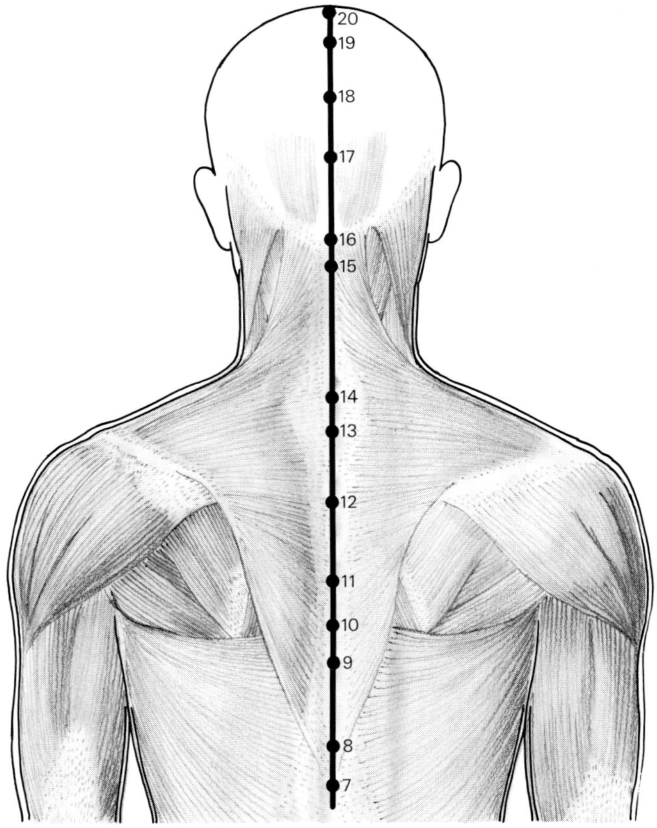
20
19
18
17
16
15
14
13
12
11
10
9
8
7

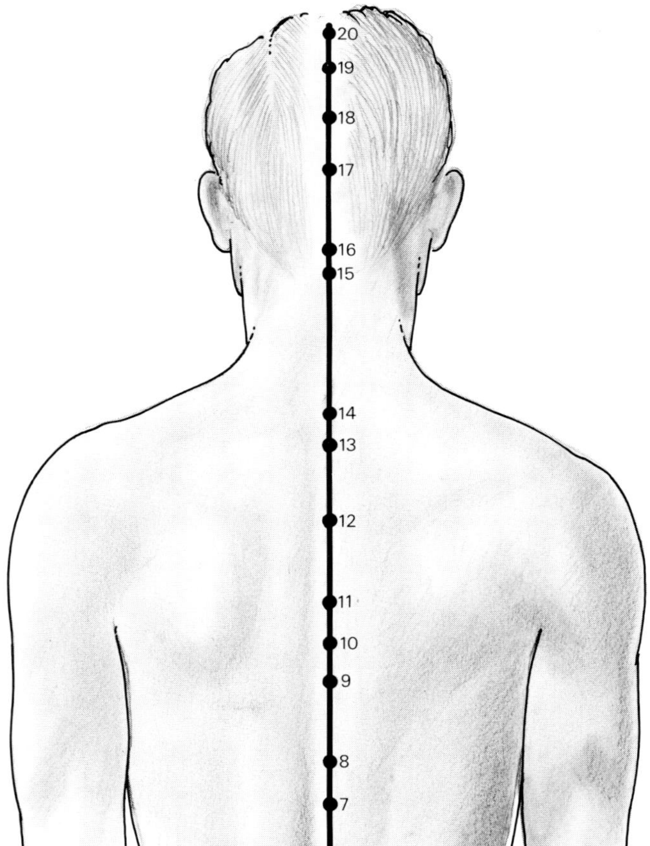
20
19
18
17
16
15
14
13
12
11
10
9
8
7

XIV **10** **Supernatural Tower** (Lingtai)

⊥ X
△ 3–7

On the posterior median line, in the depression between the sixth and seventh thoracic vertebrae.

Point of Du Mo

XIV **11** **Spirit Path** (Shentao)

⊥ X
△ 3–5

On the posterior median line, in the depression between the fifth and sixth thoracic vertebrae.

Point of Du Mo
First Aid: bites, convulsions, insensibility

XIV **12** **Body Pillar** (Shenchu)

⊥ 4
△ 5–30

On the posterior median line, in the depression between the third and fourth thoracic vertebrae.

Point of Du Mo

XIV **13** **Kiln Path** (Taotao)

⊥ 4
△ 5–10

On the posterior median line, in the depression between the first and second thoracic vertebrae.

Point of Du Mo

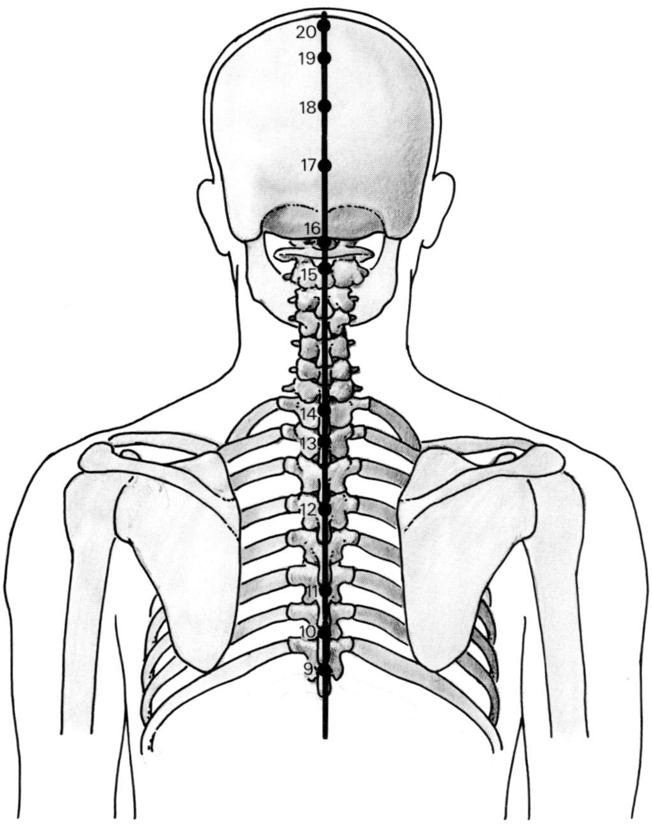
20
19
18
17
16
15
14
13
12
11
10
9

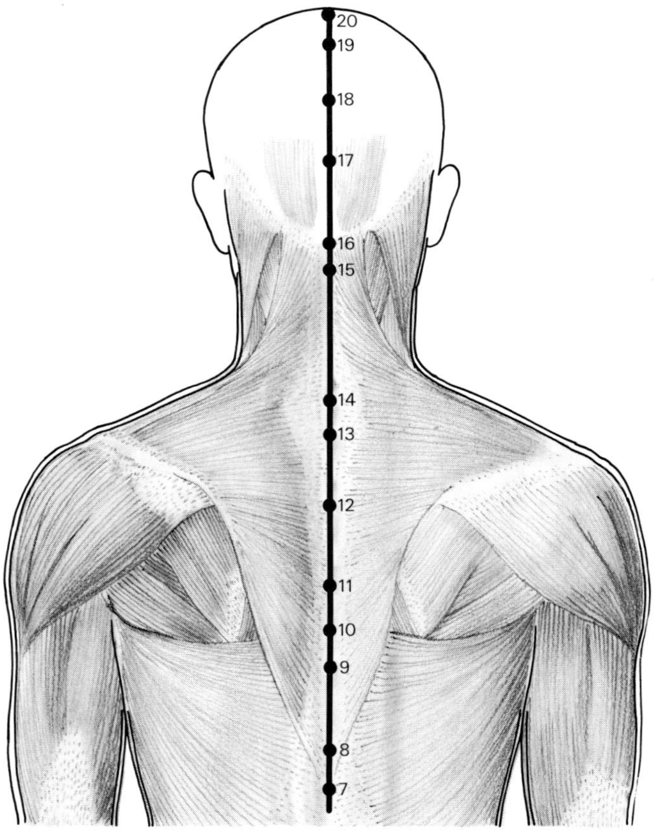
20
19
18
17
16
15
14
13
12
11
10
9
8
7

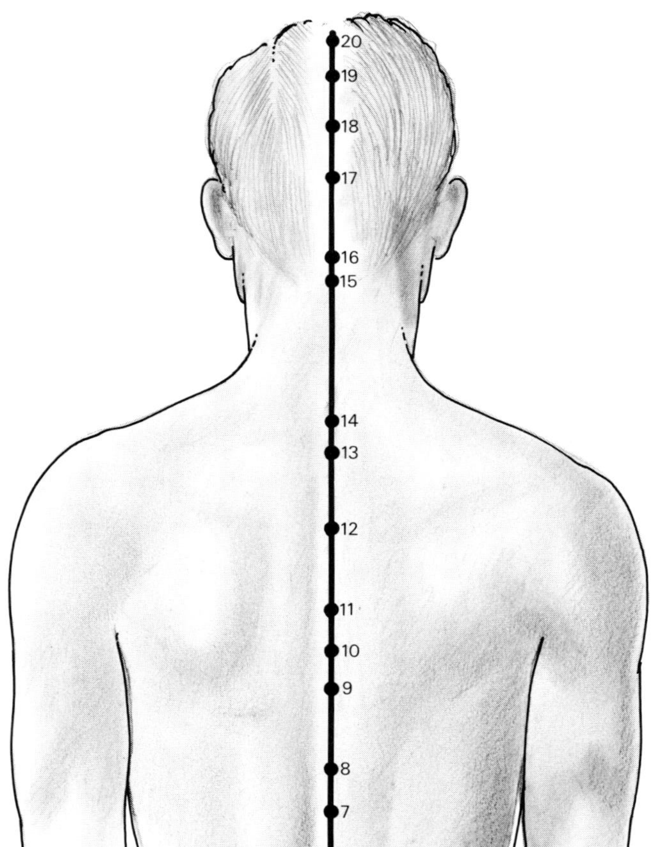
20
19
18
17
16
15
14
13
12
11
10
9
8
7

XIV **14** **Great Hammer** (Tachui)

⊥ 4 Reunion of all Yang meridians, including XIV
△ 5–15

On the posterior median line, in the depression between the seventh cervical and the first thoracic vertebrae.

Point of Du Mo
Centre Reunion General Point of Yang
First Aid: colds

XIV **15** **Gate Of Dumbness** (Yamen)

⊥ 3
△ X

On the posterior median line, in the depression between the first and second cervical vertebrae.

Point of Du Mo
Point of Yang Wei Mo
Sea of Bone Marrow

XIV **16** **Wind Palace** (Fengfu)

⊥ 3
△ X

On the median line of the head, just inferior to the base of the occipital bone, $\frac{1}{2}$ ACI superior to XIV 15.

Point of Du Mo
Point of Yang Wei Mo
Sea of Bone Marrow
Window of the Sky

XIV **17** **Brain Door** (Naohu)

⊥ X
△ X

On the median line of the head, $2\frac{1}{2}$ ACI superior to XIV 15.

Point of Du Mo

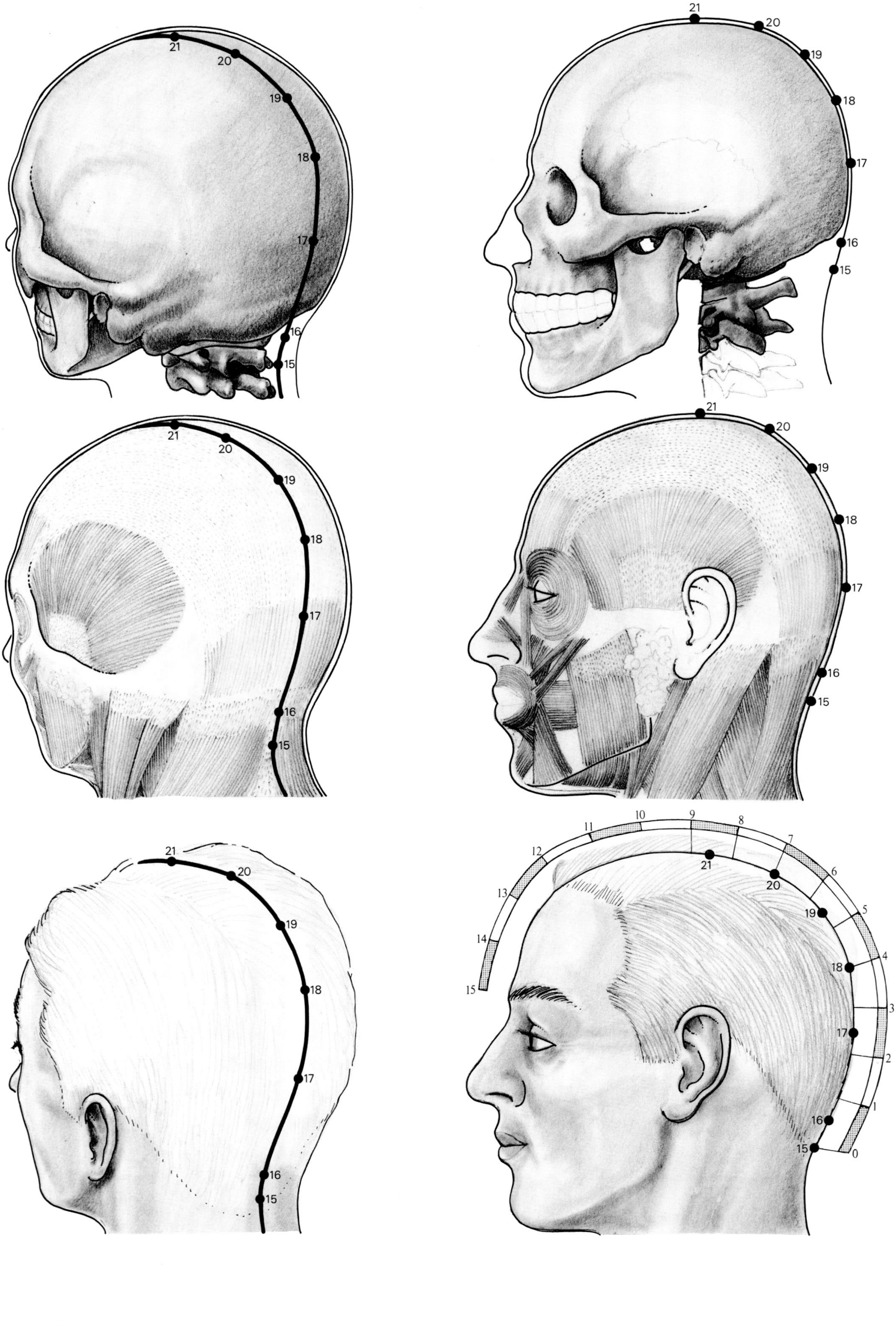
21
20
19
18
17
16
15
0
1
2
3
4
5
6
7
8
9
10
11
12
13
14
15

XIV **18** **Strength Divider** (Chiangchien)

⊥ 2
△ X

On the median line of the head, 4 ACI superior to XIV 15.

Point of Du Mo

XIV **19** **Posterior Summit** (Houting)

⊥ 3
△ 7

On the median line of the head, $5\frac{1}{2}$ ACI superior to XIV 15.

Point of Du Mo
Sea of Bone Marrow

XIV **20** **One Hundred Meetings** (Paihui)

⊥ 3
△ 7

On the median line of the head, 7 ACI superior to XIV 15.

Point of Du Mo
Sea of Bone Marrow
A point of the pattern to release the 7 Dragons on the 7 External Demons

XIV **21** **Anterior Summit** (Chienting)

⊥ 2
△ 3–7

On the median line of the head, $8\frac{1}{2}$ ACI superior to XIV 15.

Point of Du Mo

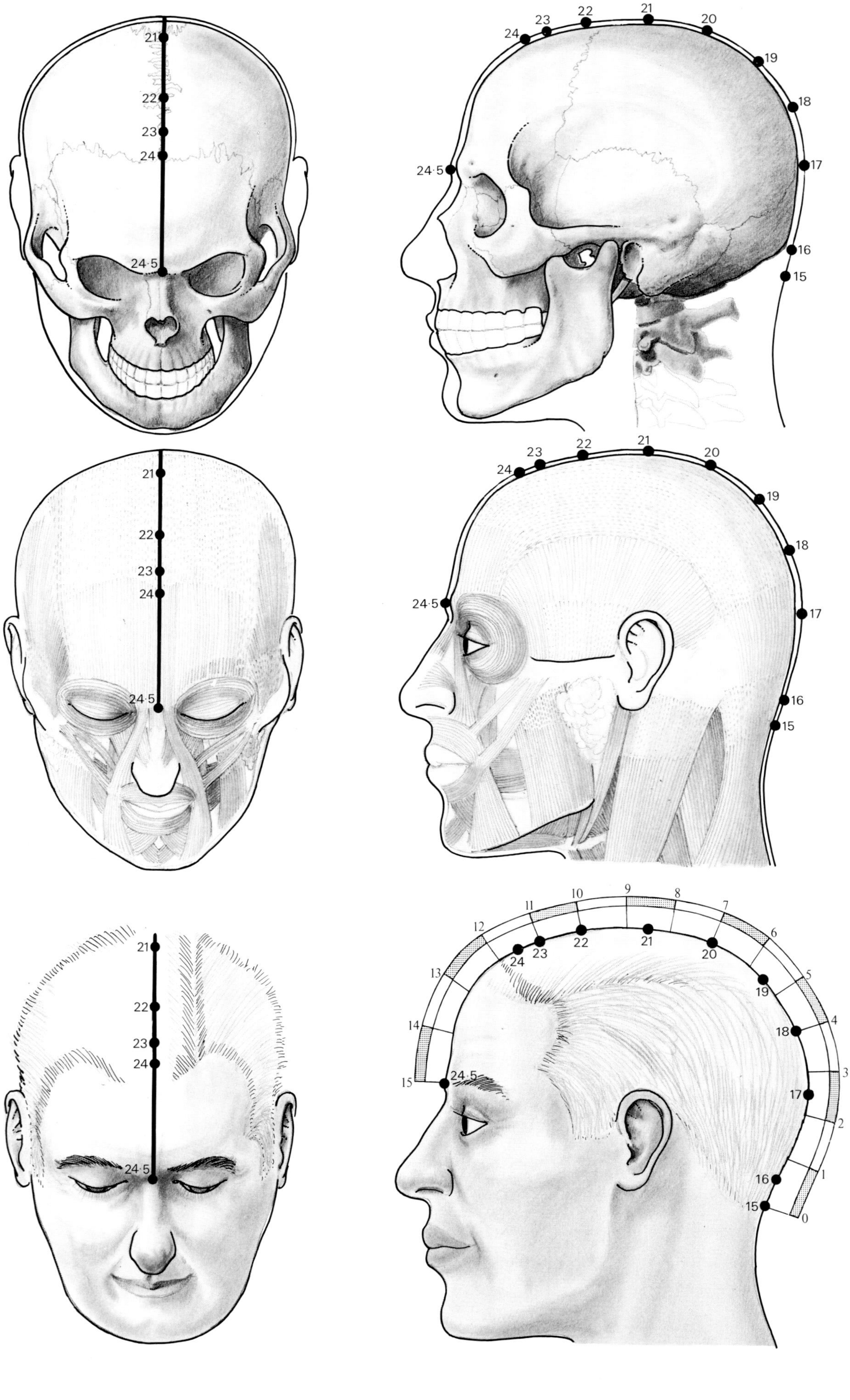
21
22
23
24
24·5
20
19
18
17
16
15
0
1
2
3
4
5
6
7
8
9
10
11
12
13
14
15

XIV **22** **Skull Meeting** (Hsinhui)

⊥ 1
△ 3

On the median line of the head, 10 ACI superior to XIV 15.

Point of Du Mo

XIV **23** **Upper Star** (Shanghsing)

⊥ 2
△ 5

On the median line of the head, 11 ACI superior to XIV 15.

Point of Du Mo

XIV **24** **Spirit Hall** (Shenting)

⊥ X
△ 5

On the median line of the head, $11\frac{1}{2}$ ACI superior to XIV 15.

Point of Du Mo

XIV **24.5**

⊥ 1–3
△ 3–5

On the anterior median line, between the medial extremities of the eyebrows, 15 ACI superior to XIV 15.

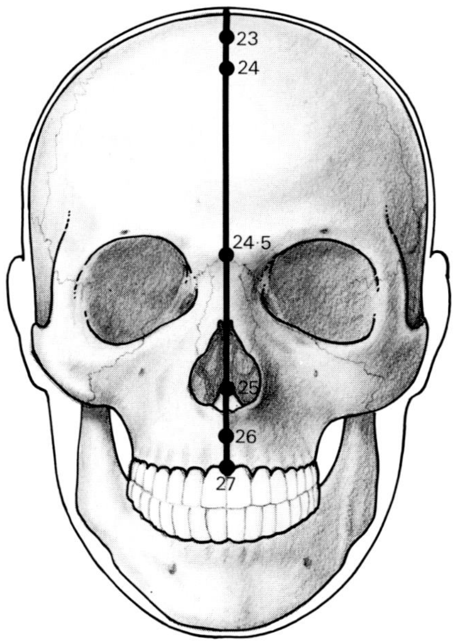
23
24
24·5
25
26
27

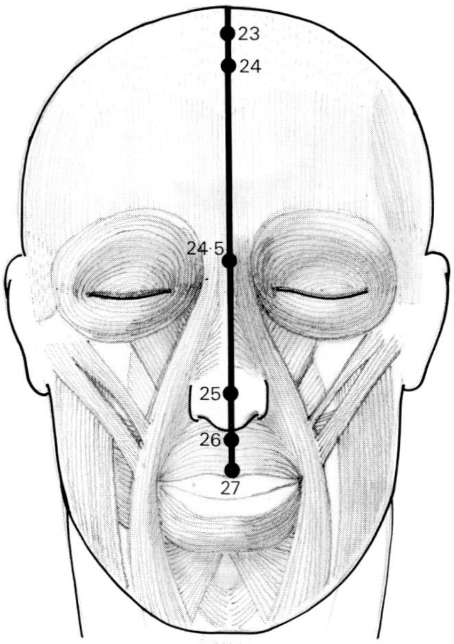
23
24
24·5
25
26
27

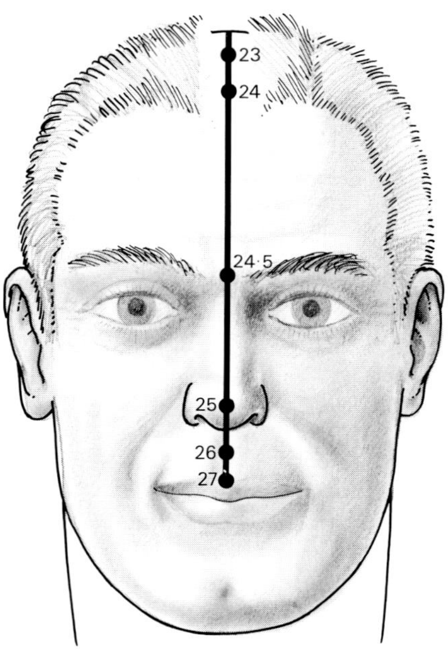
23
24
24·5
25
26
27

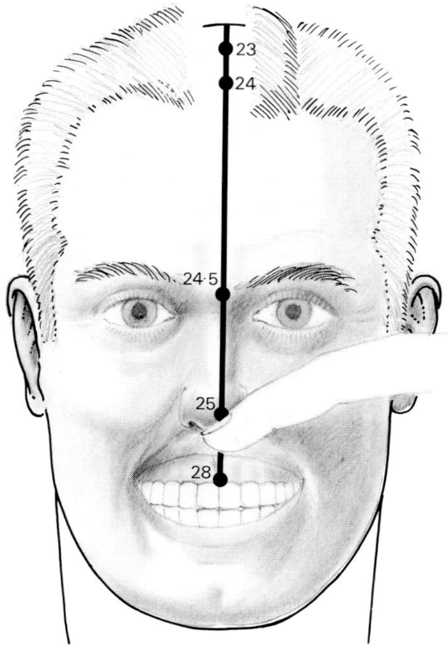
23
24
24·5
25
28

XIV **25** **Plain Bone** (Suliao)

⊥ 1–2
△ X

On the median line of the nose, at the inferior edge of the alar cartilage, just superior to the tip of the nose.

Point of Du Mo

XIV **26** **Middle Of Man** (Jenchung)

⊥ 2
△ 3

On the anterior median line, inferior to the nose, in the centre of the philtrum.

Point of Du Mo

XIV **27** **Correct Exchange** (Tuituan)

⊥ 2
△ 2

On the anterior median line, inferior to XIV 26, at the superior edge of the upper lip.

Point of Du Mo

XIV **28** **Mouth Crossing** (Yinchiao)

⊥ 2 Exit
△ X

On the upper gum, just inferior to the insertion of the frenulum of the upper lip.

Point of Du Mo

Areas for palpation

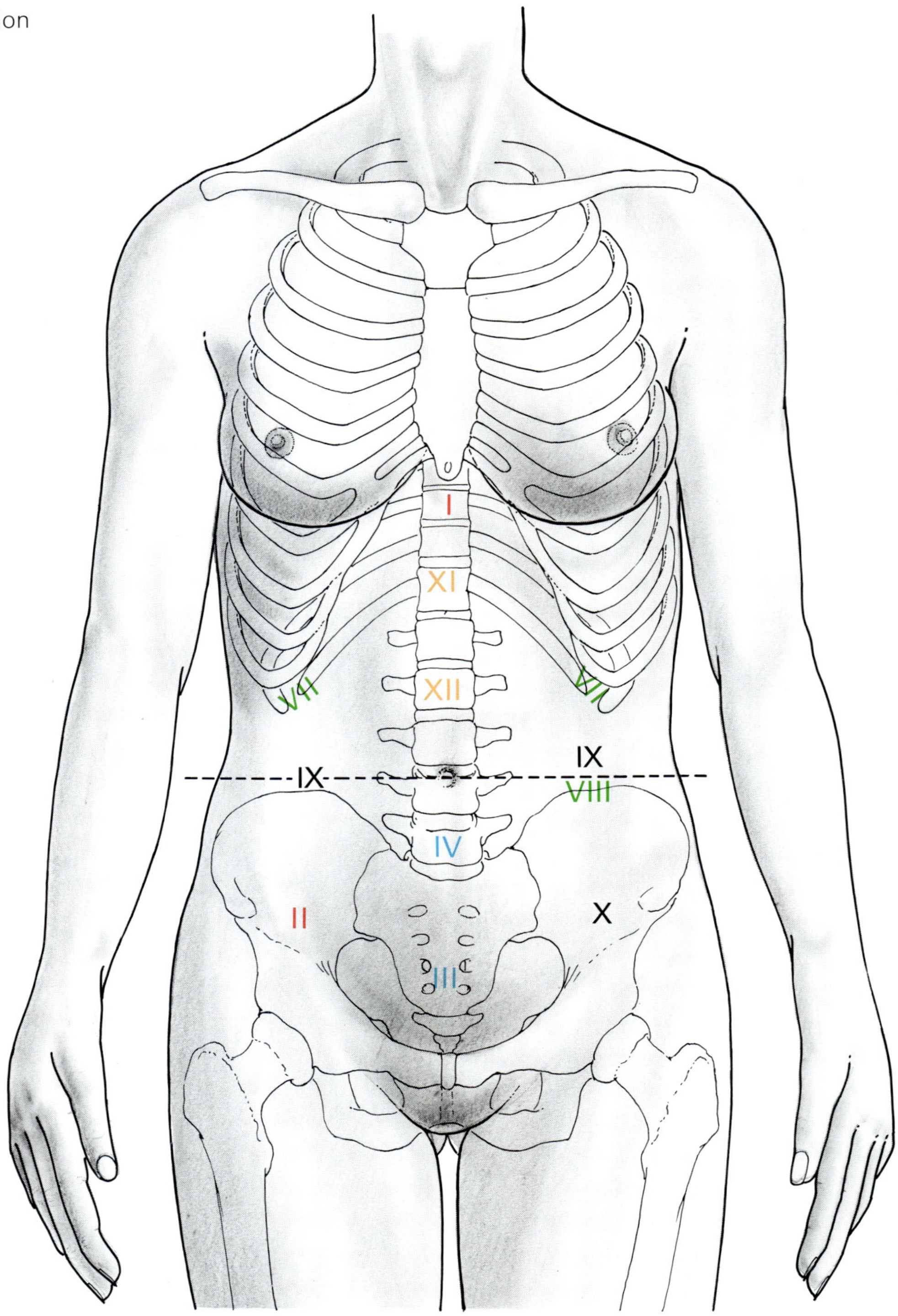

Appendix 2 Alarm Points

I	XIII 14	
II	XIII 4	
III	XIII 3	
IV	VII 25	
V	XIII 15	
VI	XIII 17	Upper Chou
	XIII 12	Middle Chou
	XIII 7	Lower Chou
	XIII 5	Main Alarm Point for whole Three Heater
VII	VII 23	
	VII 24	
VIII	VIII 14	
IX	IX 1	
X	XI 25	
XI	XIII 12	
XII	VIII 13	

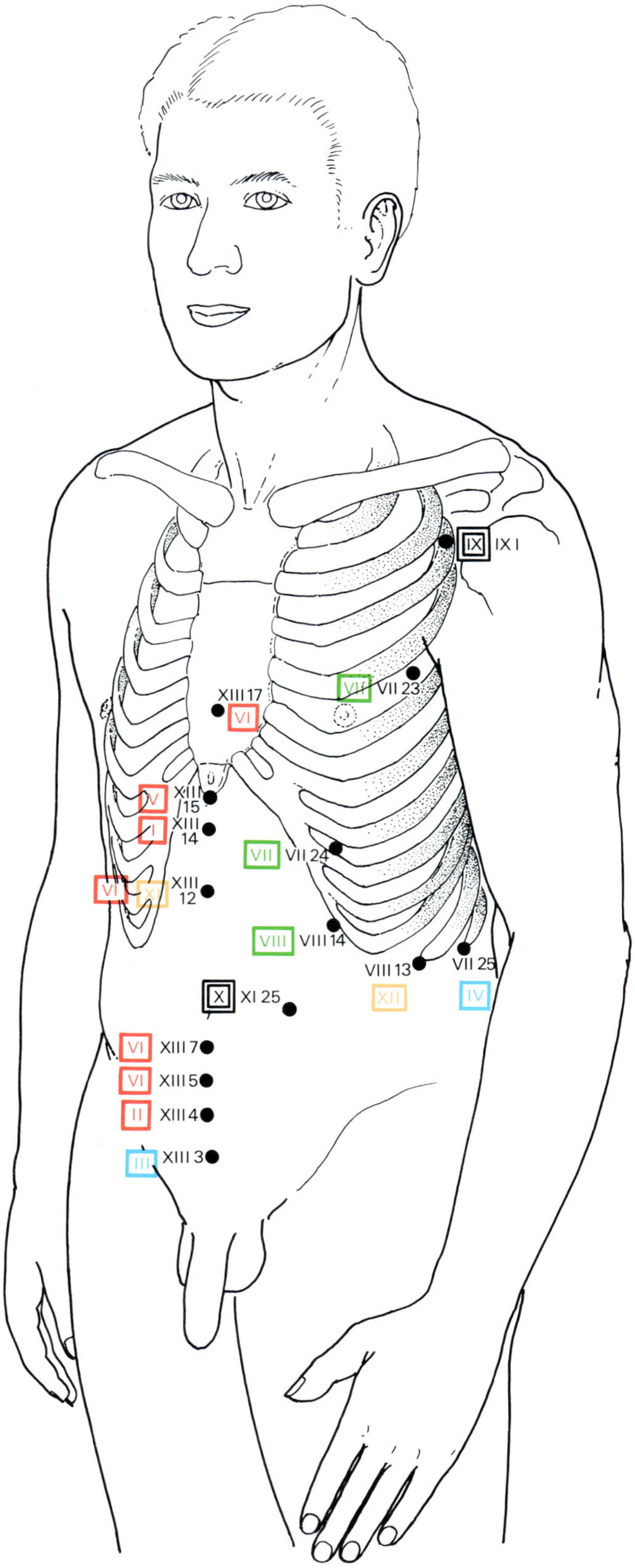

Appendix 3 Antique Points

Winter (Cheng)	*Spring* (Yung)	*Summer* (Yu)	*Late Summer* (Ching)	*Autumn* (Ho)
I 9 ● (green)	I 8 ● (red)	I 7 ● (yellow)	I 4 ○	I 3 ● (blue)
II 1 ○	II 2 ● (blue)	II 3 ● (green)	II 5 ● (red)	II 8 ● (yellow)
III 67 ○	III 66 ● (blue)	III 65 ● (green)	III 60 ● (red)	III 54 ● (yellow)
IV 1 ● (green)	IV 2 ● (red)	IV 3 ● (yellow)	IV 7 ○	IV 10 ● (blue)
V 9 ● (green)	V 8 ● (red)	V 7 ● (yellow)	V 5 ○	V 3 ● (blue)
VI 1 ○	VI 2 ● (blue)	VI 3 ● (green)	VI 6 ● (red)	VI 10 ● (yellow)
VII 44 ○	VII 43 ● (blue)	VII 41 ● (green)	VII 38 ● (red)	VII 34 ● (yellow)
VIII 1 ● (green)	VIII 2 ● (red)	VIII 3 ● (yellow)	VIII 4 ○	VIII 8 ● (blue)
IX 11 ● (green)	IX 10 ● (red)	IX 9 ● (yellow)	IX 8 ○	IX 5 ● (blue)
X 1 ○	X 2 ● (blue)	X 3 ● (green)	X 5 ● (red)	X 11 ● (yellow)
XI 45 ○	XI 44 ● (blue)	XI 43 ● (green)	XI 41 ● (red)	XI 36 ● (yellow)
XII 1 ● (green)	XII 2 ● (red)	XII 3 ● (yellow)	XII 5 ○	XII 9 ● (blue)

Appendix 4 Assembling Points

1. Hollow organs	XIII 12
2. Solid organs	VIII 13
3. Marrow	VII 39
4. Tendons	VII 34
5. Bones	III 11
6. Blood	III 17
7. Ch'i	XIII 17
8. Meridians	IX 9

Appendix 5 Associated Effect Points

Lung (IX)	III 13
Circulation-Sex (V)	III 14
Heart (I)	III 15
Governor Vessel (XIV)	III 16
Diaphragm	III 17
Liver (VIII)	III 18
Gall Bladder (VII)	III 19
Spleen (XII)	III 20
Stomach (XI)	III 21
Three Heater (VI)	III 22
Kidney (IV)	III 23
Colon (X)	III 25
Small Intestine (II)	III 27
Bladder (III)	III 28

Appendix 6 Dragons

External: XIV 20, III 11, III 23, III 61

Internal:
1. With depression:
   Master Point below XIII 15; XI 32
   Master Point between XI 36 and XI 37; XI 41

2. Without depression:
   Master Point below XIII 15; XI 25, XI 32, XI 41

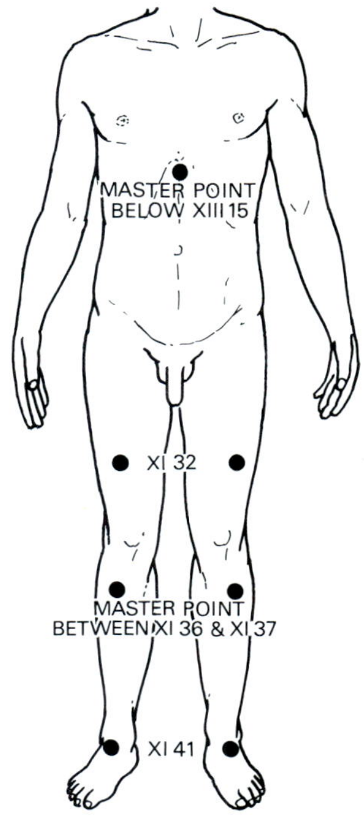

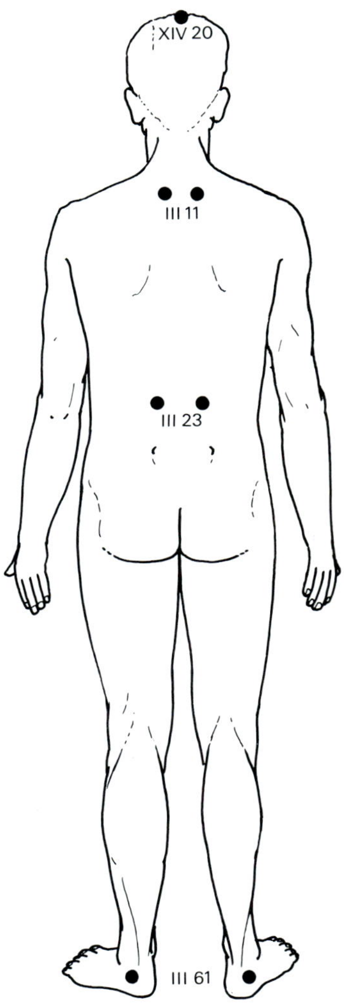

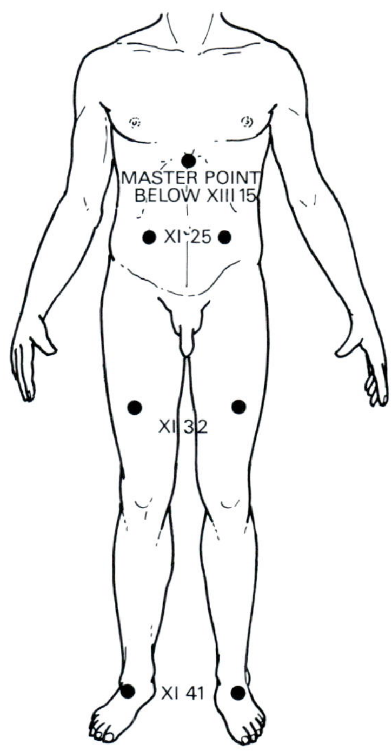

Appendix 7 Earth Points

I 7	☐	Spirit Gate	VII 34		Yang Mound Spring
II 8		Small Sea	VIII 3	☐	Supreme Rushing
III 54		Equilibrium Middle	IX 9	☐	Very Great Abyss
IV 3	☐	Greater Mountain Stream	X 11		Crooked Pond
V 7	☐	Great Mound	XI 36		Leg Three Miles
VI 10		Heavenly Well	XII 3	☐	Supreme White

1. **Yang Wei Mo** Vessel gathering the Yang

Pathway	III 63; VII 35, 29; II 10; VI 15; VII 21, 14, 13, 16, 17, 18, 19, 20; XIV 16, 15
Master Point	VI 5
Coupled Point	VII 41

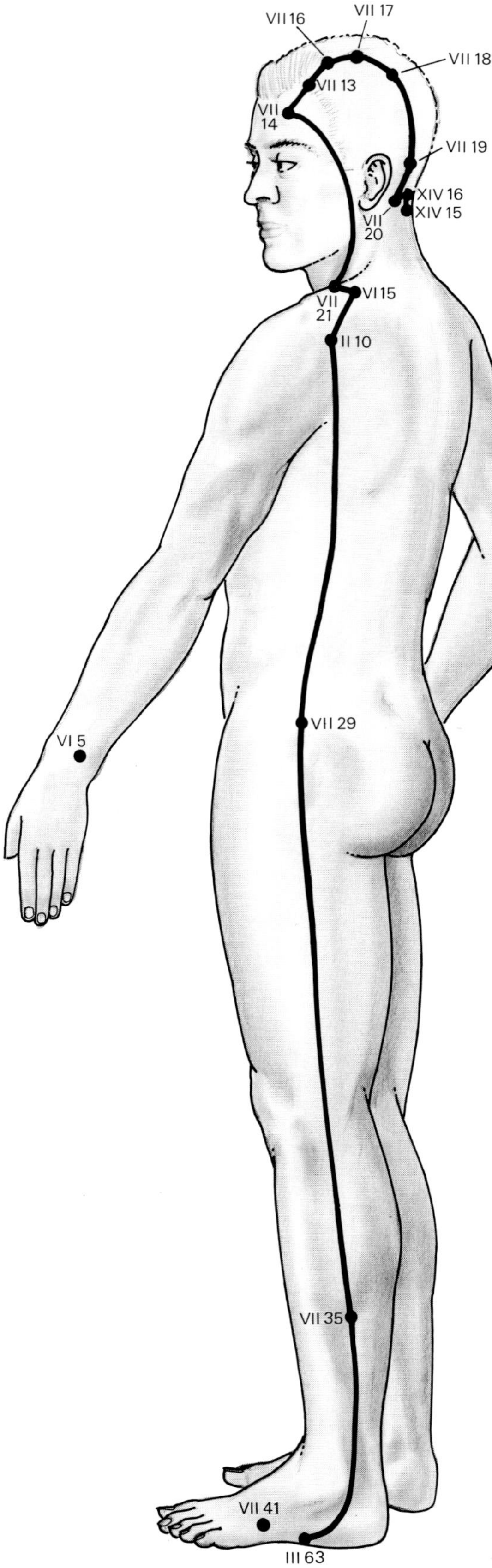

2. **Yang Qiao Mo** Yang vessel of the ankle

Pathway	III 62, 61, 59; VII 29; II 10; X 15, 16; XI 4, 3, 2, 1; III 1; VII 20
Master Point	III 62
Coupled Point	II 3

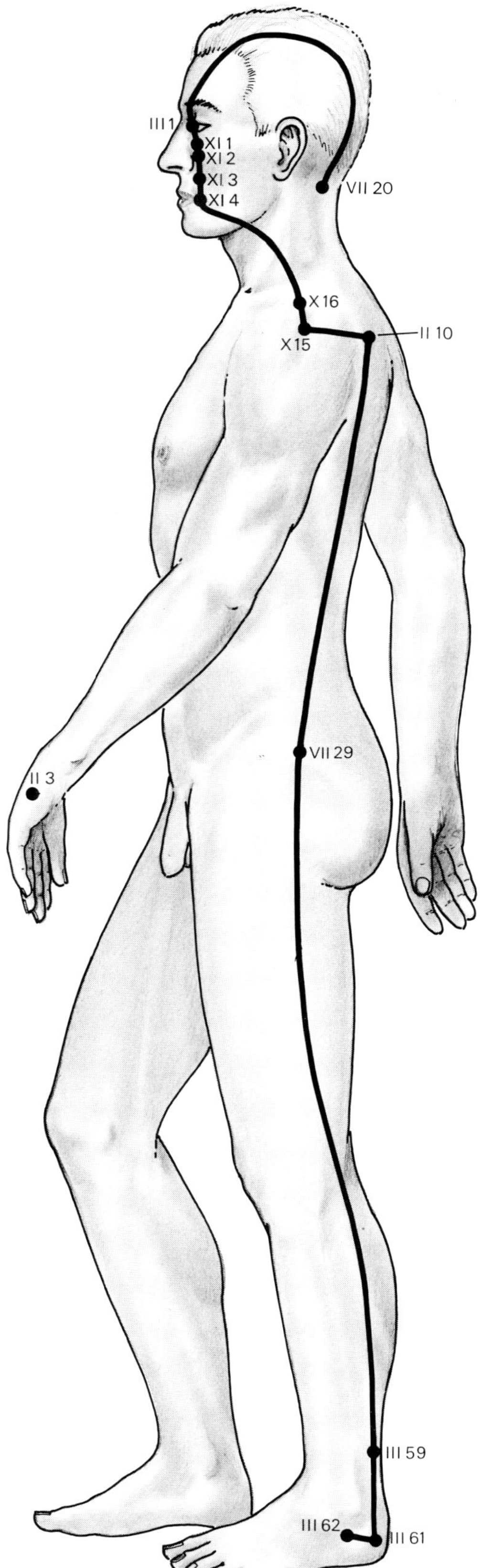

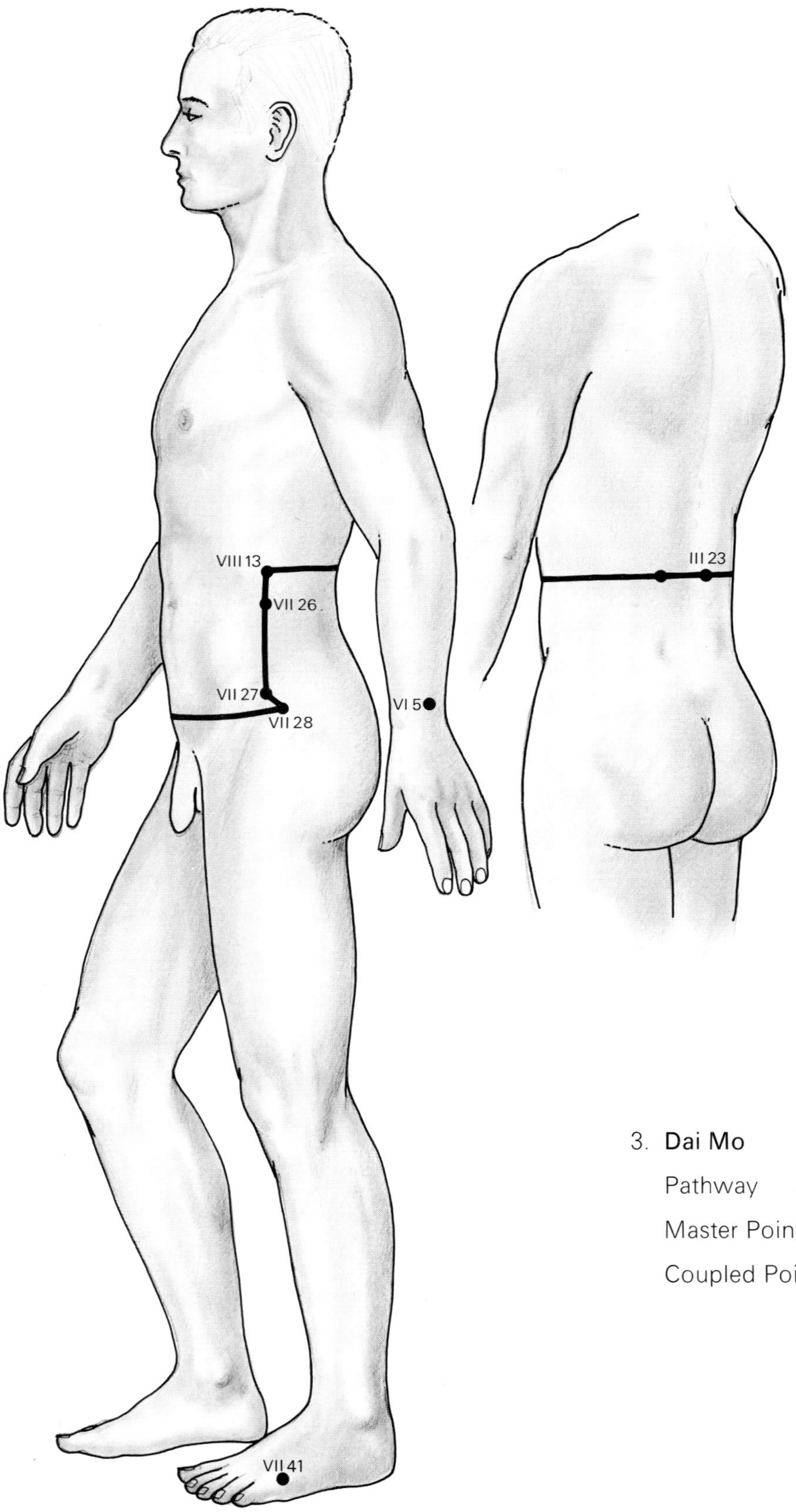

3. **Dai Mo**	Vessel of the waist
Pathway	III 23; VIII 13; VII 26, 27, 28
Master Point	VII 41
Coupled Point	VI 5

4. **Du Mo** Governor Vessel

Pathway	XIV 1–28
Master Point	II 3
Coupled Point	III 62

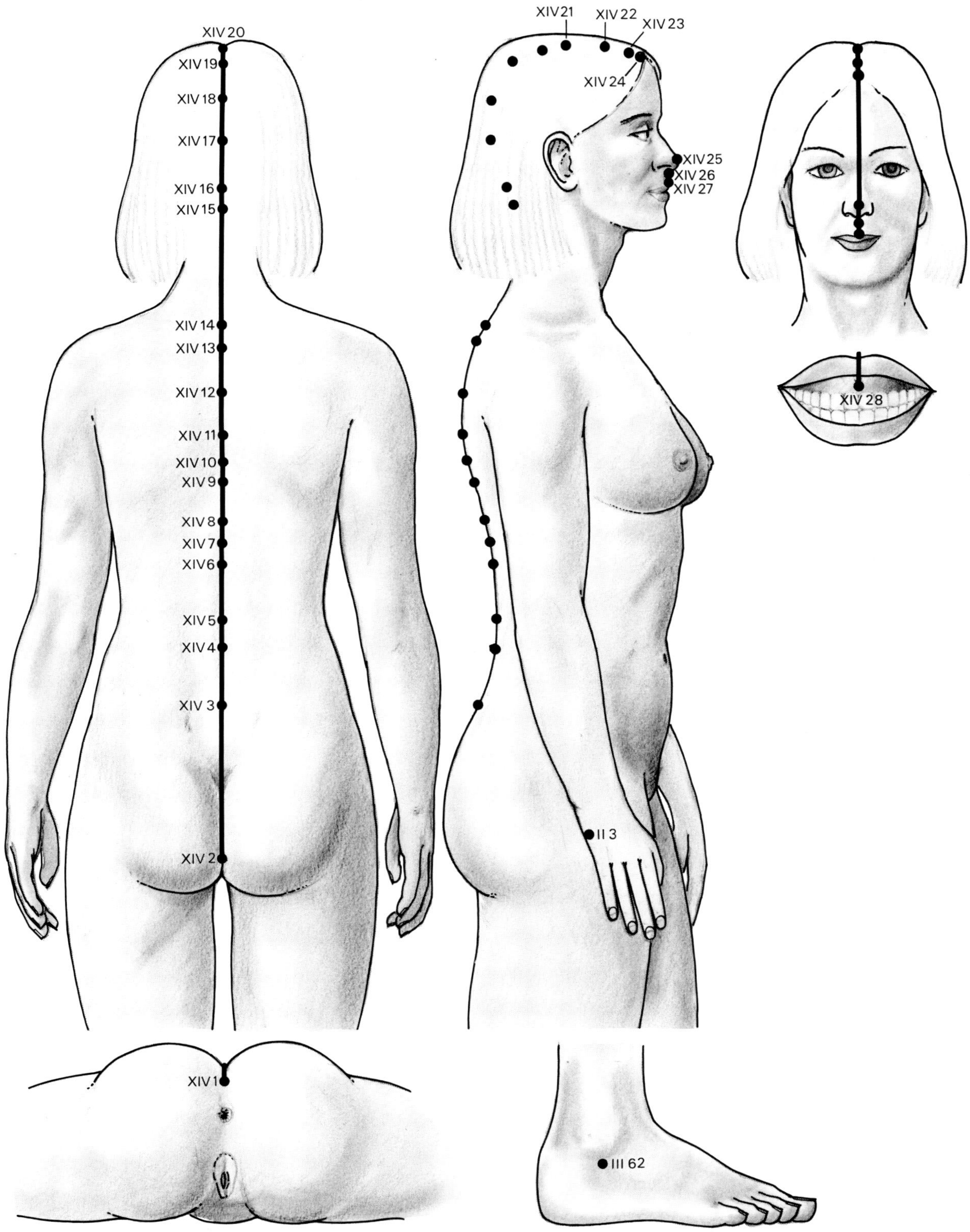

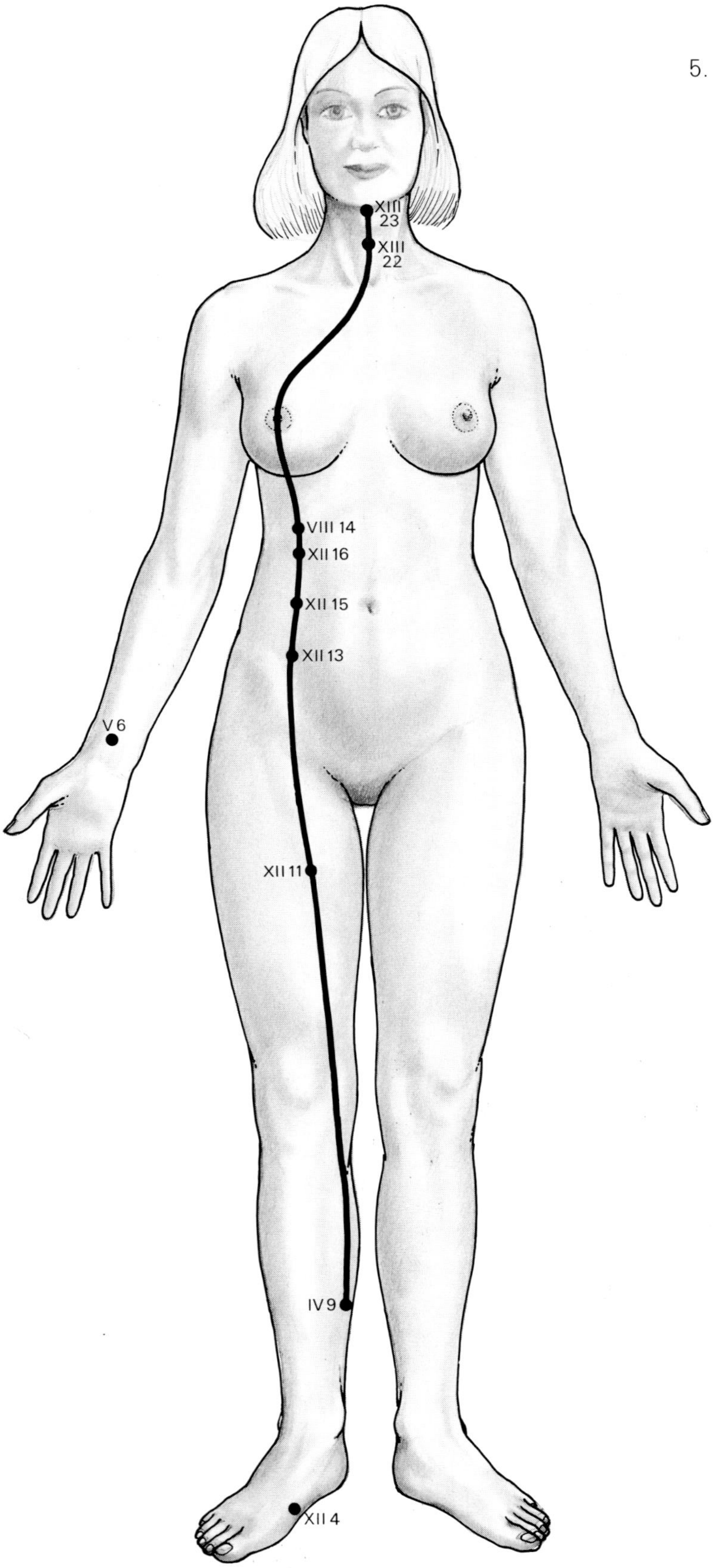

5. **Yin Wei Mo**	Vessel gathering the Yin
Pathway	IV 9; XII 11, 13, 15, 16; VIII 14; XIII 22, 23
Master Point	V 6
Coupled Point	XII 4

6. **Yin Qiao Mo** Yin vessel of the ankle

Pathway	IV 2, 6, 8; XI 12; III 1
Master Point	IV 6
Coupled Point	IX 7

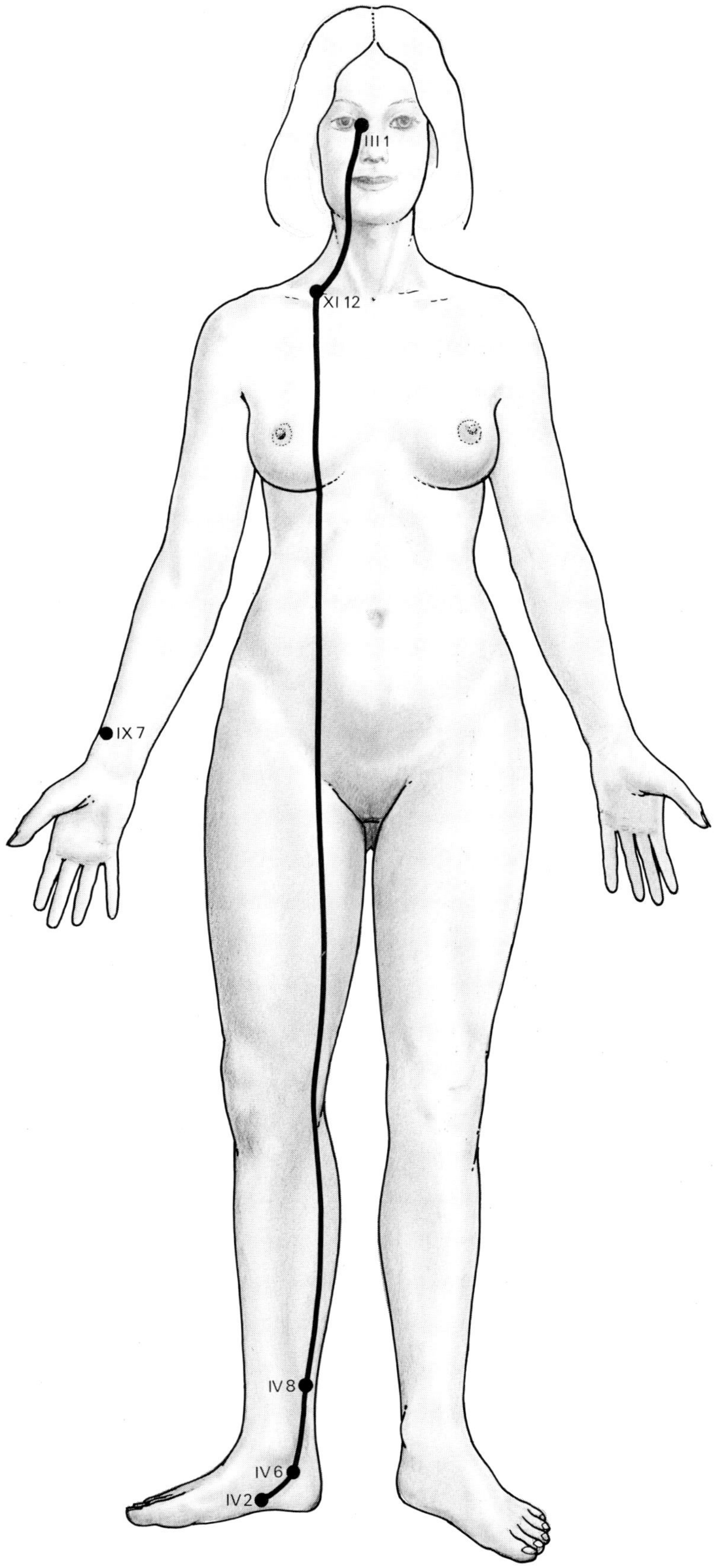

7. **Chong Mo** Vessel of the groin

Pathway	XI 30; IV 11, 12, 13, 14, 15, 16, 17, 18, 19, 20, 21; XIII 23; secondary branch XI 30; XIII 1; XIV 4
Master Point	XII 4
Coupled Point	V 6

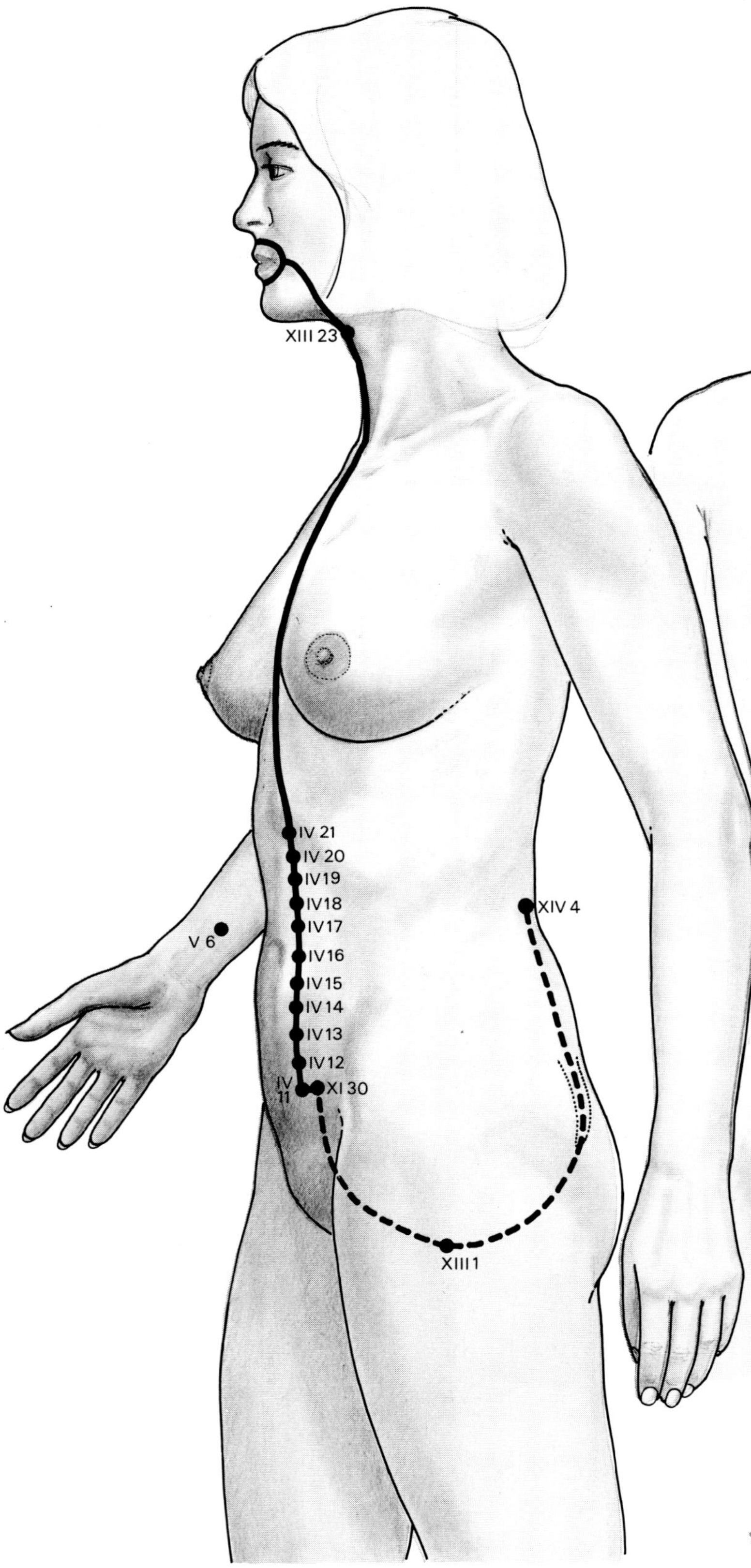

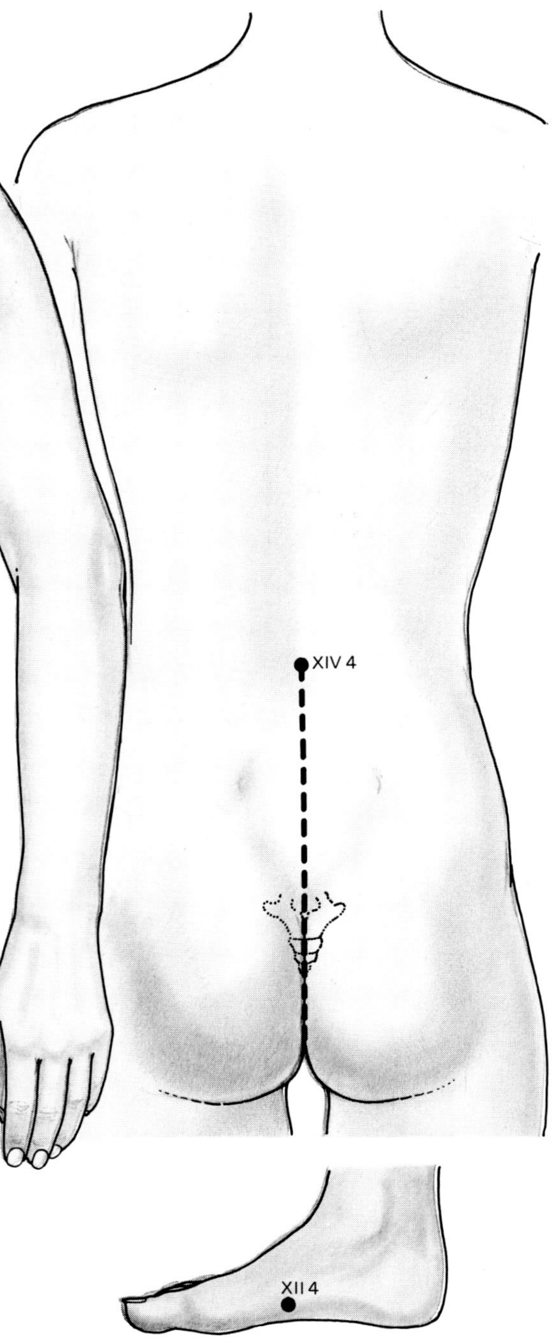

8. **Ren Mo** Conception Vessel
Pathway XIII 1–24
Master Point IX 7
Coupled Point IV 6

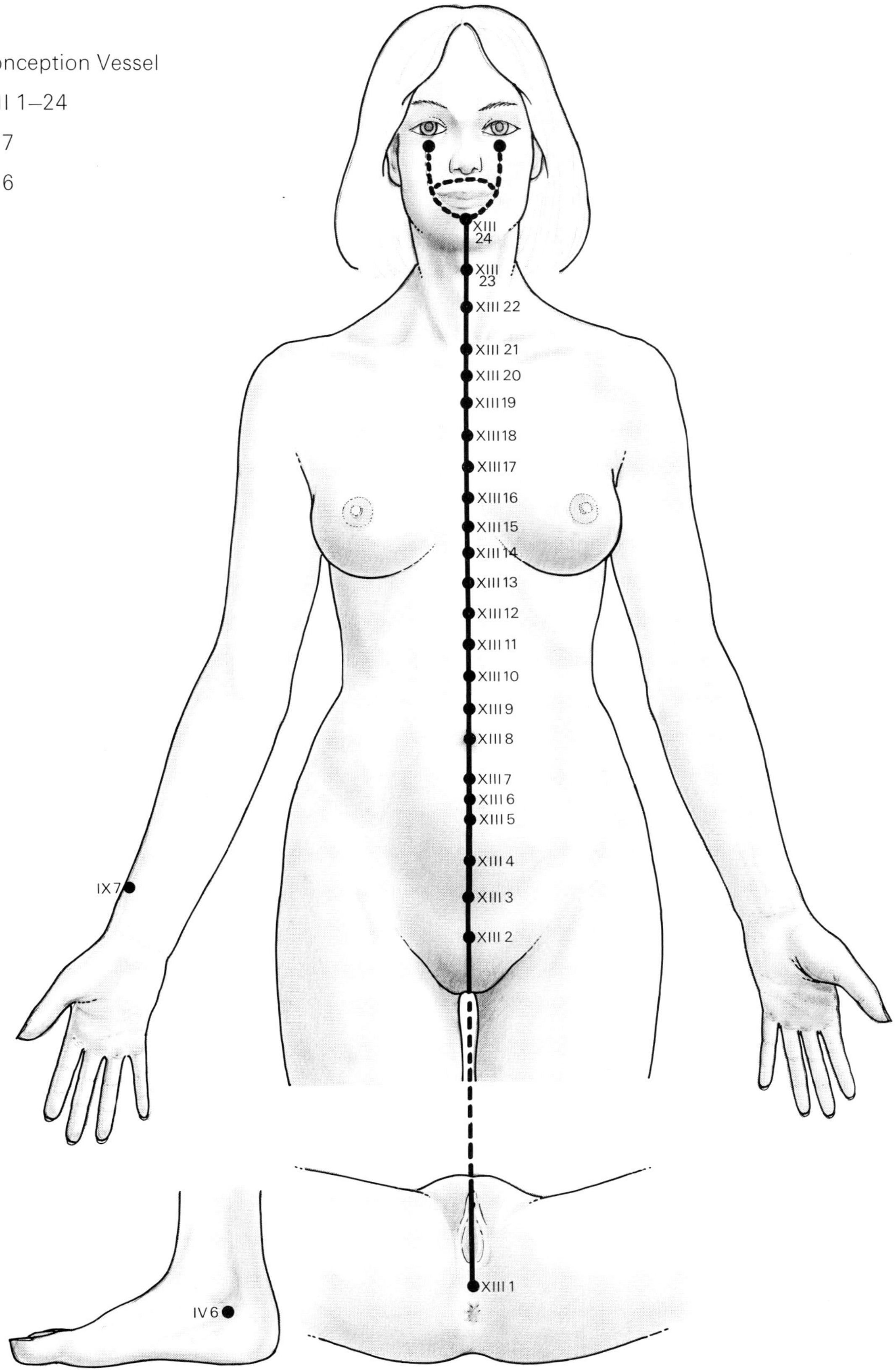

Appendix 9 Endocrine Glands, The Points of

N.B. These points must only be used in the context of five element treatment.

Thyroid	I 7	III 15	IV 7	VI 3
	X 4	XI 9	XI 10	XIII 6
	XIII 13	XIII 19	XIV 15	XIV 23
Parathyroid	III 3	III 11	III 58	V 7
	VII 30	VIII 3	XI 36	XIV 2
	XIV 15			
Adrenal	III 47	IV 7	V 7	XII 6
	XIII 10	XIII 16	XIV 6	
Pituitary	III 47	III 60	IV 11	IV 13
	VII 5	VII 37	XII 6	XIII 10
	XIII 15	XIII 16	XIII 19	
Ovaries	III 67	IV 2	IV 7	IV 13
	VII 37	VIII 3	XII 6	XIV 4
Testes	III 47	III 60	IV 11	XI 30
	XIII 3	XIII 4	XIII 5	XIV 3
	XIV 4			
Thymus	XII 2			
Pancreas	III 20	IV 3	VI 3	VIII 2
	XII 3	XIII 3		

Appendix 10 Endocrine Gland System, Direct Hormonal Application

N.B. These points must only be used in the context of five element treatment.

VI 5, VII 41: Yang Wei Mo, controls conception and birth.
Add VIII 13 when normalizing excess of gonadotrophic hormone (especially in migraine).

III 62, II 3: Yang Qiao Mo, encourages function of adrenal cortex to produce ACTH. Add III 1 to encourage production of sex hormones.

III 1 and (II 3, III 62): Du Mo plus III 1, releases small amount of ACTH immediately.

III 1 and (IV 6, IX 7): Yin Qiao Mo plus III 1, releases small amount of sex hormone immediately.

To produce an immediate, but short acting supply of cortisone: XIV 16.

Local, direct effect on adrenals: XIV 4.

Treatment to stimulate continued function of adrenal cortex and cortisone production: XII 2, XII 6, point between second and third cervical vertebrae on the Governor vessel, III 20, III 18.

Treatment to stimulate continued function of sex hormones: III 1, XIII 4, XIII 7.

Direct action on thyroid: XIII 22. Add XI 9 and IV 7.

Appendix 11 Entry Points, Exit Points

Entry Points

I 1 Utmost Source
II 1 Little Marsh
III 1 Eyes Bright
IV 1 Bubbling Spring
V 1 Heavenly Pond
VI 1 Rushing The Frontier Gate
VII 1 Orbit Bone
VIII 1 Great Esteem
IX 1 Middle Palace
X 4 Joining Of The Valleys
XI 1 Receive Tears
XII 1 Retired White
XIII 1 Meeting Of Yin
XIV 1 Long Strength

Exit Points

I 9 Little Rushing In
II 19 Listening Palace
III 67 Extremity Of Yin
IV 22 Walking On The Verandah
V 8 Palace Of Weariness
VI 22 Harmony Bone
VII 41 Foot Above Tears
VIII 14 Gate Of Hope
IX 7 Narrow Defile
X 20 Welcome Fragrance
XI 42 Rushing Yang
XII 21 Great Enveloping
XIII 24 Receiving Fluid
XIV 28 Mouth Crossing

Appendix 12 Fire Points

I 8 Lesser Palace
II 5 Yang Valley
III 60 Kunlun Mountain
IV 2 Blazing Valley
V 8 Palace Of Weariness
VI 6 Branch Ditch
VII 38 Yang Support
VIII 2 Walk Between
IX 10 Fish Region
X 5 Yang Stream
XI 41 Released Stream
XII 2 Great Capital

Appendix 13 First Aid Points

Anxiety I 7, III 60, V 9
Apoplexy III 31, IV 6, X 15
Asphyxia VIII 3, IX 9
Bee stings III 64, IV 6
Bites XIV 11
Burns III 65
Colds VI 15, XIV 14
Collapse IX 9
Concussion III 31, IV 6, IX 9, X 15, XIV 3
Convulsions II 3, IX 11, XIV 11
Cramp VIII 2, VIII 6
Cystitis III 65, IV 2
Drowning I 1, IX 1, XIII 1
Dull pains X 4
Earache II 3, VI 4, X 4
Electric shock I 7, IX 8, X 15
Exhaustion II 3, VI 3, X 15
Facial neuralgia III 60
Fainting I 1, I 7, X 4, XI 36
Food poisoning III 59, III 65, VII 40, IX 9, X 4, XI 30
Fractures III 11, III 60, VII 30, XII 2, XIV 3
Haemorrhage II 8, III 25, IV 6, VII 41, X 15
Hangover XI 45
Head injury X 15
Heart failure I 1, I 7, III 15
Hiccups III 17
Hysteria I 7
Indigestion XI 36, XI 45
Injury to testicles IV 2
Insect bites III 65
Insensibility II 3, III 31, IV 6, IX 9, IX 11, X 15, XIV 3, XIV 11
Numbness III 17
Poison III 65, VII 20, VII 40, IX 3, IX 9, X 4
Resuscitation IV 1, V 9, XIII 1
Scalds III 65
Sea sickness XIII 14
Shock I 7, IX 9, X 15
Snake bites III 31, IV 6
Spasms VIII 2, VIII 6
Spinal injury III 54, III 60, XIV 3
Sprains III 11, III 60, VII 30, XII 2, XIV 3
Sunburn III 65
Sunstroke IV 23, IX 11
Toothache X 1, X 4, XI 45
Tooth extraction I 7
Travel sickness XIII 14
Urine retention III 65, IV 2, VIII 2, VIII 6, XIII 3

Appendix 14 Forbidden Points

Heart Meridian

I 2 ⊥ Forbidden

Small Intestine Meridian

II 7 Forbidden sixth month pregnancy
II 9 △ Forbidden
II 10 Forbidden sixth month pregnancy
II 18 △ Forbidden

Bladder Meridian

III 1 △ Forbidden
III 2 △ Forbidden
III 5 △ Forbidden
III 6 △ Forbidden
III 16 ⊥ Forbidden
III 30 △ Forbidden
III 50 △ Forbidden
III 51 △ Forbidden
III 54 △ Forbidden
III 56 ⊥ Forbidden
III 62 △ Forbidden

Kidney Meridian

IV 1 Forbidden eighth month pregnancy
IV 2 Forbidden eighth month pregnancy
IV 4 Forbidden third month pregnancy
IV 7 Forbidden eighth month pregnancy
IV 11 ⊥ Forbidden

Circulation-Sex Meridian

V 1 Forbidden women
V 6 Forbidden fourth month pregnancy
V 7 △ Forbidden
V 8 Forbidden third month pregnancy

Three Heater Meridian

VI 4 △ Forbidden. Forbidden third month pregnancy
VI 8 ⊥ Forbidden
VI 10 Forbidden fourth month pregnancy
VI 16 △ Forbidden
VI 18 △ Forbidden
VI 19 ⊥ Forbidden
VI 20 ⊥ Forbidden
VI 23 △ Forbidden

Gall Bladder Meridian

VII 2 Forbidden first month pregnancy
VII 3 ⊥ Forbidden
VII 9 Forbidden fourth month pregnancy
VII 15 △ Forbidden
VII 18 ⊥ Forbidden
VII 22 △ Forbidden
VII 33 △ Forbidden
VII 34 Forbidden second month pregnancy
VII 42 △ Forbidden

Liver Meridian

VIII 12 ⊥ Forbidden

Lung Meridian

IX 3 △ Forbidden
IX 7 Forbidden sixth month pregnancy
IX 8 △ Forbidden
IX 10 △ Forbidden
IX 11 △ Forbidden. Forbidden seventh month pregnancy

Colon Meridian

X 2 Forbidden ninth month pregnancy
X 4 Forbidden first month pregnancy
X 10 Forbidden ninth month pregnancy
X 13 ⊥ Forbidden
X 19 △ Forbidden
X 20 △ Forbidden

Stomach Meridian

XI 1 △ Forbidden
XI 4 Forbidden fifth month pregnancy
XI 7 △ Forbidden
XI 8 △ Forbidden
XI 9 △ Forbidden
XI 10 △ Forbidden
XI 17 ⊥ Forbidden △ Forbidden
XI 36 Forbidden eighth month pregnancy
XI 45 Forbidden sixth month pregnancy

Appendix 14 Forbidden Points (continued)

Spleen Meridian

XII 1	△	Forbidden. Forbidden first month pregnancy
XII 2		Forbidden first month pregnancy
XII 6		Forbidden ninth month pregnancy
XII 7	△	Forbidden
XII 9	△	Forbidden

Conception Vessel Meridian

XIII 1	△	Forbidden
XIII 8	⊥	Forbidden
XIII 17	⊥	Forbidden

Governor Vessel Meridian

XIV 6	△	Forbidden		
XIV 7	⊥	Forbidden	△	Forbidden
XIV 10	⊥	Forbidden		
XIV 11	⊥	Forbidden		
XIV 15	△	Forbidden		
XIV 16	△	Forbidden		
XIV 17	⊥	Forbidden	△	Forbidden
XIV 18	△	Forbidden		
XIV 24	⊥	Forbidden		
XIV 25	△	Forbidden		
XIV 28	△	Forbidden		

Appendix 15 Four Needle Technique

	To Tonify				To Sedate			
	Tonify		Sedate		Sedate		Tonify	
I	I 9	VIII 1	I 3	IV 10	I 7	XII 3	I 3	IV 10
II	II 3	VII 41	II 2	III 66	II 8	XI 36	II 2	III 66
III	III 67	X 1	III 54	XI 36	III 65	VII 41	III 54	XI 36
IV	IV 7	IX 8	IV 3	XII 3	IV 1	VIII 1	IV 3	XII 3
V	V 9	VIII 1	V 3	IV 10	V 7	XII 3	V 3	IV 10
VI	VI 3	VII 41	VI 2	III 66	VI 10	XI 36	VI 2	III 66
VII	VII 43	III 66	VII 44	X 1	VII 38	II 5	VII 44	X 1
VIII	VIII 8	IV 10	VIII 4	IX 8	VIII 2	V 8	VIII 4	IX 8
IX	IX 9	XII 3	IX 10	V 8	IX 5	IV 10	IX 10	V 8
X	X 11	XI 36	X 5	II 5	X 2	III 66	X 5	II 5
XI	XI 41	II 5	XI 43	VII 41	XI 45	X 1	XI 43	VII 41
XII	XII 2	V 8	XII 1	VIII 1	XII 5	IX 8	XII 1	VIII 1

Appendix 16 Horary Points

I 8	●	Lesser Palace
II 5	●	Yang Valley
III 66	●	Penetrating Valley
IV 10	●	Yin Valley
V 8	●	Palace Of Weariness
VI 6	●	Branch Ditch
VII 41	●	Foot Above Tears
VIII 1	●	Great Esteem
IX 8	○	Meridian Gutter
X 1	○	Merchant Yang
XI 36	●	Leg Three Miles
XII 3	●	Supreme White

Appendix 17 Junction Points ⊖

I 5	Penetrating Inside
II 7	Upright Branch
III 58	Fly And Scatter
IV 4	Great Bell
V 6	Inner Frontier Gate
VI 5	Outer Frontier Gate
VII 37	Bright And Clear
VIII 5	Insect Ditch
IX 7	Narrow Defile
X 6	Side Passage
XI 40	Abundant Splendour
XII 4	Prince's Grandson

Appendix 18 Meeting Points

V 5 Meeting Point of the three upper Yin meridians (I:V:IX)
VI 8 Meeting Point of the three upper Yang meridians (II:VI:X)
VII 39 Meeting Point of the three lower Yang meridians (III:VII:XI)
XII 6 Meeting Point of the three lower Yin meridians (IV:VIII:XII)
VIII 13 Meeting Point of the five Yin organs
XIII 12 Meeting Point of the five Yang organs

Appendix 19 Metal Points ○

I 4 Spirit Path
II 1 Little Marsh
III 67 Extremity Of Yin
IV 7 Returning Current
V 5 The Intermediary
VI 1 Rushing The Frontier Gate
VII 44 Foot Hole Yin
VIII 4 Middle Seal
IX 8 Meridian Gutter
X 1 Merchant Yang
XI 45 Hard Bargain
XII 5 Merchant Mound

Appendix 20 Names of the Points (listed by meridian)

Heart Meridian

I 1 **Utmost Source** Chichuan
I 2 **Blue-Green Spirit** Chingling
I 3 **Little Sea** Shaohai
I 4 **Spirit Path** Lingtao
I 5 **Penetrating Inside** Tungli
I 6 **Yin Mound** Yinhsi
I 7 **Spirit Gate** Shenmen
I 8 **Lesser Palace** Shaofu
I 9 **Little Rushing In** Shaochung

Small Intestine Meridian

II 1 **Little Marsh** Shaotse
II 2 **Forward Valley** Chienku
II 3 **Back Ravine** Houhsi
II 4 **Wrist Bone** Wanku
II 5 **Yang Valley** Yangku
II 6 **Nourishing The Old** Yanglao
II 7 **Upright Branch** Chihcheng
II 8 **Small Sea** Hsiaohai
II 9 **Upright Shoulder** Chienchen
II 10 **Shoulder Blade** Naoshu
II 11 **Heavenly Ancestor** Tientsung
II 12 **Grasping The Wind** Pingfeng
II 13 **Crooked Wall** Chuyuan
II 14 **Outside The Shoulder Correspondence** Chienwaishu
II 15 **Middle Of The Shoulder Correspondence** Chienchungshu
II 16 **Heavenly Window** Tienchuang
II 17 **Heavenly Appearance** Tienjung
II 18 **Cheek Bone** Chuanliao
II 19 **Listening Palace** Tingkung

Bladder Meridian

III 1 Eyes Bright Chingming
III 2 Collect Bamboo Tsanchu
III 3 Eyebrows Rushing Meichung
III 4 Crooked Servant Chucha
III 5 Five Places Wuchu
III 6 Receive Light Chengkuang
III 7 Penetrate Heaven Tungtien
III 8 Lou End Lochueh
III 9 Jade Pillow Yuchen
III 10 Heavenly Pillar Tienchu
III 11 Great Shuttle Tachu
III 12 Wind Gate Fengmen
III 13 Lungs Correspondence Feishu
III 14 Circulation-Sex Correspondence Chuehyinshu
III 15 Heart Correspondence Hsinshu
III 16 Governor Correspondence Tushu
III 17 Diaphragm Correspondence Keshu
III 18 Liver Correspondence Kanshu
III 19 Gall Bladder Correspondence Tanshu
III 20 Spleen Correspondence Pishu
III 21 Stomach Correspondence Weishu
III 22 Three Heater Correspondence Sanchiaoshu
III 23 Kidneys Correspondence Shenshu
III 24 Sea Of Ch'i Correspondence Chihaishu
III 25 Large Intestine Correspondence Tachangshu
III 26 First Gate Correspondence Kuanyuanshu
III 27 Small Intestine Correspondence Hsiaochangshu
III 28 Bladder Correspondence Pangkuangshu
III 29 Middle Of The Backbone Correspondence Chunglushu
III 30 White Ring Correspondence Paihuanshu
III 31 Upper Sacral Bone Shangliao
III 32 Second Sacral Bone Tzuliao
III 33 Middle Sacral Bone Chungliao
III 34 Lower Sacral Bone Hsialiao
III 35 Meeting Of Yang Huiyang
III 36 Near Division Fufen
III 37 Soul Door Pohu
III 38 Rich For The Vitals Correspondence Kaohuang
III 39 Spirit Hall Shentang
III 40 Wail Of Grief Yihsi
III 41 Diaphragm Border Kekuan
III 42 Spiritual Soul Gate Hunmen
III 43 Yang Net Yangkang
III 44 Thought Dwelling Yishe
III 45 Stomach Granary Weitsang
III 46 Diaphragm Gate Of Vitality Huangmen
III 47 Ambition Room Chihshih
III 48 Womb And Heart Diaphragm Paohuang
III 49 Orderly Frontier Chihpien
III 50 Receive And Support Chengfu
III 51 Prosperous Gate Yinmen
III 52 Floating Reserve Fuhsi
III 53 Equilibrium Yang Weiyang
III 54 Equilibrium Middle Weichung
III 55 Uniting Yang Hoyang
III 56 Supporting Muscles Chengchin
III 57 Supporting Mountain Chengshan
III 58 Fly And Scatter Feiyang
III 59 Foot Bone Yang Fuyang
III 60 Kunlun Mountain Kunlun
III 61 Servant's Aide Pushen
III 62 Extended Meridian Shenmo
III 63 Golden Gate Chinmen
III 64 Capital Bone Chingku
III 65 Bone Binder Shuku
III 66 Penetrating Valley Tsu tungku
III 67 Extremity Of Yin Chihyin

Kidney Meridian

IV 1 Bubbling Spring Yungchuan
IV 2 Blazing Valley Janku
IV 3 Greater Mountain Stream Taihsi
IV 4 Great Bell Tachung
IV 5 Water Spring Shuichuan
IV 6 Illuminated Sea Chaohai
IV 7 Returning Current Fuliu
IV 8 Exchange Pledges Chiaohsin
IV 9 Building Guest Chupin
IV 10 Yin Valley Yinku
IV 11 Transverse Bone Hengku
IV 12 Great Brightness Taho
IV 13 Door Of Infants Tzuhu
IV 14 Four Full Szuman
IV 15 Middle Flowing Out Chungchu
IV 16 Vitals Correspondence Huangshu
IV 17 Merchant Crooked Shangchu
IV 18 Stone Border Shihkuan
IV 19 Yin Capital Yintu
IV 20 Through The Valley Fu tungku
IV 21 Dark Gate Yumen
IV 22 Walking On The Verandah Pulang
IV 23 Spirit Seal Shenfeng
IV 24 Spirit Burial Ground Linghsu
IV 25 Spirit Storehouse Shentsang
IV 26 Amidst Elegance Yuchung
IV 27 Store House Shufu

Circulation-Sex Meridian

V 1 Heavenly Pond Tienchih
V 2 Heavenly Spring Tienchuan
V 3 Crooked Marsh Chutse
V 4 Gate Of Ch'i Reserve Hsimen
V 5 The Intermediary Chienshih
V 6 Inner Frontier Gate Neikuan
V 7 Great Mound Taling
V 8 Palace Of Weariness Laokung
V 9 Rushing Into The Middle Chungchung

Three Heater Meridian

VI 1 **Rushing The Frontier Gate** Kuanchung
VI 2 **Fluid Secretion Gate** Yehmen
VI 3 **Middle Islet** Chungchu
VI 4 **Yang Pond** Yangchih
VI 5 **Outer Frontier Gate** Waikuan
VI 6 **Branch Ditch** Chihkou
VI 7 **Assembly Of Ancestors** Huitsung
VI 8 **Three Yang Junction** Sanyanglo
VI 9 **Fourth Gutter** Szutu
VI 10 **Heavenly Well** Tienching
VI 11 **Pure Cold Abyss** Chinglengyuan
VI 12 **Relax And Joy** Hsiaolo
VI 13 **Shoulder Meeting** Naohui
VI 14 **Shoulder Bone** Chienliao
VI 15 **Heavenly Bone** Tienliao
VI 16 **Heavenly Window** Tienyu
VI 17 **Wind Screen** Yifeng
VI 18 **Feeding Meridians** Chimo
VI 19 **Skull Breathing** Luhsi
VI 20 **Small Angle Of Ear** Chuehsun
VI 21 **Ear Gate** Erhmen
VI 22 **Harmony Bone** Holiao
VI 23 **Silk Bamboo Hollow** Szuchukung

Gall Bladder Meridian

VII 1 **Orbit Bone** Tungtzuliao
VII 2 **Hearing Assembly** Tinghui
VII 3 **Upper Pass** Shangkuan
VII 4 **Loathsome Jaws** Hanyen
VII 5 **Suspended Skull** Hsuanlu
VII 6 **Suspended Regulator** Hsuanli
VII 7 **Crooked Hair On The Temples** Chupin
VII 8 **Flowing Valley** Shuaiku
VII 9 **Heaven Rushing** Tienchung
VII 10 **Floating White** Fupai
VII 11 **Head Hole Yin** Tou chiaoyin
VII 12 **Final Bone** Wanku
VII 13 **Root Spirit** Penshen
VII 14 **Yang White** Yangpai
VII 15 **Head Above Tears** Tou linchi
VII 16 **Eye Window** Muchuang
VII 17 **Upright Living** Chengying
VII 18 **Receiving Spirit** Chengling
VII 19 **Brain Hollow** Naokung
VII 20 **Wind Pond** Fengchih
VII 21 **Shoulder Well** Chienching
VII 22 **Armpit Abyss** Yuanyeh
VII 23 **Neglected Muscles** Chechin
VII 24 **Sun And Moon** Jihyueh
VII 25 **Capital Gate** Chingmen
VII 26 **Girdle Vessel** Taimo
VII 27 **Five Pivots** Wushu
VII 28 **Binding Path** Weitao
VII 29 **Dwelling In The Bone** Chuliao
VII 30 **Jumping Circle** Huantiao
VII 31 **Wind Market** Fengshih
VII 32 **Middle Ditch** Chungtu
VII 33 **Knee Yang Border** Tsu yangkuan
VII 34 **Yang Mound Spring** Yanglingchuan
VII 35 **Yang Crossing** Yangchiao
VII 36 **Outer Mound** Waichiu
VII 37 **Bright And Clear** Kuangming
VII 38 **Yang Support** Yangfu
VII 39 **Hanging Cup** Hsuanchung
VII 40 **Wilderness Mound** Chiuhsu
VII 41 **Foot Above Tears** Tsu linchi
VII 42 **Earth Five Meetings** Tiwuhui
VII 43 **Valiant Stream** Hsiahsi
VII 44 **Foot Hole Yin** Tsu chiaoyin

Liver Meridian

VIII 1 **Great Esteem** Tatun
VIII 2 **Walk Between** Hsingchien
VIII 3 **Supreme Rushing** Taichung
VIII 4 **Middle Seal** Chungfeng
VIII 5 **Insect Ditch** Likou
VIII 6 **Middle Capital** Chungtu
VIII 7 **Knee Border** Hsikuan
VIII 8 **Crooked Spring** Chuchuan
VIII 9 **Yin Wrapping** Yinpao
VIII 10 **Five Miles** Tsu wuli
VIII 11 **Yin Angle** Yinlien
VIII 12 **Hasty Pulse** Chimo
VIII 13 **Chapter Gate** Changmen
VIII 14 **Gate Of Hope** Chimen

Lung Meridian

IX 1 **Middle Palace** Chungfu
IX 2 **Cloud Gate** Yunmen
IX 3 **Heavenly Palace** Tienfu
IX 4 **Valiant White** Hsiapai
IX 5 **Outside Marsh** Chihtse
IX 6 **Greatest Hole** Kungtsui
IX 7 **Narrow Defile** Liehchueh
IX 8 **Meridian Gutter** Chingchu
IX 9 **Very Great Abyss** Taiyuan
IX 10 **Fish Region** Yuchi
IX 11 **Little Merchant** Shaoshang

Colon Meridian

X 1 Merchant Yang Shangyang
X 2 Second Interval Erhchien
X 3 Third Interval Sanchien
X 4 Joining Of The Valleys Hoku
X 5 Yang Stream Yanghsi
X 6 Side Passage Pienli
X 7 Warm Current Wenliu
X 8 Lower Side Hsialien
X 9 Upper Angle Shanglien
X 10 Arm Three Miles Shou sanli
X 11 Crooked Pond Chuchih
X 12 Elbow Bone Chouliao
X 13 Arm Five Miles Shou wuli
X 14 Outer Bone Of The Arm Pinao
X 15 Shoulder Joint Chienyu
X 16 Great Bone Chuku
X 17 Heavenly Vessel Tienting
X 18 Support And Rush Out Futu
X 19 Grain Bone Holiao
X 20 Welcome Fragrance Yinghsiang

Stomach Meridian

XI 1 Receive Tears Chengchi
XI 2 Four Whites Szupai
XI 3 Great Cheekbone Chuliao
XI 4 Earth Granary Titsang
XI 5 Great Welcome Taying
XI 6 Mandible Wheel Chiache
XI 7 Lower Passage Hsiakuan
XI 8 Head Tied Touwei
XI 9 People Welcome Jenying
XI 10 Water Rushing Out Shuitu
XI 11 Ch'i Cottage Chishe
XI 12 Broken Bowl Chuehpen
XI 13 Ch'i Door Chihu
XI 14 Storehouse Kufang
XI 15 Room Screen Wuyi
XI 16 Breast Window Yingchuang
XI 17 Centre Of The Breasts Juchung
XI 18 Root Of The Breasts Juken
XI 19 Not At Ease Pujung
XI 20 Receiving Fullness Chengman
XI 21 Bridge Gate Liangmen
XI 22 Border Gate Kuanmen
XI 23 Great Oneness Taiyi
XI 24 Lubrication Food Gate Huajoumen
XI 25 Heavenly Pivot Tienshu
XI 26 Outside Mound Wailing
XI 27 Great Might Tachu
XI 28 Water Path Shuitao
XI 29 The Return Kueilai
XI 30 Ch'i Rushing Chichung
XI 31 Thigh Border Pikuan
XI 32 Prostrate Hare Futu
XI 33 Yin Market Yinshih
XI 34 Beam Mound Liangchiu
XI 35 Calf Nose Tupi
XI 36 Leg Three Miles Tsu sanli
XI 37 Upper Great Void Shangchuhsu
XI 38 Branch Opening Tiaokou
XI 39 Lower Great Void Hsiachuhsu
XI 40 Abundant Splendour Fenglung
XI 41 Released Stream Chiehhsi
XI 42 Rushing Yang Chungyang
XI 43 Sinking Valley Hsienku
XI 44 Inner Courtyard Neiting
XI 45 Hard Bargain Litui

Spleen Meridian

XII 1 Retired White Yinpai
XII 2 Great Capital Tatu
XII 3 Supreme White Taipai
XII 4 Prince's Grandson Kungsun
XII 5 Merchant Mound Shangchiu
XII 6 Three Yin Crossing Sanyinchiao
XII 7 Leaky Valley Louku
XII 8 Earth Motivator Tichi
XII 9 Yin Mound Spring Yinlingchuan
XII 10 Sea Of Blood Hsuehhai
XII 11 Basket Gate Chimen
XII 12 Rushing Gate Chungmen
XII 13 Official Residence Fushe
XII 14 Abdomen Knot Fuchieh
XII 15 Great Horizontal Taheng
XII 16 Abdomen Sorrow Fuai
XII 17 Food Drain Shihtou
XII 18 Heavenly Stream Tienhsi
XII 19 Chest Region Hsiunghsiang
XII 20 Encircling Glory Choujung
XII 21 Great Enveloping Tapao

Conception Vessel Meridian

XIII 1 Meeting Of Yin Huiyin
XIII 2 Crooked Bone Chuku
XIII 3 Utmost Middle Chungchi
XIII 4 First Gate Kuanyuan
XIII 5 Stone Gate Shihmen
XIII 6 Sea Of Ch'i Chihai
XIII 7 Yin Crossing Yinchiao
XIII 8 Spirit Deficiency Shenchueh
XIII 9 Water Division Shuifen

Appendix 20 Names of the Points (listed by meridian, continued)

XIII 10 **Lower Duct** Hsiawan
XIII 11 **Established Mile** Chienli
XIII 12 **Middle Duct** Chungwan
XIII 13 **Upper Duct** Shangwan
XIII 14 **Great Deficiency** Chuchueh
XIII 15 **Dove Tail** Chiuwei
XIII 16 **Middle Hall** Chungting
XIII 17 **Within The Breast** Shanchung
XIII 18 **Jade Court** Yutang
XIII 19 **Purple Palace** Tzukung
XIII 20 **Flower Covering** Huakai
XIII 21 **Pearl Jade** Hsuanchi
XIII 22 **Heaven Rushing Out** Tientu
XIII 23 **Angle Spring** Lienchuan
XIII 24 **Receiving Fluid** Chengchiang

Governor Vessel Meridian

XIV 1 **Long Strength** Changchiang
XIV 2 **Loins Correspondence** Yaoshu
XIV 3 **Loins Yang Border** Yao yangkuan
XIV 4 **Gate Of Life** Mingmen
XIV 5 **Suspended Pivot** Hsuanshu
XIV 6 **Middle Of The Spine** Chichung
XIV 7 **Middle Pivot** Chungshu
XIV 8 **Contracted Muscle** Chinso
XIV 9 **Utmost Yang** Chihyang
XIV 10 **Supernatural Tower** Lingtai
XIV 11 **Spirit Path** Shentao
XIV 12 **Body Pillar** Shenchu
XIV 13 **Kiln Path** Taotao
XIV 14 **Great Hammer** Tachui
XIV 15 **Gate Of Dumbness** Yamen
XIV 16 **Wind Palace** Fengfu
XIV 17 **Brain Door** Naohu
XIV 18 **Strength Divider** Chiangchien
XIV 19 **Posterior Summit** Houting
XIV 20 **One Hundred Meetings** Paihui
XIV 21 **Anterior Summit** Chienting
XIV 22 **Skull Meeting** Hsinhui
XIV 23 **Upper Star** Shanghsing
XIV 24 **Spirit Hall** Shenting
XIV 25 **Plain Bone** Suliao
XIV 26 **Middle Of Man** Jenchung
XIV 27 **Correct Exchange** Tuituan
XIV 28 **Mouth Crossing** Yinchiao

Appendix 21 Names of the Points (listed alphabetically)

Abdomen Knot XII 14 Fuchieh
Abdomen Sorrow XII 16 Fuai
Abundant Splendour XI 40 Fenglung
Ambition Room III 47 Chihshih
Amidst Elegance IV 26 Yuchung
Angle Spring XIII 23 Lienchuan
Anterior Summit XIV 21 Chienting
Armpit Abyss VII 22 Yuanyeh
Arm Five Miles X 13 Shou wuli
Arm Three Miles X 10 Shou sanli
Assembly Of Ancestors VI 7 Huitsung
Back Ravine II 3 Houhsi
Basket Gate XII 11 Chimen
Beam Mound XI 34 Liangchiu
Binding Path VII 28 Weitao
Bladder Correspondence III 28 Pangkuangshu
Blazing Valley IV 2 Janku
Blue-Green Spirit I 2 Chingling
Body Pillar XIV 12 Shenchu
Bone Binder III 65 Shuku
Border Gate XI 22 Kuanmen
Brain Door XIV 17 Naohu
Brain Hollow VII 19 Naokung
Branch Ditch VI 6 Chihkou
Branch Opening XI 38 Tiaokou
Breast Window XI 16 Yingchuang
Bridge Gate XI 21 Liangmen
Bright And Clear VII 37 Kuangming
Broken Bowl XI 12 Chuehpen
Bubbling Spring IV 1 Yungchuan
Building Guest IV 9 Chupin
Calf Nose XI 35 Tupi
Capital Bone III 64 Chingku
Capital Gate VII 25 Chingmen
Centre Of The Breasts XI 17 Juchung
Chapter Gate VIII 13 Changmen
Cheek Bone II 18 Chuanliao
Chest Region XII 19 Hsiunghsiang
Ch'i Cottage XI 11 Chishe
Ch'i Door XI 13 Chihu
Ch'i Rushing XI 30 Chichung
Circulation-Sex Correspondence III 14 Chuehyinshu

Cloud Gate IX 2 Yunmen
Collect Bamboo III 2 Tsanchu
Contracted Muscle XIV 8 Chinso
Correct Exchange XIV 27 Tuituan
Crooked Bone XIII 2 Chuku
Crooked Hair On The Temples VII 7 Chupin
Crooked Marsh V 3 Chutse
Crooked Pond X 11 Chuchih
Crooked Servant III 4 Chucha
Crooked Spring VIII 8 Chuchuan
Crooked Wall II 13 Chuyuan
Dark Gate IV 21 Yumen
Diaphragm Border III 41 Kekuan
Diaphragm Gate Of Vitality III 46 Huangmen
Diaphragm Correspondence III 17 Keshu
Door Of Infants IV 13 Tzuhu
Dove Tail XIII 15 Chiuwei
Dwelling In The Bone VII 29 Chuliao
Ear Gate VI 21 Erhmen
Earth Five Meetings VII 42 Tiwuhui
Earth Granary XI 4 Titsang
Earth Motivator XII 8 Tichi
Elbow Bone X 12 Chouliao
Encircling Glory XII 20 Choujung
Equilibrium Middle III 54 Weichung
Equilibrium Yang III 53 Weiyang
Established Mile XIII 11 Chienli
Exchange Pledges IV 8 Chiaohsin
Extended Meridian III 62 Shenmo
Extremity Of Yin III 67 Chihyin
Eyebrows Rushing III 3 Meichung
Eyes Bright III 1 Chingming
Eye Window VII 16 Muchuang
Feeding Meridians VI 18 Chimo
Final Bone VII 12 Wanku
First Gate XIII 4 Kuanyuan
First Gate Correspondence III 26 Kuanyuanshu
Fish Region IX 10 Yuchi
Five Miles VIII 10 Tsu wuli
Five Pivots VII 27 Wushu
Five Places III 5 Wuchu
Floating Reserve III 52 Fuhsi
Floating White VII 10 Fupai
Flower Covering XIII 20 Huakai
Flowing Valley VII 8 Shuaiku
Fluid Secretion Gate VI 2 Yehmen
Fly And Scatter III 58 Feiyang
Food Drain XII 17 Shihtou
Foot Above Tears VII 41 Tsu linchi
Foot Bone Yang III 59 Fuyang
Foot Hole Yin VII 44 Tsu chiaoyin
Forward Valley II 2 Chienku
Four Full IV 14 Szuman
Four Whites XI 2 Szupai
Fourth Gutter VI 9 Szutu
Gall Bladder Correspondence III 19 Tanshu
Gate Of Ch'i Reserve V 4 Hsimen
Gate Of Dumbness XIV 15 Yamen
Gate Of Hope VIII 14 Chimen
Gate Of Life XIV 4 Mingmen
Girdle Vessel VII 26 Taimo
Golden Gate III 63 Chinmen
Governor Correspondence III 16 Tushu
Grain Bone X 19 Holiao
Grasping The Wind II 12 Pingfeng
Great Bell IV 4 Tachung
Great Bone X 16 Chuku
Great Brightness IV 12 Taho
Great Capital XII 2 Tatu
Great Cheekbone XI 3 Chuliao
Great Deficiency XIII 14 Chuchueh
Great Enveloping XII 21 Tapao
Great Esteem VIII 1 Tatun
Great Hammer XIV 14 Tachui
Great Horizontal XII 15 Taheng
Great Might XI 27 Tachu
Great Mound V 7 Taling
Great Oneness XI 23 Taiyi
Great Shuttle III 11 Tachu
Great Welcome XI 5 Taying
Greater Mountain Stream IV 3 Taihsi
Greatest Hole IX 6 Kungtsui
Hanging Cup VII 39 Hsuanchung
Hard Bargain XI 45 Litui
Harmony Bone VI 22 Holiao
Hasty Pulse VIII 12 Chimo
Head Above Tears VII 15 Tou linchi
Head Hole Yin VII 11 Tou chiaoyin
Head Tied XI 8 Touwei
Hearing Assembly VII 2 Tinghui
Heart Correspondence III 15 Hsinshu
Heaven Rushing VII 9 Tienchung
Heaven Rushing Out XIII 22 Tientu
Heavenly Ancestor II 11 Tientsung
Heavenly Appearance II 17 Tienjung
Heavenly Bone VI 15 Tienliao
Heavenly Palace IX 3 Tienfu
Heavenly Pillar III 10 Tienchu
Heavenly Pivot XI 25 Tienshu
Heavenly Pond V 1 Tienchih
Heavenly Spring V 2 Tienchuan
Heavenly Stream XII 18 Tienhsi
Heavenly Vessel X 17 Tienting
Heavenly Well VI 10 Tienching
Heavenly Window II 16 Tienchuang
Heavenly Window VI 16 Tienyu
Illuminated Sea IV 6 Chaohai
Inner Courtyard XI 44 Neiting
Inner Frontier Gate V 6 Neikuan
Insect Ditch VIII 5 Likou
The Intermediary V 5 Chienshih
Jade Court XIII 18 Yutang

Jade Pillow III 9 Yuchen
Joining Of The Valleys X 4 Hoku
Jumping Circle VII 30 Huantiao
Kidneys Correspondence III 23 Shenshu
Kiln Path XIV 13 Taotao
Knee Border VIII 7 Hsikuan
Knee Yang Border VII 33 Tsu yangkuan
Kunlun Mountain III 60 Kunlun
Large Intestine Correspondence III 25 Tachangshu
Leaky Valley XII 7 Louku
Leg Three Miles XI 36 Tsu sanli
Lesser Palace I 8 Shaofu
Listening Palace II 19 Tingkung
Little Marsh II 1 Shaotse
Little Merchant IX 11 Shaoshang
Little Rushing In I 9 Shaochung
Little Sea I 3 Shaohai
Liver Correspondence III 18 Kanshu
Loathsome Jaws VII 4 Hanyen
Loins Correspondence XIV 2 Yaoshu
Loins Yang Border XIV 3 Yao yangkuan
Long Strength XIV 1 Changchiang
Lou End III 8 Lochueh
Lower Duct XIII 10 Hsiawan
Lower Great Void XI 39 Hsiachuhsu
Lower Passage XI 7 Hsiakuan
Lower Sacral Bone III 34 Hsialiao
Lower Side X 8 Hsialien
Lubrication Food Gate XI 24 Huajoumen
Lungs Correspondence III 13 Feishu
Mandible Wheel XI 6 Chiache
Meeting Of Yang III 35 Huiyang
Meeting Of Yin XIII 1 Huiyin
Merchant Crooked IV 17 Shangchu
Merchant Mound XII 5 Shangchiu
Merchant Yang X 1 Shangyang
Meridian Gutter IX 8 Chingchu
Middle Capital VIII 6 Chungtu
Middle Ditch VII 32 Chungtu
Middle Duct XIII 12 Chungwan
Middle Flowing Out IV 15 Chungchu
Middle Hall XIII 16 Chungting
Middle Islet VI 3 Chungchu
Middle Of Man XIV 26 Jenchung
Middle Of The Backbone Correspondence III 29 Chunglushu
Middle Of The Shoulder Correspondence II 15 Chienchungshu
Middle Of The Spine XIV 6 Chichung
Middle Palace IX 1 Chungfu
Middle Pivot XIV 7 Chungshu
Middle Sacral Bone III 33 Chungliao
Middle Seal VIII 4 Chungfeng
Mouth Crossing XIV 28 Yinchiao
Narrow Defile IX 7 Liehchueh
Near Division III 36 Fufen
Neglected Muscles VII 23 Chechin
Not At Ease XI 19 Pujung
Nourishing The Old II 6 Yanglao
Official Residence XII 13 Fushe
One Hundred Meetings XIV 20 Paihui
Orbit Bone VII 1 Tungtzuliao
Orderly Frontier III 49 Chihpien
Outer Bone Of The Arm X 14 Pinao
Outer Frontier Gate VI 5 Waikuan
Outer Mound VII 36 Waichiu
Outside Marsh IX 5 Chihtse
Outside Mound XI 26 Wailing
Outside The Shoulder Correspondence II 14 Chienwaishu
Palace Of Weariness V 8 Laokung
Pearl Jade XIII 21 Hsuanchi
Penetrate Heaven III 7 Tungtien
Penetrating Inside I 5 Tungli
Penetrating Valley III 66 Tsu tungku
People Welcome XI 9 Jenying
Plain Bone XIV 25 Suliao
Posterior Summit XIV 19 Houting
Prince's Grandson XII 4 Kungsun
Prosperous Gate III 51 Yinmen
Prostrate Hare XI 32 Futu
Pure Cold Abyss VI 11 Chinglengyuan
Purple Palace XIII 19 Tzukung
Receive And Support III 50 Chengfu
Receive Light III 6 Chengkuang
Receive Tears XI 1 Chengchi
Receiving Fluid XIII 24 Chengchiang
Receiving Fullness XI 20 Chengman
Receiving Spirit VII 18 Chengling
Relax And Joy VI 12 Hsiaolo
Released Stream XI 41 Chiehhsi
Retired White XII 1 Yinpai
Return, The XI 29 Kueilai
Returning Current IV 7 Fuliu
Rich For The Vitals Correspondence III 38 Kaohuang
Room Screen XI 15 Wuyi
Root Of The Breasts XI 18 Juken
Root Spirit VII 13 Penshen
Rushing Gate XII 12 Chungmen
Rushing Into The Middle V 9 Chungchung
Rushing The Frontier Gate VI 1 Kuanchung
Rushing Yang XI 42 Chungyang
Sea Of Blood XII 10 Hsuehhai
Sea Of Ch'i XIII 6 Chihai
Sea Of Ch'i Correspondence III 24 Chihaishu
Second Interval X 2 Erhchien
Second Sacral Bone III 32 Tzuliao
Servant's Aide III 61 Pushen
Shoulder Blade II 10 Naoshu
Shoulder Bone VI 14 Chienliao
Shoulder Joint X 15 Chienyu
Shoulder Meeting VI 13 Naohui
Shoulder Well VII 21 Chienching
Side Passage X 6 Pienli
Silk Bamboo Hollow VI 23 Szuchukung

Sinking Valley XI 43 Hsienku
Skull Breathing VI 19 Luhsi
Skull Meeting XIV 22 Hsinhui
Small Angle Of Ear VI 20 Chuehsun
Small Intestine Correspondence III 27 Hsiaochangshu
Small Sea II 8 Hsiaohai
Soul Door III 37 Pohu
Spirit Burial Ground IV 24 Lingshu
Spirit Deficiency XIII 8 Shenchueh
Spirit Gate I 7 Shenmen
Spirit Hall III 39 Shentang
Spirit Hall XIV 24 Shenting
Spirit Path I 4 Lingtao
Spirit Path XIV 11 Shentao
Spirit Seal IV 23 Shenfeng
Spirit Storehouse IV 25 Shentsang
Spiritual Soul Gate III 42 Hunmen
Spleen Correspondence III 20 Pishu
Stomach Correspondence III 21 Weishu
Stomach Granary III 45 Weitsang
Stone Border IV 18 Shihkuan
Stone Gate XIII 5 Shihmen
Store House IV 27 Shufu
Storehouse XI 14 Kufang
Strength Divider XIV 18 Chiangchien
Sun And Moon VII 24 Jihyueh
Supernatural Tower XIV 10 Lingtai
Support And Rush Out X 18 Futu
Supporting Mountain III 57 Chengshan
Supporting Muscles III 56 Chengchin
Supreme Rushing VIII 3 Taichung
Supreme White XII 3 Taipai
Suspended Pivot XIV 5 Hsuanshu
Suspended Regulator VII 6 Hsuanli
Suspended Skull VII 5 Hsuanlu
Thigh Border XI 31 Pikuan
Three Heater Correspondence III 22 Sanchiaoshu
Third Interval X 3 Sanchien
Three Yang Junction VI 8 Sanyanglo
Three Yin Crossing XII 6 Sanyinchiao
Thought Dwelling III 44 Yishe
Through The Valley IV 20 Fu tungku
Transverse Bone IV 11 Hengku
Uniting Yang III 55 Hoyang
Upper Angle X 9 Shanglien
Upper Duct XIII 13 Shangwan
Upper Great Void XI 37 Shangchuhsu
Upper Pass VII 3 Shangkuan
Upper Sacral Bone III 31 Shangliao
Upper Star XIV 23 Shanghsing
Upright Branch II 7 Chihcheng
Upright Living VII 17 Chengying
Upright Shoulder II 9 Chienchen
Utmost Middle XIII 3 Chungchi
Utmost Source I 1 Chichuan
Utmost Yang XIV 9 Chihyang
Valiant Stream VII 43 Hsiahsi
Valiant White IX 4 Hsiapai
Very Great Abyss IX 9 Taiyuan
Vitals Correspondence IV 16 Huangshu
Wail Of Grief III 40 Yihsi
Walk Between VIII 2 Hsingchien
Walking On The Verandah IV 22 Pulang
Warm Current X 7 Wenliu
Water Division XIII 9 Shuifen
Water Path XI 28 Shuitao
Water Rushing Out XI 10 Shuitu
Water Spring IV 5 Shuichuan
Welcome Fragrance X 20 Yinghsiang
White Ring Correspondence III 30 Paihuanshu
Wilderness Mound VII 40 Chiuhsu
Wind Gate III 12 Fengmen
Wind Market VII 31 Fengshih
Wind Palace XIV 16 Fengfu
Wind Pond VII 20 Fengchih
Wind Screen VI 17 Yifeng
Within The Breast XIII 17 Shanchung
Womb And Heart Diaphragm III 48 Paohuang
Wrist Bone II 4 Wanku
Yang Crossing VII 35 Yangchiao
Yang Mound Spring VII 34 Yanglingchuan
Yang Net III 43 Yangkang
Yang Pond VI 4 Yangchih
Yang Stream X 5 Yanghsi
Yang Support VII 38 Yangfu
Yang Valley II 5 Yangku
Yang White VII 14 Yangpai
Yin Angle VIII 11 Yinlien
Yin Capital IV 19 Yintu
Yin Crossing XIII 7 Yinchiao
Yin Market XI 33 Yinshih
Yin Mound I 6 Yinhsi
Yin Mound Spring XII 9 Yinlingchuan
Yin Valley IV 10 Yinku
Yin Wrapping VIII 9 Yinpao

Appendix 22 Reunion Points

Reunion points are those where pathways intersect; they include entry, exit, junction and meeting points.

		I	II	III	IV	V	VI	VII	VIII	IX	X	XI	XII	XIII	XIV
I	1	×											×		
I	5	×	×												
I	9	×	×												
II	1	×	×												
II	7	×	×												
II	12		×				×	×							
II	18		×				×	×							
II	19		×	×			×	×							
III	1		×	×			×	×				×			
III	11			×				×							
III	12			×											×
III	31			×				×							
III	33			×				×							
III	58			×	×										
III	67			×	×										
IV	1			×	×										
IV	4			×	×										
IV	22				×	×									
V	1				×	×									
V	5	×				×				×					
V	6					×	×								
V	8					×	×								
VI	1					×	×								
VI	5					×	×								
VI	8		×				×				×				
VI	13						×				×				
VI	17						×	×							
VI	20						×	×							
VI	22						×	×							
VII	1		×				×	×							
VII	3							×				×			
VII	4						×	×				×			
VII	5						×	×				×			
VII	6							×				×			
VII	8			×				×							
VII	9			×				×							
VII	10			×				×							
VII	11			×				×							
VII	12			×				×							
VII	14						×	×							
VII	21						×	×							
VII	24							×					×		
VII	30			×				×							
VII	37							×	×						
VII	39			×				×				×			
VII	41							×	×						
		I	II	III	IV	V	VI	VII	VIII	IX	X	XI	XII	XIII	XIV

		I	II	III	IV	V	VI	VII	VIII	IX	X	XI	XII	XIII	XIV
VIII	1							×	×						
VIII	5							×	×						
VIII	13	×			×			×	×	×			×		
VIII	14								×	×			×		
IX	1								×	×			×		
IX	7									×	×				
X	4									×	×				
X	6									×	×				
X	20										×	×			
XI	1										×	×		×	
XI	5							×				×			
XI	6							×				×			
XI	12		×				×	×			×	×			
XI	25										×	×			
XI	30							×				×			
XI	40											×	×		
XI	42											×	×		
XII	1											×	×		
XII	4											×	×		
XII	6				×				×				×		
XII	12								×				×		
XII	13								×				×		
XII	21	×											×		
XIII	1													×	×
XIII	2								×					×	
XIII	3			×	×				×				×	×	
XIII	4		×		×				×			×	×	×	
XIII	5						×							×	
XIII	7				×	×	×							×	
XIII	9									×				×	
XIII	10												×	×	
XIII	11		×							×		×	×	×	
XIII	12		×	×		×	×	×		×	×	×		×	
XIII	13		×							×		×		×	
XIII	14	×												×	
XIII	15					×								×	
XIII	17	×	×		×	×	×							×	
XIII	24											×		×	×
XIV	1				×			×	×					×	×
XIV	13			×											×
XIV	14		×	×			×	×			×	×			×
XIV	17			×											×
XIV	20		×	×				×	×		×	×			×
XIV	23			×				×							×
XIV	24			×								×			×
XIV	26										×	×			×
XIV	28											×		×	×
		I	II	III	IV	V	VI	VII	VIII	IX	X	XI	XII	XIII	XIV

Appendix 23 Seas and Oceans

The Sea of Nourishment: XI 30; XI 36

The Sea of Energy: XIII 17; III 10; XI 9

The Sea of Blood: III 11; XI 37; XI 39

The Sea of Bone Marrow: XIV 15; XIV 16; XIV 19; XIV 20

Appendix 24 Sedation Points

I 7	●	Spirit Gate
II 8	●	Small Sea
III 65	●	Bone Binder
IV 1	●	Bubbling Spring
V 7	●	Great Mound
VI 10	●	Heavenly Well
VII 38	●	Yang Support
VIII 2	●	Walk Between
IX 5	●	Outside Marsh
X 2	●	Second Interval
XI 45	○	Hard Bargain
XII 5	○	Merchant Mound

Appendix 25 Source Points □

I 7	●	Spirit Gate
II 4		Wrist Bone
III 64		Capital Bone
IV 3	●	Greater Mountain Stream
V 7	●	Great Mound
VI 4		Yang Pond
VII 40		Wilderness Mound
VIII 3	●	Supreme Rushing
IX 9	●	Very Great Abyss
X 4		Joining Of The Valleys
XI 42		Rushing Yang
XII 3	●	Supreme White

Appendix 26 Three Chou

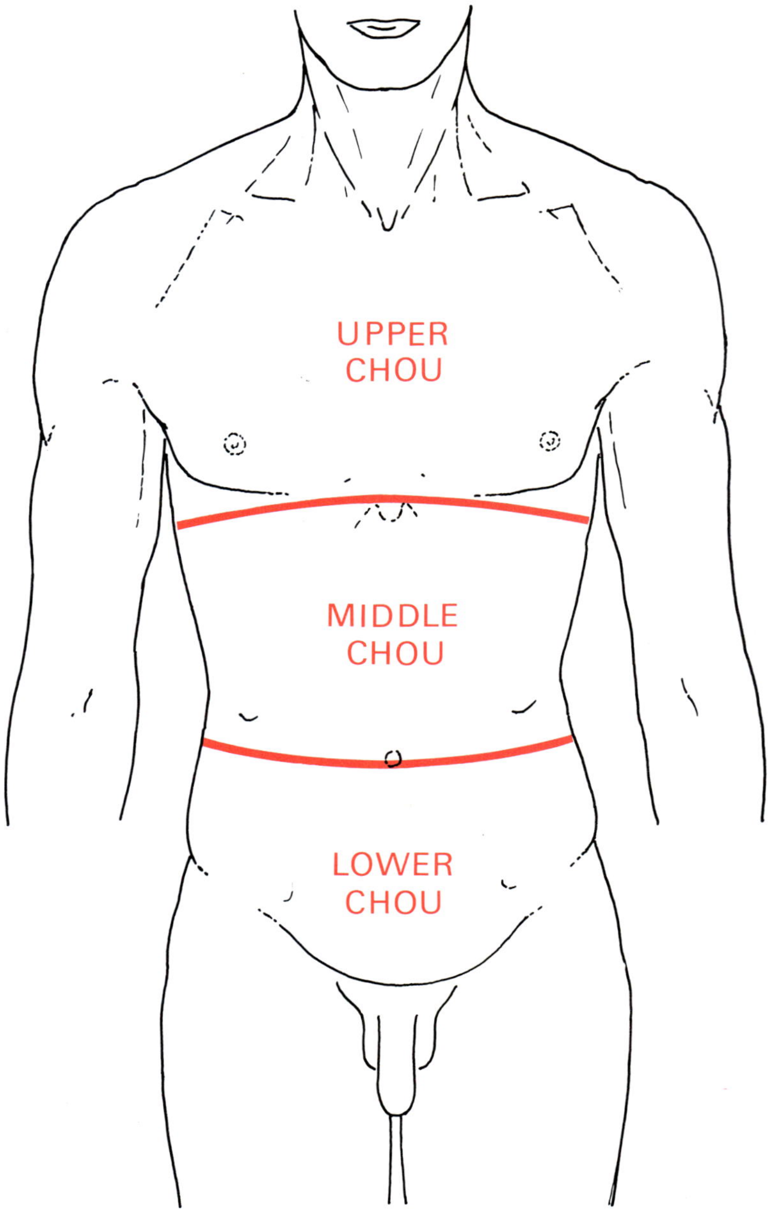

Appendix 27 Tonification Points

I	9	●	Little Rushing In
II	3	●	Back Ravine
III	67	○	Extremity Of Yin
IV	7	○	Returning Current
V	9	●	Rushing Into The Middle
VI	3	●	Middle Islet
VII	43	●	Valiant Stream
VIII	8	●	Crooked Spring
IX	9	●	Very Great Abyss
X	11	●	Crooked Pond
XI	41	●	Released Stream
XII	2	●	Great Capital

Appendix 28 Water Points ●

I	3	Little Sea
II	2	Forward Valley
III	66	Penetrating Valley
IV	10	Yin Valley
V	3	Crooked Marsh
VI	2	Fluid Secretion Gate
VII	43	Valiant Stream
VIII	8	Crooked Spring
IX	5	Outside Marsh
X	2	Second Interval
XI	44	Inner Courtyard
XII	9	Yin Mound Spring

Appendix 29 Windows of the Sky

II 16 Heavenly Window
II 17 Heavenly Appearance
III 10 Heavenly Pillar
V 1 Heavenly Pond
VI 16 Heavenly Window
IX 3 Heavenly Palace
X 18 Support And Rush Out
XI 9 People Welcome
XIII 22 Heaven Rushing Out
XIV 16 Wind Palace

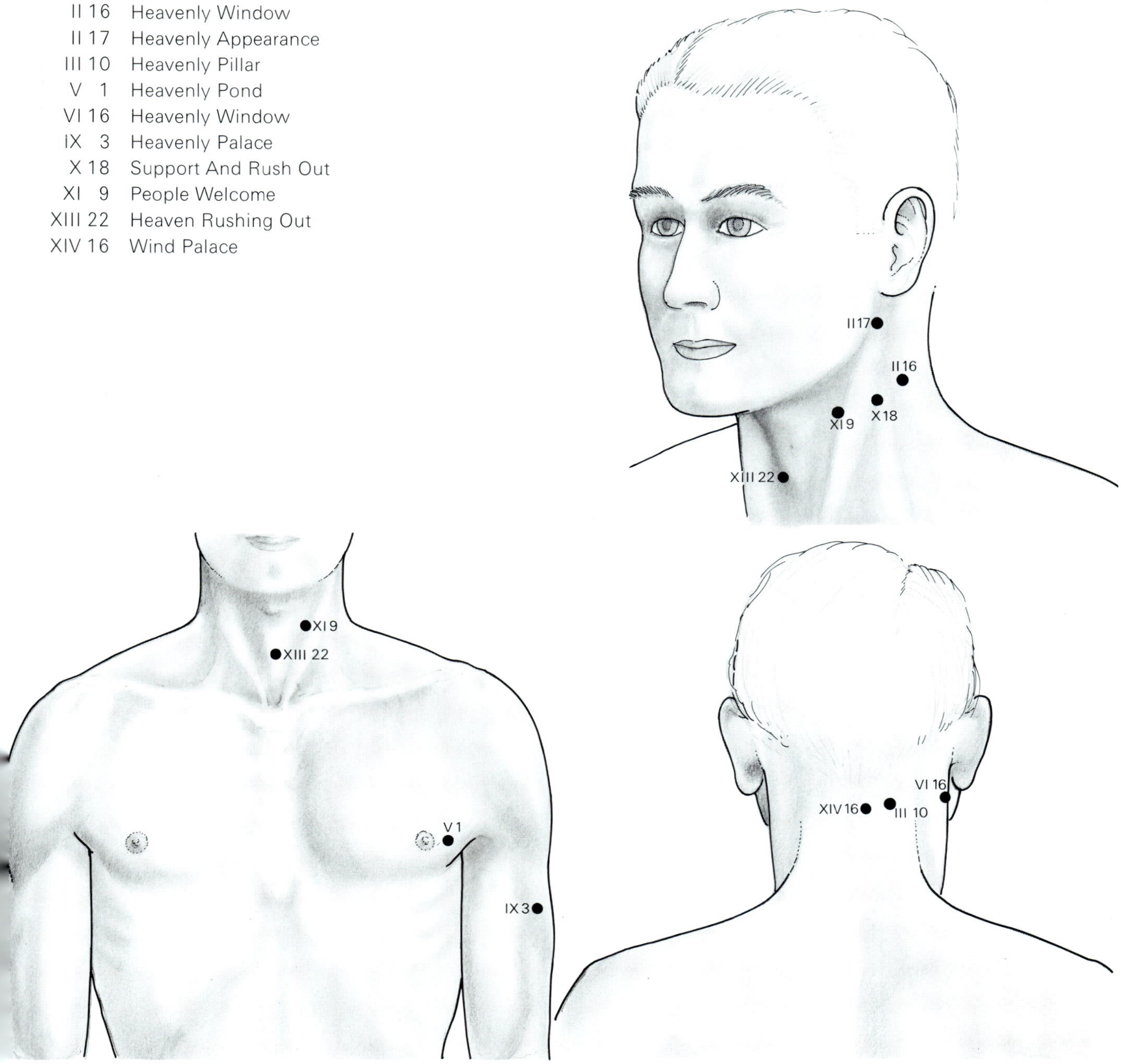

Appendix 30 Wood Points

I 9 Little Rushing In
II 3 Back Ravine
III 65 Bone Binder
IV 1 Bubbling Spring
V 9 Rushing Into The Middle
VI 3 Middle Islet
VII 41 Foot Above Tears
VIII 1 Great Esteem
IX 11 Little Merchant
X 3 Third Interval
XI 43 Sinking Valley
XII 1 Retired White

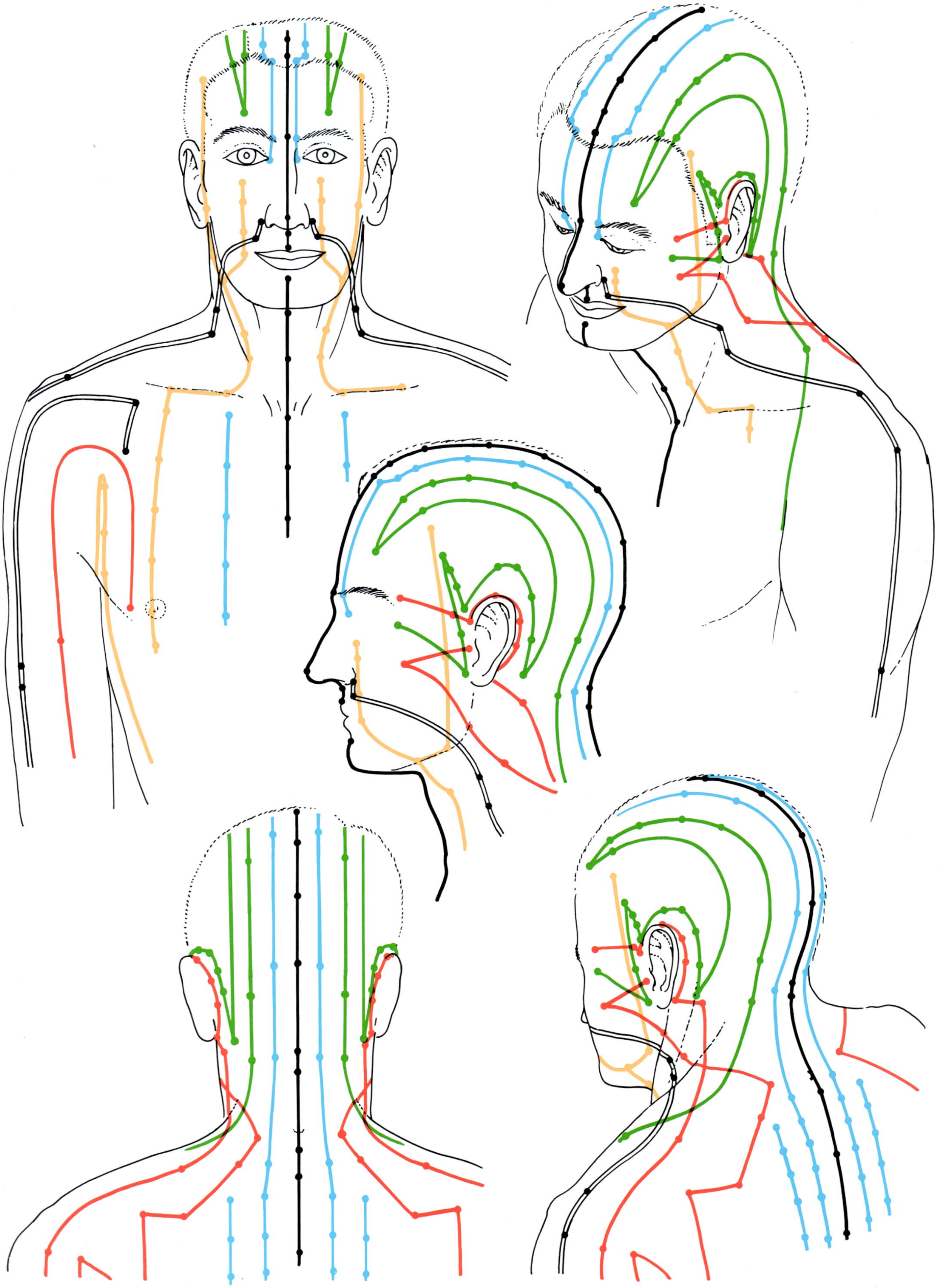

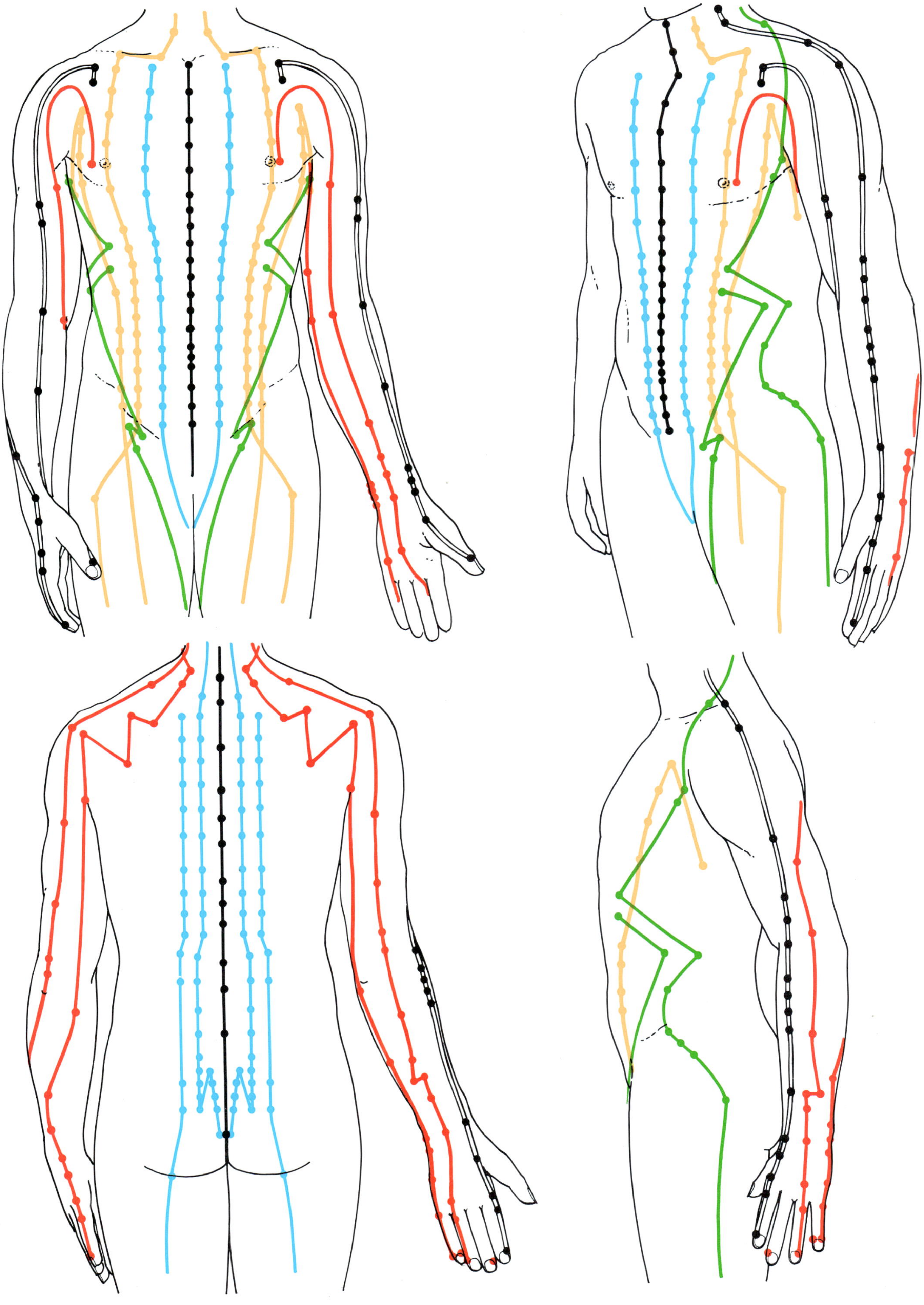

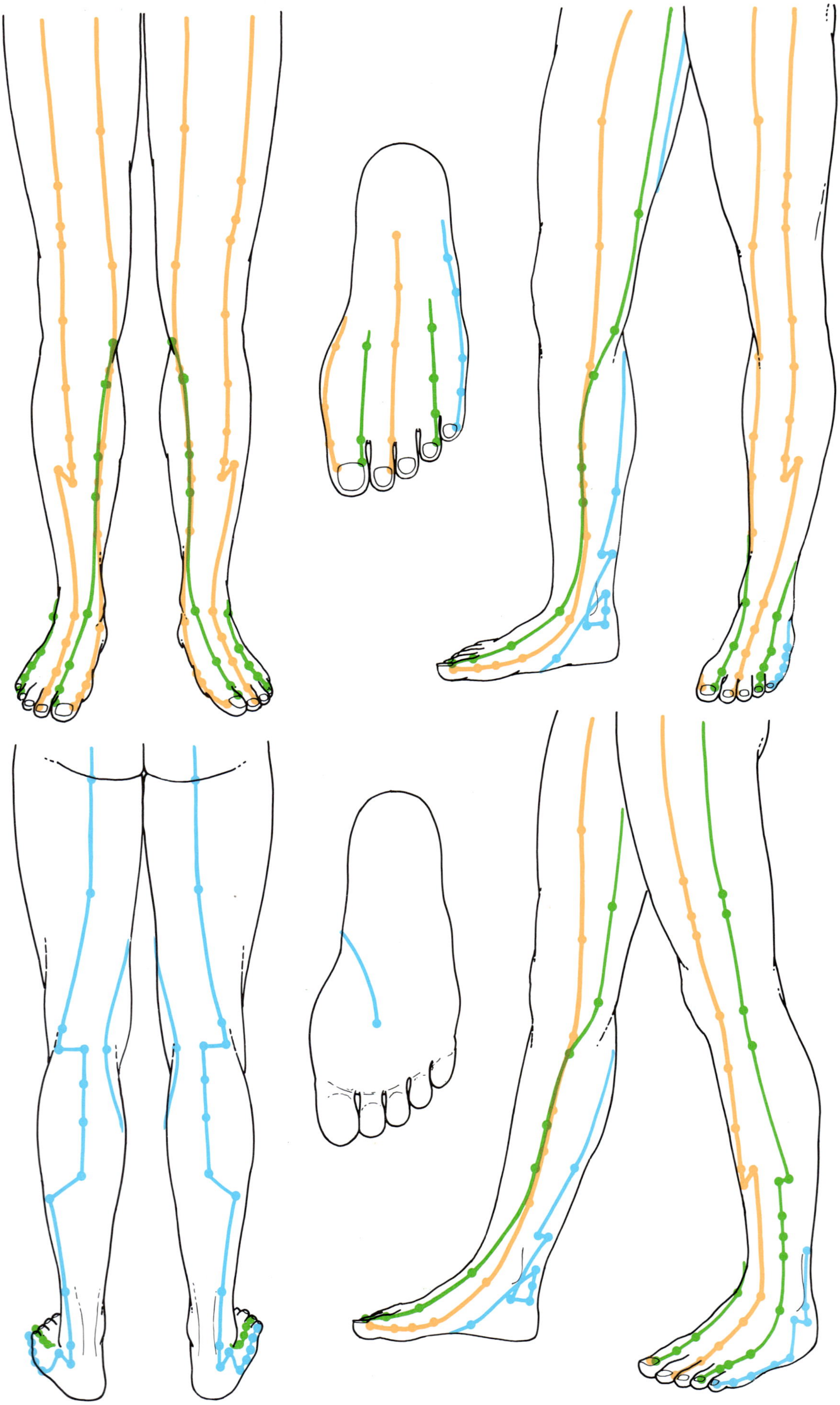

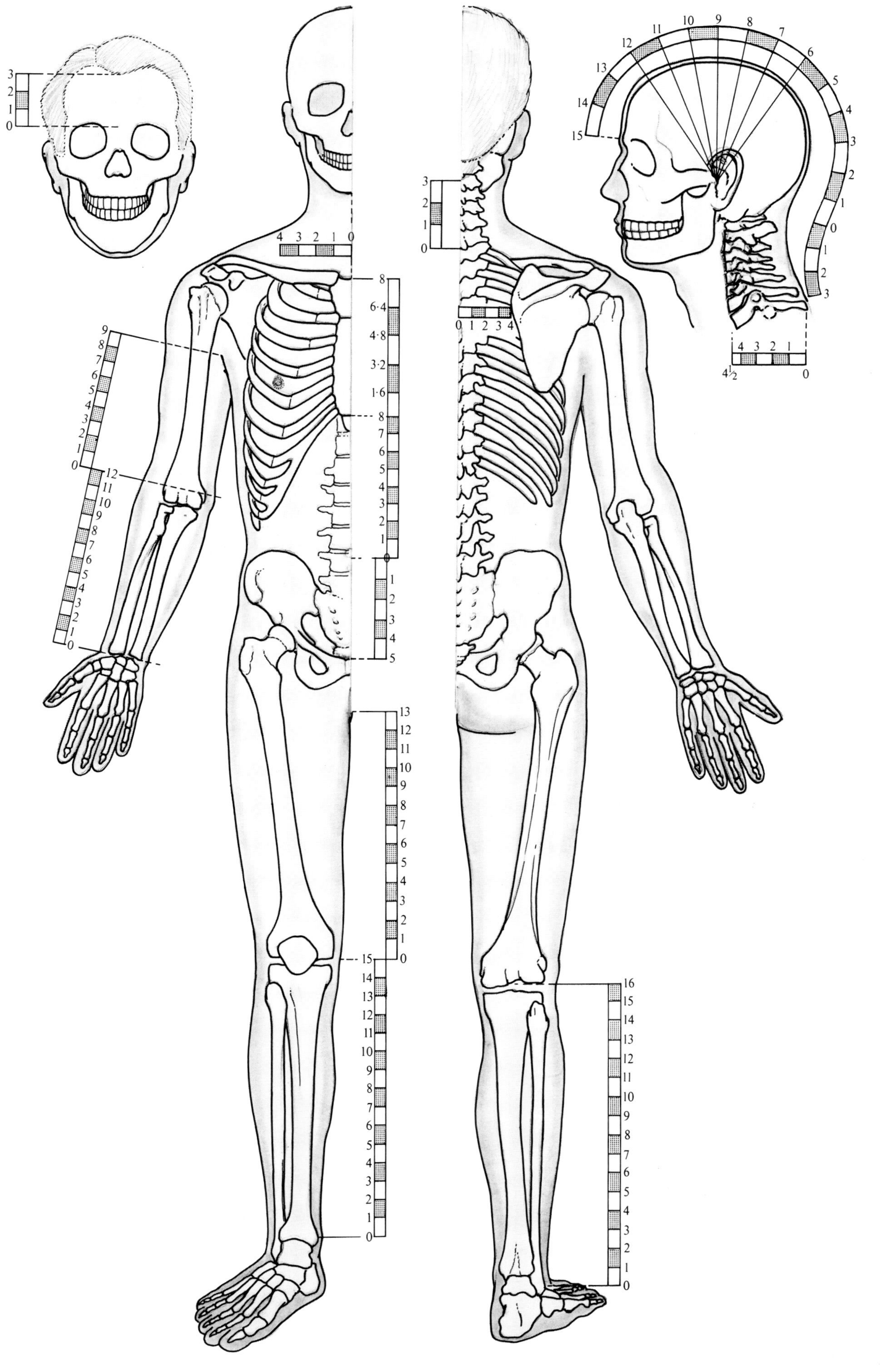

Index of Appendices

Italic bold numerals refer to illustrations; roman bold numerals indicate text references